Margherita Spagnuolo Lobb
Nancy Amendt-Lyon (eds.)

Creative License

The Art of Gestalt Therapy

Springer-Verlag Wien GmbH

Margherita Spagnuolo Lobb
Istituto di Gestalt, Siracusa, Italy

Nancy Amendt-Lyon
Austrian Association for Group Psychotherapy
and Group Dynamics, Vienna, Austria

Financial support was given by the *Bundesministerium für Bildung,
Wissenschaft und Kultur*, Vienna

© 2003 Springer-Verlag Wien
Originally published by Springer-Verlag Wien New York in 2003

Cover illustration: © Lotte Lyon
Typesetting: Composition & Design Services, Minsk 220027, Belarus
Printing: Druckerei Theiss GmbH, A-9431 St. Stefan im Lavanttal
Printed on acid-free and chlorine-free bleached paper
With 7 partly coloured Figures
CIP data applied for
SPIN: 10803780

ISBN 978-3-211-83901-0   ISBN 978-3-7091-6023-7 (eBook)
DOI 10.1007/978-3-7091-6023-7

To our children,
with whom we continue to learn

Preface

The time is ripe, more than fifty years after the publication of the magnum opus by Perls, Hefferline & Goodman, to publish a book on the topic of creativity in Gestalt therapy. The idea for this book was conceived in March 2001, on the island of Sicily, at the very first European Conference of Gestalt Therapy Writers of the *European Association for Gestalt Therapy*. Our starting point was an article on art and creativity in Gestalt therapy, which was presented there by one of the editors, and illuminated by a vision, held by the other editor, of bringing together colleagues from around the world to contribute to a qualified volume on the subject of creativity within the realm of Gestalt therapy. We wanted to continue the professional discourse internationally and capture the synergetic effects of experienced colleagues' reflections on various aspects of our chosen subject. Moreover, we intended to explore how the theoretical reflection of one's practice can inspire effective interventions and, vice versa, how the discussion of practical experiences can shape new theoretical directions.

Hence, our aim in this book is to create a forum on the concept of creativity in Gestalt therapy. We do not intend to hermeneutically define the concept, but rather to rethink it as a group, giving voice to a number of prominent practitioners of Gestalt therapy who, over the last few decades, have put creativity at the center of their work. Since it is a fundamental concept in our approach, we are aware that this is a complex matter, one that would imply, in some sense, a rewriting of the epistemological principles of Gestalt therapy itself. To find our direction in the meaning of the Gestalt therapeutic concept of creativity, it is essential to reflect on the fact that we are distinguishing between the adjective and the noun, as in "creative adjustment" and "creativity". On the one hand, the word "creativity" is inspiring and intriguing, especially when linked to a method of psychotherapy; on the other hand, this word has undergone such inflation in our language, that any attempt to define it ends in a tangle of semantic confusions from which it is difficult to extricate oneself. In practice, we readily attach the adjective "creative" to any event that we simply want to define in line with the spirit of our approach or that is capable of surprising us positively. Thus, the lack of an epistemological definition of creativity in our approach easily leads to its abuse, if not misuse. A main purpose of this book is therefore to be a starting point: once the syntax of the concept of creativity has been clarified, a series of contributions follow which, taken together, enable us to reread Gestalt creativity in society – our own – which has changed radically.

The Gestalt approach is particularly known and admired for its diversified spectrum of psychotherapeutic interventions, including artistic materials and methods from the fine and performing arts. This characteristic appeal of the method, which Joseph Zinker once aptly referred to as the permission to be creative, applies to both practitioners and their clientele. The focus of the present volume is on the creative process within the therapeutic relationship, on that which happens in-between. We intend to explore the interaction of individuals in the field with which they are inextricably interwoven. Creative process is a function of the field! It appears to be a stroke of fate that our project was "born" in Sicily, an island that has integrated disparate cultures for thousands of years and has exemplified in a classic manner the unique results of highly productive mutual stimulation and assimilation.

Our inspiration for editing this challenging book is couched in the conviction that Gestalt therapy has something unique to offer and that this unique something is the *creative license* that we, as practitioners, enjoy in our work and that can be derived from our theory. The concept of creativity is an integral part of our anthropology, which holds that being creative is synonymous with normality in human nature. Creativity characterizes the individual's spontaneous adjustment to his or her environment. While deliberating the justified questions of what particular characteristics distinguish Gestalt therapy from other schools of psychotherapy and of how they relate to our themes of creativity, aesthetics, and diversity in therapeutic interventions, several concepts came to mind.

Historically, the first one is the concept of *dental aggression*, which Fritz Perls, in collaboration with his wife, Laura, put forth in *Ego, Hunger and Aggression*, marking a revolutionary change in psychoanalytic thinking at that time. Dental aggression emphasized the productive role that aggression plays in the interactions in which a person, inextricably part of his or her environmental field, is involved. Founded on the careful observations that Laura Perls made while nursing and weaning her own children, dental aggression is seen as a developmental and life-affirming, rather than destructive, ability.

A second concept specific to Gestalt therapy is that of *creative adjustment*, which holds that an individual in his or her field strives to achieve the best possible results within the given situation. Under certain circumstances, these organism-environmental field interactions may result in symptoms and suffering into which the energy and the spontaneous flow of the figure/ground process of a person have been misguided and locked, instead of reaching their originally intended targets of contact-making. In this light, symptoms are seen as the individual's creative solutions to difficult situations. Gestalt therapy focuses on allowing and supporting the spontaneous flow of energy held captive in the symptom to be redirected toward the proper target of contact-making, and on experimenting with alternative relational patterns.

Described poignantly by Laura Perls, the three "E's" of Gestalt therapy comprise the third concept. She claimed that Gestalt therapists may include a tremendous variety of therapeutic interventions in their work as long as these are *existential, experiential*, and *experimental*, provided that adequate support for the experiment can be mobilized. Thus, it is necessary to work phenomenologically, organizing recognized patterns into meaningful wholes, to be present-centered, and to spontaneously create custom-tailored experiments that will support figure formation within therapeutic interactions. In turn, these interventions must be organized and enacted so that the patient can experience them holistically: i.e., not merely cognitively, but also senso-motorically and emotionally.

A fourth and closely related concept is the notion of *style*. Laura Perls suggested that there are as many styles of Gestalt therapy as there are Gestalt therapists, and she encouraged therapists to assimilate into their therapeutic work talents, skills, and interests that have influenced their lives. Reflecting on our work with patients, she went on to say that those who have style – those who have found their unique way of being in the world (a reference therefore to self-actualization) – no longer require therapy.

Fifth is the concept of *dialogic relationship* in psychotherapy, as described by Martin Buber in *I and Thou*. Issues of what we traditionally refer to as transference and countertransference are brought into the here-and-now and dealt with in the present. The present life contexts of both the therapist and patient are taken into account. The therapeutic stance intentionally supports the *presence* of the therapist and his or her selective authenticity when interacting with each patient.

A sixth relevant concept is the use of *polarities*, derived from Salomo Friedlaender's philosophical theory of creative indifference. Just as related opposites can be derived from the fertile void between them, so too are our personalities comprised of many polar traits, which are often split off from awareness or subjectively unevenly experienced. Gestalt therapy adheres to the notion that attending to the fertile void allows for creative integration of these seemingly unrelated poles.

A seventh and final concept for our purpose refers to the creative quality of *ego function*: deliberately identifying with or alienating from certain parts of the organism/environmental field. To Otto Rank we owe the concept of creative will and the revolutionizing of the psychological perspective on the artist. In his view, the artist is considered the one who succeeds in running the risk of identifying himself as distinct from the masses, and who thus successfully deals with the fullness of existence, thanks to his courage of believing in life despite the awareness of his mortality.

Creativity, traditionally seen as a special gift of remarkable and exceptional personalities, is considered in Gestalt therapy to be a quality of spontaneous adaptation in interpersonal processes, as well as an important ingredient of healthy social living. It is our belief that the current role of the concept of creativity in the helping professions needs to be re-discovered. What contribution can present-day therapists make to this post-modern society, subject as it is to processes of fragmentation and complexity that render it impossible to recognize oneself in pre-established points of reference, and constantly oblige us to find new solutions for ever-new problems, including those solutions that imply fundamental choices, such as conceiving a child or sharing life space with a partner? In a word, how do we today view the application of creative adjustment to the problems of our society? How is this an-thropological and clinical principle of Gestalt therapy regarded and applied by contemporary Gestalt therapists?

In presenting this book, we wish to open up a path on which all travelers might find themselves, in its attractions and in its voids, and perhaps come to contribute, one day, fresh tracks along our road. Clearly, this book is ad-dressed not only to professional psychotherapists, but also to all those who make art and curiosity about human nature an important aspect of their lives. The path of creativity is one that many travel. Supporting human cre-ativity is a sort of mission inherent in many professions, above all the artist's, which bequeaths to all humanity a powerful message capable of advancing the growth of the human race precisely by provoking upheaval. Yet it is also the teacher's – for it is the teacher to whom we entrust that most delicate of tasks, the education of tomorrow's men and women –, the counselor's, called to stimulate processes of creative adjustment in groups faced with critical life situations, *and* the politician's, whose choices should be inspired by aesthetic rather than economic aims. And finally, of course, the profession of the psy-chotherapist, whose function may be defined as "intimately political".

We would like to thank the participants of the first European Conference of Gestalt Therapy Writers in 2001, who encouraged our project from the be-ginning. We are deeply indebted to our copyeditor, Laurie Cohen, for her in-valuable help with the preparation of the manuscripts. Our husbands, Mario Lobb and Gerhard Amendt, who patiently watched vacations and weekends melt into weeks of editorial work, deserve our heartfelt thanks for their sup-port and encouragement. Collaborating as editors, which has been a cre-ative adjustment in itself, also deserves our proud acknowledgement.

Syracuse and Vienna, March 2003   Margherita Spagnuolo Lobb
                                                 Nancy Amendt-Lyon

Contents

Part I
The Emergence of the Creative Field

Part II
The Challenge of Defining Creative Concepts

Part III
Connecting Theory and Practice: Case Examples

Part IV
A Taste of the Field in Practice

Authors' Addresses

Nancy Amendt-Lyon

Kundmanngasse 13/23
A-1030 Vienna
Austria
amendtlyon@aon.at

Daniel J. Bloom

35 West Ninth Street
New York, NY 10011
USA
djbnyc@nyc.rr.com

Todd Burley

1900 Royalty Dr., Suite 210
Pomona, CA 91767
USA
T1burley@cs.com

Sandra Cardoso Zinker

P.O. Box 861
Wellfleet, MA 02667
USA
sandrazinker@aol.com

Ludwig Frambach

Ottensooser Weg 1
D-91207 Lauf/Pegnitz
Germany
projekt.spiritualitaet@ejn.de

Ruella Frank

124 West 93rd Street #2C
New York 10025
USA
ruellafrank@nyc.rr.com

Carl Hodges

80 Cranberry Street
Brooklyn, NY 11201
USA
cwhvosge@aol.com

Richard Kitzler

140 West 16th Street, Apt. 2E
New York, NY 10011
USA
lycidas@earthlink.net

Edward J. and Barbara Lynch

Southern Connecticut State University
New Haven, CT
USA
EJ52@aol.com

Sonia March Nevis

PO Box 515
South Wellfleet, MA 02663
USA
smnevis@aol.com

Joseph Melnick

17 South St.
Portland, ME 04101
USA
gestaltrev@aol.com

Michael Vincent Miller

863 Massachusetts Avenue – Suite 54
Cambridge, MA 02139
USA
mvmiller39@aol.com

Bertram Müller

Cranachstr. 32
D-40235 Düsseldorf
Germany
bmueller@tanzhaus-nrw.de

Edwin C. Nevis

PO Box 515
South Wellfleet, MA 02663
USA
ECNevis@aol.com

Malcolm Parlett

The Coach House
Nether Skyborry, Knighton
Powys LD7 1TW
United Kingdom
malcolm.parlett@virgin.net

Giuseppe Sampognaro

Via Gela, 68
96100 Siracusa
Italy
dmmksa@tin.it

Antonio Sichera

Via Carlo Papa, 29
97015 Modica (RG)
Italy
asichera@unict.it

Margherita Spagnuolo Lobb

Via San Sebastiano, 38
96100 Siracusa
Italy
training@gestalt.it

Daniel N. Stern

14, Ch. de Clairejoie
CH-1225 Chène-Bourg
Geneva
Switzerland

Gordon Wheeler

66 Orchard St.
Cambridge, MA 02140
USA
gicpress@aol.com

Joseph C. Zinker

P.O. Box 861
Wellfleet, MA 02667
USA
jczink@aol.com

Introduction

Margherita Spagnuolo Lobb and Nancy Amendt-Lyon

We have approached the topic of creativity in Gestalt therapy from four directions:

Part I. *The Emergence of the Creative Field* deals with new theoretical reflections on the ability to promote creative processes. Nancy Amendt-Lyon presents the idea that creative processes are triggered in the no man's land of the contact boundary, and she gives an overview of those theoretical principles that guide our being creative in practice. Daniel Stern, known for his infant research, indirectly confirms Gestalt therapy's core theory with a revolutionary view on what makes the change happen in psychotherapy, and he challenges Gestalt therapists with his concept of implicit knowledge. Leading classical Gestalt therapy theory toward a most vital post-modern perspective, Margherita Spagnuolo Lobb explores the contribution of Gestalt therapy to Stern's theory, relying on the common concept of improvisational co-creation. Continuing the idea of life as an art of improvising, Malcolm Parlett presents five creative abilities, which he defines as the adaptive and spontaneous response to living in this world. Daniel Bloom shows how the core concepts of Gestalt therapy (contact boundary, contact, self, creative adjustment) are *per se* aesthetic values, and he provocatively favors the contribution of American pragmatism to the development of Gestalt therapy over that of Gestalt psychology. Referring to recent neuroscience research, Todd Burley shows how creativity is a phenomenon relying on the entire human brain and how this whole process always differs from one person to the other.

Part II. *The Challenge of Defining Creative Concepts* explores different levels of defining creativity in Gestalt therapy. It starts with a chapter by Antonio Sichera, a philosopher, who clarifies a syntactical problem inherent in *Gestalt Therapy* about the use of creativity as an essential attribute of the experience of contact rather than as a noun; Sichera proceeds from this basis to an analysis of dreams and art. Richard Kitzler narrates how creativity was experienced when Gestalt therapy was first established in New York. Ludwig Frambach offers an account of Salomo Friedlaender's theory of creative indifference, which decisively influenced Fritz Perls' concept of polarities

and the notion of a fertile void that bears the possibility of differentiation between interrelated poles in constant tension. Bertram Müller explains how
Otto Rank's concept of creative will has influenced the foundations of Gestalt therapy theory, closing the first four contributions devoted to a definition of our history. The next three authors approach creativity with regard to
yet further aspects of interrelatedness. Joseph Zinker focuses on how the
beauty inherent in human relationships is an aspect that therapists ought to
bring forth with their patients. Michael Vincent Miller portrays the attitude
of commitment as an aesthetic and therapeutic value that artists' ways of
working can teach us. Gordon Wheeler maps out how creativity develops
within the context of contact-withdrawal experience and human evolution.

Part III. *Connecting Theory and Practice: Case Examples* presents three
contributions which, through the description of clinical examples, demonstrate the importance of this fertile interchange in our professional practice.
Ruella Frank describes two clients' developmental bodily and relational patterns from a phenomenological perspective. Sandra Cardoso-Zinker relates
how a therapist can support the spontaneous emergence of creative adjustment with a child in session. Depicting memorable moments experienced
with individual patients and a training group, Nancy Amendt-Lyon demonstrates how the fruitful interchange between theory and practice inspires
her.

Part IV. *A Taste of the Field in Practice* gathers a few possibilities for applying Gestalt therapeutic concepts of creativity to specific clinical settings.
Joseph Melnick and Sonia March Nevis present their method of developing
creativity in long-term intimate relationships, explaining how it plays an
important role in sustaining couples' vitality and growth. Edward and
Barbara Lynch focus on the creative forces at work within the family therapeutic system and encourage us to appreciate how these creative forces include both the attempt to remedy disturbances in the field and the spontaneous effort to create new solutions. Carl Hodges presents his model of
working with groups as one relevant aspect of the research that the New
York Institute for Gestalt Therapy has accomplished in the last two decades.
Similarly, Margherita Spagnuolo Lobb presents her method for addressing
psychosis, both in private and in public psychiatric institutions, which resulted from the research carried out in her institute. Giuseppe Sampognaro
provides a new technique for working creatively in psychiatric institutions:
the psychoportrait. The book closes with a contribution by Edwin Nevis,
who, starting with a pragmatic analysis of successfully developing large organizations, describes Gestalt therapy's perspective on dealing with the six
most prominent obstacles to creativity in organizations.

It is with pleasure and gratitude that we present the contributions from acknowledged practitioners who solidly represent contemporary Gestalt therapy in Europe and the United States. This representation bridges divides
among various schools of our method and reflects the lively, present-day discourse among them.

Part I
The Emergence of the Creative Field

Toward a Gestalt Therapeutic Concept for Promoting Creative Process

Nancy Amendt-Lyon

Merely encouraging play and artistic production as a therapist, or working with a patient who exhibits exceptional artistic talents, does not adequately define creativity within the therapeutic relationship. A more appropriate definition of this type of creativity must include interpersonal aspects, such as the daring, creative interaction, or that which happens in the no man's land between us. This implies venturing beyond self-expression as an end in itself and entering the dynamics of the fertile complexity within the therapeutic relationship. Creative interchange can best be encouraged in Gestalt therapy when those involved in the therapeutic process are productively curious and willing to experiment; as a consequence, the chances for optimal results with the givens of the situation are much higher. Drawing from my experience as a therapist, I have realized that achieving this goal implies the use of precisely those individually designed experiments that both take the uniqueness of each patient into account and require the therapist to dare to take creative leaps. My aim is to make a passionate plea for the spontaneous development of "custom-made" interventions that risk articulating something novel, unexpected, or outright eccentric, be it in individual, couples, or group therapy. Only these unique "experiments", born out of the process of the therapeutic relationship, can stimulate the liveliness, innovation, and meaningfulness necessary to call them creative in the Gestalt therapeutic sense of the word.

The multitude of therapeutic interventions in Gestalt therapy is one of its most distinguishing characteristics. This professional freedom to design "custom-made" interventions with an abundance of media and materials, together with my constant fascination with the unique life stories of my patients, have kept my interest in realms of creativity and the creative process active for many years. When attempting to define the subject of creative process within Gestalt therapy, let us first consider the process of contact between individuals over time and the development of relationships – specific styles and ways of being in the world with others as part of the organism/environmental field – as creative expression in relationship. The anthropological position of Gestalt therapy holds that humans tend to organize their experiences into meaningful, structured, and organized wholes, and that this creative activity is the basis for healthy functioning. Good contact between individuals can be seen as an aesthetic activity, meaningfully organized, well-integrated, and appropriate to the demand characteristics of the field. Thus, the personal styles of individuals interacting with each other develop into interpersonal relationships that have varying degrees of aesthetic qualities.

With regard to the therapeutic relationship, promoting creative process depends not least upon therapists' perception of their patients' sensory strengths. In this vein, therapists have "good form" in mind when addressing themselves to their patients and choosing a mode of communication. Recent neuroscience research confirms that neither the minds nor the bodies of two persons work in exactly the same way.[1] Inasmuch as no two brains function identically, we are required as therapists to distinguish the sensory strengths of our patients. Some orient themselves well visually in terms of images, shapes, colors, and designs; some attend readily to auditory signals; and some are particularly receptive to spatial modes of communication and need interaction involving directions, movement, and space. Others communicate easily in metaphoric terms or enjoy playing with figures of speech. Yet the use of metaphors and verbal imagery may not have the intended effect on a person, whereas movement – such as gestures, facial expressions, and group "sculptures" – will. Having discovered in which sensory mode a patient's strength lies, it is advisable for a therapist to direct interventions to the patient's preferred way of experiencing. An important aspect of the art of Gestalt therapy lies in successfully addressing the particular sensory strengths of our patients and matching them with appropriate therapeutic interventions. This is a prerequisite for what I colloquially call "picking up the patient where he or she is". A further aspect is having the diagnostic knowledge necessary to assess the patient's developmental level, major conflicts, and ways of dealing with interpersonal problems. This requires not only the creative work of configuring all the patterns and elements of information available into a whole picture that makes sense, but also the willingness to reconfigure these elements repeatedly as the diagnostic-therapeutic process progresses. Should our patients not react favorably to our interventions, then we may be addressing them in a sensory mode to which they are slow to react or with which they cannot deal properly. Assuming that cognition and emotions are inseparable processes, I concur with Burley's statement that creativity is a phenomenon relying on the entire human brain, with differing emphasis, depending on whether the activity involved is one of composing music, writing, dancing, or painting (Burley, 1998, p. 133).

I. Practice-Related Theoretical Influences

The practice-related theoretical influences that I call to mind for the effective application of artistic methods and materials in Gestalt therapy are de-

---

[1] See Todd Burley's chapter in this volume.

rived from the tradition of the founders of Gestalt therapy (F. and L. Perls, Goodman), the "pioneers" of Gestalt therapy using artistic methods and materials in the United States (Rhyne, Zinker, Polster, Oaklander, Rapp), and compatible psychotherapeutic approaches to creativity. To paraphrase Kurt Lewin, who claimed that nothing is as practical as a good theory, sixteen influences, which I will first summarize and then describe in detail, are offered as markers for orientation (see Table 1). These overlapping and interrelated influences begin with the application of such principles of Gestalt theory as figure/background, the principles of good Gestalt, *prägnanz*, and closure; they also deal with perception as an active process. These principles themselves imply a process-oriented approach in working with artistic methods. A further influence involves productive thinking, considered by some to be analogous to creative adjustment. Productive or "independent" thinking allows us to understand the relationship between figure and background, give meaning to our experiences, and gain insight into the implications of our actions. To this end, we search for "good form" in the sense of an aesthetic self-expression and our own uniquely appropriate style, which should always be seen within relationships. Another influence involves the process of creative adjustment, which aims for the transformation of the familiar into something novel and valuable. Gestalt therapy's process-oriented diagnostic approach supports the concept of perceiving and understanding. Over and above the products of creative expression, our focus is directed to the process through which it came to be. Acknowledging the interwovenness of cognition and emotion helps us understand the relationship between figure and background, which is what we refer to as meaning. Behavior patterns and patterns of emotional states and their location within the context of our present life begin to emerge. Another influence on creative therapeutic practice involves reconfiguring or restructuring the field in search of good form. Reorganizing familiar, chronically poorly-configured elements into something novel and valuable, and therefore beautiful, reflects the embeddedness of Gestalt therapy in field theory. When familiar elements in the field are reconfigured, and the new configuration suddenly makes sense and seems to "fit", then the impact of an insightful "aha" experience reflects the forces of the field. Additional influences are related to the ability to appreciate personal meaning and achieve individual style as developmental goals in a culture of rapidly changing mass fads and increasing complexity. Also, attending to the isomorphism or structural relatedness between internal experience and external expression has deepened my connection between the practice and theory of Gestalt therapy. Practicing process-oriented diagnosis and engaging in dialogic relationship during all phases of the therapeutic process also underscore that which emerges between therapist and patient. Describing interpersonal behavior patterns, modes of sensing, thinking, and feeling, symptoms and disturbances as well as strengths and resources generates our working hypotheses. Process-oriented diagnosis can be metaphorically described as a number of temporary stops one makes along a journey. Diagnosis can thus be viewed as particular styles or ways of being in the world with others, of varying duration. The life context, interpersonal pat-

Table 1. An Overview of Influences on Creative Therapeutic Intervention in Gestalt Therapy

- Stimulating Productive Thinking, Insight and Creative Adjustment
- Applying Principles of Gestalt Theory
- Reorganizing the Field in Search of "Good Form"
- Taking a Process-Oriented Approach
- Perceiving and Understanding
- Addressing the Structural Relatedness between Expression and Experience
- Finding Personal Meaning within the Context of One's Life
- Transforming the Familiar into Something Novel and Valuable
- Risk-Taking and Allowing Surprises
- Using Humor, Metaphors, and Parapraxes Productively
- Having Knowledge of the Indications and Counterindications of Using Various Methods and Materials
- Engaging in Dialogic Relationship
- Practicing Process-Oriented Diagnosis
- Facilitating Authentic Self-Expression and Unique Style within Relationship
- Creating Potential Space for Playful Experiences between Therapist and Patient
- Being Personally Familiar with Materials and Methods

terns, and immediate emotional responses of the therapist (i.e., counter-transference) are an integral part of this diagnostic process and influence creative therapeutic practice as well. The potential space for playful experiences within the therapeutic relationship, a further influence, enables authentic self-expression, whose meaning is jointly found in the life context of the person involved. By creating an atmosphere in which impulses can unfold and develop, Gestalt therapy can facilitate the ability of human beings to engage playfully and creatively with one another. When therapeutic interaction facilitates the authentic expression of inner experiences with artistic materials, the dynamics of that which exists "between" therapist and patient is influenced. Participating in this process makes it something beyond mere self-expression. Creative expression within relationship implies a relational field, co-creations, and mutual dependencies. It happens between two or more persons. A final influence involves being personally familiar with the materials and methods I use. This familiarity is a prerequisite for appreciating the possible attractiveness of materials and the effects that they can have on others. The resources of having had my own experience with the repercussions and risks of materials have been essential in applying them effectively.

II. Developing Aesthetic and Creative Dimensions of Gestalt Therapy

The initial phase in the development of Gestalt therapy reflects its withdrawal from the drive theory of classical psychoanalysis and the development of an approach which can appreciate the comprehensive expression of a human being on different levels of experience. Looking back on the cultural interests and activities of Fritz and Laura Perls, it comes as no surprise that the founders of Gestalt therapy, through an abundance of media and materials, stimulated and inspired creative expression in their students and patients. Fritz Perls worked in plays directed by Max Reinhardt, integrated elements of Moreno's psychodrama into his new psychotherapeutic method, and loved to dramatize. German Expressionism and modern literature had a strong influence on both Perls.[2] Although he received more acknowledgment as a social critic and philosopher, Paul Goodman wrote in various genres, and his literary style is obvious in the theoretical part of our basic text on Gestalt therapy: "But the contrary of neurotic verbalizing is various and creative speech; it is neither scientific semantics nor silence; it is poetry" (Perls F et al., 1951, p. 321). Laura Perls encouraged Gestalt therapists to apply a broad range of techniques in their interventions, depending of course upon their own personal and professional experiential background (see Perls L, 1971, 1978, 1989). Her prerequisite was that their work adhere to the three "E's" of Gestalt therapy: it is existential-phenomenological, experiential, and experimental, provided that adequate support for the experiment is available.

Although Laura Perls considered the name *Gestaltung Therapie* more appropriate, because the term *Gestaltung* describes a process, not something that is static, such as a fixed gestalt, the new approach was named Gestalt therapy. Laura Perls not only depicted *Gestalt* as a philosophic and aesthetic concept (Kitzler et al., 1982, p. 13), she also deplored the narrow backgrounds that some psychotherapists had and that limited their practice of therapy. She claimed that many interpersonal phenomena, which are designated as pathological or psychotic, are often not understood or cannot be accessed by certain therapists (Kurdirka and Perls, 1982, p. 32): "Psychotherapy is as much an art as it is a science. The intuition and immediacy of the artist are as necessary for the good therapist as a scientific education" (Perls L and Rosenfeld, 1982, p. 27). Laura Perls also suggested that good therapists are good artists, too, even though they are not known as artists or considered to be artistic. Therefore, a background and continuing experience in the arts as an influence on a psychotherapist broadens his or her communicative abilities and deepens his or her understanding of many aspects of personalities. This influential role of the arts, enhancing the therapist's insight into human nature, is manifested in Gestalt therapy's emphasis on intuitively comprehending essentials and the process approach. In practice, this implies, for instance, the art of grasping the larger picture, zooming in on a detail and putting it into perspective, perceiving a situation from various and contrasting viewpoints, acquiring a sense of atmospheres and moods, imagining what it is like to "slip into the skin" of another person, and delighting in the incredible uniqueness of every human being.

---

[2] Srekovic offers a detailed and lively account of the history and development of Gestalt therapy in German: Geschichte und Entwicklung der Gestalttherapie. In: Fuhr R, Srekovic M, Gremmler-Fuhr M (eds) (1999) Handbuch der Gestalttherapie. Hogrefe, Göttingen, pp 673–683.

III. Contributions from the Pioneers

Within the limits of this article, it is neither possible to duly describe the most significant, creative practitioners and theorists with respect to this aspect of Gestalt therapy, to whom I refer as the pioneers in the United States, nor to fully acknowledge the most important theoretical influences on the founders of Gestalt therapy. In the present article, I will instead introduce several outstanding colleagues who have paved the way for a better understanding of the creative aspects of Gestalt therapy.[3] One of the most stimulating pioneers is Janie Rhyne (1971, 1973, 1980, 1996; Vich and Rhyne, 1967), whose *Gestalt art experience*, the term she coined to describe her approach, gives us guidelines for the use of art materials in exploring one's own (and others') individually unique qualities. Her emphasis lies on expanding and deepening perception through the creation of forms with art materials and on understanding the visual messages which these forms convey. Rhyne's approach is guided by laws of Gestalt psychology (*prägnanz*, closure, figure formation, similarity, and proximity), as well as the conviction that our perception is influenced by actual needs, experiences, and individual personalities. Crucial to the therapists' task is their skill in transferring the insights and realizations of the entire process onto the way patients structure and experience life and relationships. Rhyne encourages Gestalt therapists to activate sensory memories more effectively by nonverbal, sensory experiences, such as movement and body awareness, as well as working with art materials, as opposed to intervening solely on a verbal level. Playfully, and with many examples of his own artistry, Joseph Zinker (1971, 1973, 1977) warns psychotherapists about the pitfalls of stereotyped, repetitive exercises, and he strongly advocates the spontaneous creation of custom-made experiments. Considering Gestalt therapy to be creative process in itself, Zinker sums up his position with the basic tenet that Gestalt therapy is "permission to be creative" (1974, p. 75). Erving Polster's (1987) fascination with the life stories of his patients reminds us of the commonalities between writers and psychotherapists. He argues that the therapist's appropriate acknowledgment of the material of a patient's life as being unique and interesting has curative qualities. Using writers' perspectives and a number of dramatic techniques, therapists can help patients to recognize the wonders of their own novel of life, opening up a satisfying and effective way of dealing with narratives. Violet Oaklander (1978, 1979) demonstrates a phenomenological approach to working with children and adolescents in the field of art and creative expression. She reminds psychotherapists to focus on the consequences of their patients' behavior and to use artistic material as a catalyst, rather than as a means to an end in itself. Oaklander advocates the development of one's personal therapeutic style and preferences for materials. *Gestalt Art Therapy*, as practiced by Elaine Rapp (1980; Leedy and Rapp, 1973), reveals an existential perspective that explores the relationship be-

---

[3] For detailed overviews of the historical development and theoretical foundations of the creative aspects of Gestalt therapy, the interested reader is referred to Amendt-Lyon 1999, 2001a, b.

tween a person and his or her environment through a broad spectrum of experiments with formable materials. The unique artistic creation is regarded as a symbol with personal meaning to be communicated.[4] Rapp finds that creative growth (i.e., health) can occur when this communication with one's environment is meaningfully processed, and she encourages the cooperation of therapists from various expressive disciplines.

A summary of the contributions to theory and practice from the founders and pioneers of Gestalt therapy would include treating the term *gestalt* as an aesthetic concept, searching for "good form" in the sense of behavioral and emotional expression that is fitting or adequate to the interpersonal situation, discovering and accepting one's own style, transforming or reconfiguring familiar elements into new and valuable information, and experimenting with novel, unaccustomed behavior.

During the past fifty years, in addition to the founders of Gestalt therapy and the pioneers in the United States, numerous Gestalt therapists in the United States and Europe have used a wide range of artistic materials in their awareness training and promotion of creativity based on Gestalt therapy theory. Their focus on the promotion of creative behavior and on the creative aspects of psychotherapeutic interventions have led to a number of valuable guidelines. These well-tried guidelines include: alternating between verbal and nonverbal expressive forms, such as painting or pantomime; alternately using the dominant and nondominant hand in drawing – for example, working with self-portraits drawn with each hand, respectively; stressing the need for space to play in the therapeutic situation, such as experimenting with new behaviors or enacting fantasies in the safe environment of the therapist's office; remembering the parallels between the creative and therapeutic processes, especially the need for chaos and disorganization of the poorly organized field before reorganization can take place and appropriate, "good form" can emerge; playing with and integrating polarities, such as reowning those personality aspects that an individual is accustomed to delegate to a partner instead of embodying him- or herself; and, describing an experience in one particular sense medium in terms of another medium, for instance, dancing a dream or painting one's present mood. In the field of art as well as in psychotherapy, the goal is to bring something novel into the foreground in order for a new configuration to emerge out of the transformation or reorganization of the old elements. "The word 'information'", Arnheim reminds us, "taken literally, means to give form; and form needs structure" (quoted in Miller, 1980, p. 88). Human nature's tendency to form and transform familiar elements and thus bring about new information, and to transform one's own experiences in the world in a way that allows for processing and integration, are reflected in both the worlds of art and psychotherapeutic practice. Through the act of creating something unique and meaningful, we give form to human experience.

---

[4] Compare Groddeck (1990, pp. 122–128) on the issue of illness as the symbolic vital expression of a human being.

IV. Toward a Gestalt Therapeutic Concept
for Promoting Creative Process

In exploring the development of the aesthetic and creative dimensions of Gestalt therapy, I have been led to numerous interrelated influences on creative therapeutic process. For better comprehension of their interrelated aspects, some will be grouped together for discussion. I intend to discuss the Gestalt therapeutic substantiation of these influences as well as authors from other therapeutic orientations who do not contradict Gestalt philosophy in these topics and, moreover, who complement the Gestalt approach with essential aspects. My aim is to present a Gestalt therapeutic concept for promoting creative interpersonal expression and process. This approach is incompatible with technique-oriented, often categorical perspectives of working with artistic materials that ignore the subjectivity and interrelational aspects of the process. Also, this concept must be distinguished from those therapeutic approaches that merely use artistic media as a welcome means of livening up stagnant therapeutic interactions without reflecting them within the framework of Gestalt therapy theory. Even worse, these approaches use methods gleaned from Gestalt therapy as "techniques" for creative expression, stripped of their theoretical basis, in order to loosen up or satisfy the supposed needs of patients or clients. This is often attempted to make their method appear more attractive than the rather ascetic demands of more verbally oriented therapeutic methods.

A. Stimulating Productive Thinking, Insight, and Creative Adjustment

The concept presently offered begins with the relationship between Wertheimer's concept of productive thinking and the Gestalt therapeutic concept of creative adjustment. Laura Perls unequivocally claimed how essential the teachings of Gestalt psychology were for the development of Gestalt therapy: "Anyone who wants fully to understand Gestalt therapy would do well to study Wertheimer on productive thinking, Lewin on the incomplete gestalt and the crucial importance of interest for gestalt formation, and Kurt Goldstein on the organism as an indivisible totality" (Perls L, 1978, p. 33).

In a similar vein, Portele (1996) saw a close relationship between Wertheimer's concept of productive thinking and what F. Perls and Goodman termed creative adjustment. Productive thinking strives for the kind of intellectual independence that requires insight, holistic perception, and bestowal of meaning. Among the laws of Gestalt theory that are crucially important to this process are (1) the principle of *prägnanz*, which holds that percepts take the best form possible under the given circumstances, and (2) the tendency toward making good gestalten, as exemplified by the organization of the field pressing for the greatest clarity and simplicity possible under the given conditions. When our productive thinking process, which adheres to the demand characteristics of the situation, is blocked, and we cannot process the information we get from our environment appropriately, structural blindness, lack of perspicuity, panic reactions resulting from impatience, or confusion as a result of obtrusive and incomplete ways of thinking, as well as functional fixedness, may arise (Wertheimer, 1964, pp. 226–235). Likewise, creative adjustment is a holistic process within the organism/environmental field, involving interrelated sensory, motor, emotional, and intellectual aspects. Striving for the "good gestalt", creative adjustment involves letting go of chronically dysfunctional behavior patterns, using one's perceptual functions and available resources optimally in the interchange with the given circumstances of one's present life, implying also insight and the bestowal of new meaning.

For example, I engaged an extremely intellectual adult patient, suffering from panic reactions and irrational fears when home alone in the evening, in a two-chair dialogue between his fears and his logic. He had indefatigably attempted to avoid the uncomfortable situation of being alone, hoping that this would solve his panic reactions. He also tried to elicit a magic formula from me that would intellectually dissolve the cause of the fears. In the role of his fears, he was speechless, without muscle tone. At this point in our therapeutic process, I dared to slip into the role of his irrational fears and gave voice to my fantasies, appealing to his logical role: "You need to feel me! I am the only part of your life which cannot be rationally explained or calculated! You can't pretend I am not here! I want you to see me, hear me! I am part of you, and I make sense! Don't try to cut me off!" He began to shake, drop his head, and weep silently. When he emerged from this emotional state, he looked me straight in the face and claimed: "This is a turning point for me. I want to accept the fears now, but I don't know how to do it." The acknowledgment of a disowned aspect of himself was an important step toward integration.

B. Applying the Principles of Gestalt Theory, and Reorganizing the Field in Search of "Good Form"

Stressing the significance of Gestalt psychology theory for the Gestalt approach, Wallen (1971), suggested three basic tasks that serve as guidelines for Gestalt therapeutic interventions:

"First, to break up the patient's chronically poorly organized field. The patient has certain standard ways of perceiving or acting in relationship to a need. The Gestalt therapist isolates portions of this field so that the self-regulating tendency of the neurotic can be broken up into smaller subunits. This eventually will permit the reorganization of both the motor field and the perceptual field. Also the Gestalt therapist works to heighten each emerging figure. (...) The therapist works to unblock the impulse so that it can organize the field" (Wallen, 1971, pp. 12–13).

Thus the therapist and patient engage in making the patient's ability to control himself a matter of intentional choice, adhering to the tenet of responsibility in Gestalt therapy. Allowing familiar elements to be mixed up, reweighted, and reconfigured results in new meaning as well as in different mutual influences between the parts and the whole.

When a patient grumbled about having had all kinds of mishaps during summer break, I noticed how she clenched her fists while speaking, checking an impulse. I suggested that we work on the nagging tone of her voice in conjunction with the aggression she was directing toward herself by clenching her fists instead of directly addressing her anger. By amplifying her tone and experimenting with a firm rubber ball in each hand, her anger toward me about having taken a six-week summer break could finally be expressed.

C. Perceiving and Understanding, and Taking a Process-Oriented Approach

The interactive process between perception and comprehension can be promoted by implementing methods and materials from expressive arts. Perceiving and understanding the figure and background, the directed tensions, and the interplay of forces that a person presents, and locating them within the life context of this individual – in short, helping to make sense out of the givens – are essential aspects of the therapeutic task.

A patient suffering from disabling dizziness and panic attacks could gain insight into the function of her symptoms by role-playing a trialogue with two aunts. Used to sitting slumped, not exhaling, and pressing her voice into unnaturally high octaves, she was surprised to feel particularly comfortable in the role of one of the aunts. In this role, in which her posture and breathing nearly collapsed, the function of her persistent symptoms slowly became clear, as she disclosed with obvious satisfaction: "Now you are one of us! We all suffer from the same symptoms, and now we can fully accept you as one of the women in our family. Stay this way!" The process through which her dysfunctional patterns developed could be experienced, and she became aware of how she was maneuvering herself into her persistent symptoms.

D. Addressing the Structural Relatedness between Experience and Expression, and Finding Personal Meaning within the Context of One's Life

"Recent psychological thinking, then, encourages us to call vision a creative activity of the human mind. Perceiving accomplishes at the sensory level what in the realm of reasoning is known as understanding. Every man's eyesight anticipates in a modest way the justly admired capacity of the artist to produce patterns that validly interpret experience by means of organized form. Eyesight is insight" (Arnheim, 1974, p. 46).

Arnheim holds that the expression of a creation lies in the perceptual qualities of its stimulus pattern. His concept of isomorphism proposes a structural kinship between this stimulus pattern and the expression which it conveys (ibid., p. 450): a perceptual expression is inherent in every clearly formed object or process. The structural relatedness between internal experience and external expression may take the form of a metaphor, symbol, or tangible creation. One of the examples that Arnheim offers for this should ring a bell with most Gestalt therapists: he mentions a person who cannot swallow, because there once was something in his or her life which could not be "swallowed whole". Following this train of thought, I have found evidence for structural kinship between patients' creations and their present emotional state. The challenging therapeutic task, then, involves helping the perception and awareness of the phenomena that these creations express emerge. It is exactly this "in-between us", this relationship between therapist and patient, which forms the context in which a figure can emerge from a background. Consolidating our work implies reacting to the creative process in its entirety. For instance, with a painting, by attending to the interaction of the forms and their directions, to that which has become figure and background, to the patterns, to the relations and isolations, to the colors and their significance, as well as reflecting the affective states, breathing, and thoughts or fantasies while painting, and understanding what this process signifies within the therapeutic relationship and the patient's life outside therapy.

In other words, the therapeutic relationship involves jointly reflecting what has been experienced during the creative process. During the processing part of these sessions, we concentrate on the personal meaning and implications of these newly acquired realizations within the patient's life context. This involves understanding patterns, connections, and repetitions as well as bringing the future into the here-and-now and discussing what we expect to happen next and how the patient intends to deal with these insights in the near future.

E. Transforming the Familiar into Something New and Valuable, Risk-Taking and Allowing Surprises, and Using Humor, Metaphors and Parapraxes Productively

My approach to the creative aspects of the therapeutic relationship has benefited tremendously from Albert Rothenberg, who examined the creative operations of successful psychotherapeutic practice. Whereas a common definition of "creativity" is "the capacity or state of bringing something into being", Rothenberg defines creative process and creativity as "the state, capacities, and conditions of bringing forth entities or events that are *both* new and valuable" (Rothenberg, 1988, p. xiii).

Rothenberg's study focussed not only on creative processes in patients, but also on therapists' creative ways of working. He encourages therapists not merely to stimulate creative activities in their patients, but also to engage in their own creative doing and daring within the therapeutic relationship. This functions as a model or identification figure for the patient. The two creative operations that Rothenberg describes in detail relate to all sensory modalities and operate with the productive integration of two different or even antithetical objects or ideas. The first, the homospatial process, "consists of actively conceiving two or more discrete entities occupying the same space, a conception leading to the articulation of new identities" (ibid., p. 7), whereas the second, the "Janusian process, consists of actively conceiving two or more opposites or antitheses simultaneously" (ibid., p. 11). These approaches to productive integration may remind Gestalt therapists of the processes of inclusion, the therapeutic task of attempting to be simultaneously aware of oneself and of another person (Yontef, 1993) and our established methods for working with polarities. Since my therapeutic style is highlighted by the use of humor, metaphors, and what are commonly known as Freudian slips, I fully embrace Rothenberg's reflections on their role in therapeutic interventions. Effectively using metaphor, humor (paradox and irony), and parapraxes demonstrates the psychotherapeutic art of connecting the concrete with the abstract, stimulating the imagination, and deepening appreciation. Moreover, this practice reveals the readiness of the therapist to be an identification figure by trusting one's intuition and willingly taking the risk of articulating one's realizations in an unfamiliar way. New meanings for the conflicts and dysfunctions of the patient emerge spontaneously, accompanied by the feeling of surprise and sudden realization. Advances in cognition and emotion go hand in hand. Rothenberg also offers a moving account of the interrelationship of the creative psychotherapeutic process and the interventions that arise out of empathic understanding. He notes that the act of giving to others is a characteristic of creative activities, reminding us of the essence of the helping professions (see Rothenberg, 1988, p. 185).

F. Practicing Process-Oriented Diagnosis, Having Knowledge of the Indications and Counterindications for Using Various Methods and Materials, and Engaging in Dialogic Relationship

Handling the indications and counterindications of specific materials and methods for particular disorders and disturbances categorically presents more of a hindrance than helpful support for a therapist who is attempting to promote creative expression and interaction. Just as Gestalt therapy takes a process-oriented approach to diagnosis, which encompasses the search for meaning in the patient's unique interpersonal patterns and dialogic relationship (e.g. Yontef, 1993; Staemmler, 1999), this process-oriented approach is also applicable when using artistic materials and methods. The process-oriented diagnosis takes a number of factors into account, including the patient's as well as the therapist's personality structure, the patient's interpersonal relationship patterns and unresolved conflicts, and the dynamics of the therapeutic interaction.

There are infinite ways of dealing with the difficulties and sufferings of a human being. The effectiveness of therapeutic intervention depends on the skills available to create the appropriate atmosphere and work together in whatever medium has been chosen. Which medium or method is indeed chosen depends upon such factors as the present problems with which a patient is struggling; the problem-solving strategies of the therapist; the availability of time, room, and costs; the attractiveness of certain materials to the patient and therapist; the situations and phases in treatment that are particularly conducive to using artistic materials; and, the influence of such external factors as in-patient or out-patient treatment. Also, the risk factors involved when using these media must be taught and taken seriously (see Franzke, 1989, pp. 221–259).

There is neither one single method that represents a cure-all nor such a thing as *the* one and only technique as a remedy for a specific dysfunction or symptom. In practice, it becomes evident that different materials have very different degrees of attractiveness to and effects on different patients. The challenging task of the therapist is to learn the art and science of offering means for creative expression by "picking patients up" at their present cognitive and emotional whereabouts, facilitating an atmosphere where playful exchange is possible, and finding an adequate means for this form of interpersonal communication.

For example, a young patient, obsessed about receiving the recognition of his mother for his achievements at the university, had used up most of one session with reports on his scholastic performance to date. His narrative, however, was devoid of emotional involvement, and I noticed that I was becoming bored and impatient. As this was a pattern we had previously experienced together, I decided to change our medium of communication in an effort to contact the avoided emotional aspects of his narrative. I sat down on the carpet and grabbed a plastic ball that makes noises like a human voice when rolled. As it came rolling toward him, he began to giggle, and he appeared relieved, rolling it back to me with force. Then I took a stuffed animal, a cuddly, yellow crocodile, and answered him by using the crocodile as a hand puppet and uttering nonsense syllables. He dropped to the carpet himself and reached for a monkey hand puppet, with which he answered me. After a buoyant joust and lots of laughter, he grinned sheepishly and said: "It feels good not to have to impress you like my mother."

G. Creating Potential Space for Playful Experiences between Therapist and Patient, and Facilitating Authentic Self-Expression and Unique Style within Relationship

In general, playful experiences allow a person to anticipate the realities of life and the demands upon him- or herself within the context of their life. Therapeutic methods that have integrated such creative and practicing techniques offer an important approach to children, adolescents, and adults. In this aspect, the perspectives of Winnicott, the child psychoanalyst, and of F. Perls on the goal of therapy are quite compatible:

"Psychotherapy takes place in the overlap of two areas of playing, that of the patient and that of the therapist. Psychotherapy has to do with two people playing together. The corollary of this is that where playing is not possible, then the work done by the therapist is directed towards bringing the patient from a state of not being able to play into a state of being able to play. (...) It is in playing and only in playing that the individual child or

adult is able to be creative and to use the whole personality, and it is only in being creative that the individual discovers the self" (Winnicott, 1999, pp. 38, 54).

"Creativity and adjustment are polar, they are mutually necessary" (Perls F
et al., 1951, p. 231). Perls and Goodman, in their description of creative adjustment and progressive integration, compared creative artists with children, calling particular attention to the structure of art-working and children's play and proposing that the same middle mode of acceptance and
growth also operates in creative adjustment in general (ibid., pp. 245–6). The
tenet that spontaneity can be considered evidence of curative insight appears compatible also with Winnicott's approach.

H. Being Personally Familiar with Materials and Methods

Yet another fundamental requirement for therapists applying artistic methods is to have sufficient experience themselves with the materials and methods they offer. Being personally familiar with the methods used not only enables better appreciation for the ways in which the patients may experience
and react to them, but also sensitizes therapists to the dangers of overstimu-
lation and insufficient processing of what has been experienced by the patient. When therapists draw from their own experience, they become aware
not only that the same material can have varying degrees of attraction for
one and the same person during different phases of therapy, but also that the
same material, such as clay, can stimulate the desire to knead it energetically as proof of one's own vitality as well as trigger off repulsive reactions
and fears of getting dirty and losing control.

V. Conclusion

It has been my intention to present creatively practiced Gestalt therapy as a
science as well as an art. Allowing theory to influence my practice and vice
versa, I have felt more stimulated and have found the results to be more effective. Thus I am motivated to trust my judgment and intuition and to explore with patients the "in-between" with a certain degree of risk. By facilitating novel, valuable reorganizations of familiar givens, it is the element of
surprise, the unexpected viewpoint or feedback, which can effect more
change by promoting awareness in our patients than a mere repetition of
what they expect from us. The fact that methods taken from expressive arts
have, in some cases, been used in Gestalt therapy without theoretical reflection, either as *art for art's sake*, loosening up the therapeutic process when it
is sluggish, as a means of allowing Gestalt therapy to appear to be "nourishing" in comparison to more ascetic methods, or even as an adventure-prom-
ising and practical "auxiliary technique", is deplorable.[5] Superficial use of

---

[5] Compare Schreyoegg A (1991) Supervision. Ein Integratives Modell. Junfermann,
Paderborn.

artistic materials or Gestalt therapeutic interventions appears to reflect the misconception of Gestalt therapy which Laura Perls (1978) and Isadore From (1984) discussed. Implementing certain methods and media without basing them in the theory to which they belong does not reflect professional seriousness. Good theory generates good practice, and vice versa. In this vein, I whole-heartedly make a case for teaching the theoretical foundations of working with creative processes and artistic materials to Gestalt trainees and encouraging their unique therapeutic style. Judging from my own experiences as a therapist and supervisor, it is my conviction that understanding and appreciating the relationship between theory and practice will inspire therapists and trainees with respect to their own creative processes as well as their interactions with patients. It makes for enjoyable and satisfying work.[6]

References

Amendt-Lyon N (1999) Kunst und Kreativität in der Gestalttherapie. In: Fuhr R, Srekovic M, Gremmler-Fuhr M (eds) Handbuch der Gestalttherapie. Hogrefe, Göttingen, pp 857–877

Amendt-Lyon N (2001a) Art and creativity in Gestalt therapy. Gestalt Review 5(4): 225–248

Amendt-Lyon N (2001b) "No risk, no fun!" A reply to commentaries. Gestalt Review 5(4): 272–275

Arnheim R (1974) Art and visual perception: A psychology of the creative eye. U of Calif Press, Berkeley Los Angeles

Burley T (1998) Minds and brains for Gestalt therapists. Gestalt Review 2(2): 131–142

Franzke E (1989) Der Mensch und sein Gestaltungserleben. Psychotherapeutische Nutzung kreativer Arbeitsweisen. 3., korr. Auflage. Hans Huber, Bern Stuttgart Toronto

Groddeck G (1990) Krankheit als Symbol. Schriften zur Psychosomatik. Fischer, Frankfurt/M

From I (1984) Reflections on Gestalt therapy after thirty-two years of practice: A requiem for Gestalt. Gestalt J VII(1): 4–12

Kitzler R, Perls L, Stern M (1982) Retrospects and prospects: A trialogue between Laura Perls, Richard Kitzler and E. Mark Stern. Voices 18(2): 5–22

Kurdirka N, Perls L (1982) A talk with Laura Perls about the therapist and the artist. Voices 18(2): 29–37

Leedy J, Rapp E (1973) Poetry therapy and some links to art therapy. Art Psychotherapy 1: 145–151

Miller MV (1980) Notes on art and symptoms. Gestalt J III(1): 86–98

Oaklander V (1979) A Gestalt therapy approach with children through the use of art and creative expression. In: Marcus EH (ed) Gestalt therapy and beyond: An integrated mind-body approach. Meta, California, pp 235–247

Oaklander V (1988) Windows to our children. A Gestalt therapy approach to children and adolescents. Gestalt J Press, Highland, New York

Perls F (1948) Theory and technique of personality integration. In: Stevens JO (ed) (1977) gestalt is. Bantam, New York, pp 44–69

Perls F, Hefferline R, Goodman P (1951) Gestalt therapy: Excitement and growth in the human personality. Dell, New York

---

[6] The author is deeply indebted to Marc Erismann for his theoretical inspiration.

Perls L (1971) Two instances of Gestalt therapy. In: Pursglove P (ed) Recognitions in Gestalt therapy. Harper Colophon, New York Evanston San Francisco London, pp 42–63

Perls L (1978) Concepts and misconceptions of Gestalt therapy. Voices 14(3): 31–36

Perls L (1989) Leben an der Grenze. Köln, Edition Humanistische Psychologie

Perls L, Rosenfeld E (1982) A conversation between Laura Perls and Edward Rosenfeld. Voices 18(2): 22–29

Polster E (1987) Every person's life is worth a novel. WW Norton, New York

Portele H (1996) Max Wertheimer. Gestalttherapie 10(2): 4–13

Rapp E (1980) Gestalt art therapy in groups. In: Ronall R, Feder B (eds) Beyond the hot seat. Brunner/Mazel, New York, pp 86–104

Rhyne J (1971) The Gestalt art experience. In: Fagan J, Shepherd IL (eds) Gestalt therapy now. Theory techniques applications. Harper & Row, New York Evanston San Francisco London, pp 274–284

Rhyne J (1973) The Gestalt approach to experience, art, and art therapy. Amer J of Art Therapy 12(4): 237–248

Rhyne J (1980) Gestalt psychology/Gestalt therapy: Forms/contexts. Gestalt J III(1): 76–84

Rhyne J (1996) The Gestalt art experience. Patterns that connect. Magnolia Street Publishers, Chicago

Rothenberg A (1988) The creative process of psychotherapy. WW Norton, New York London

Staemmler F (1999) Verstehen und Verändern – Dialogisch-prozessuale Diagnostik. In: Fuhr R, Srekovic M, Gremmler-Fuhr M (eds) Handbuch der Gestalttherapie. Hogrefe, Göttingen, pp 673–682

Vich M, Rhyne, J (1967) Psychological growth and the use of art materials: Small group experiments with adults. J of Humanistic Psych 7(1): 163–170

Wallen R (1971) Gestalt therapy and Gestalt psychology. In: Fagan J, Shepherd IL (eds) Gestalt therapy now. Theory techniques applications. Harper & Row, New York Evanston San Francisco London, pp 8–13

Wertheimer M (1964) Produktives Denken. Kramer, Frankfurt a. M

Winnicott DW (1999) Playing and Reality. Routledge, London New York

Yontef G (1993) Awareness, dialogue & process. Essays on Gestalt therapy. Gestalt J Press, Highland, New York

Zinker J (1971) Dreamwork as theatre. Voices 7(2): 18–21

Zinker J (1973) Gestalt therapy is permission to be creative. A sermon in praise of the use of experiment in Gestalt therapy. Voices 9(4): 75

Zinker J (1977) Creative process in Gestalt therapy. Brunner/Mazel, New York

On the Other Side of the Moon: The Import of Implicit Knowledge for Gestalt Therapy[1]

Daniel N. Stern and the Boston Change Process Study Group[2]

Thank you, Margherita and Giovanni. Actually, I guess this is our third meeting. We seem to have met through the literature before Palermo,[3] which was a sort of preparing the territory. When we met in Palermo, I think that the three of us fell in love with each other. So the real reason why I'm here is to continue our affair. In fact, like most lovers, we're going to have many disagreements, and that will be the fun part to talk about, I think.

What I'm going to address in part during this seminar is "the other side of the moon", because we all accept that the relationship is important and that it is primary over the content. These are not the two sides of the moon we're talking about. I want to talk about the implicit knowledge that never has to become verbalized and that plays a huge role in the context and in how people change in psychotherapy. Many psychotherapies use nonverbal techniques, but the remarkable role of the non-explicit or the implicit and how it really works is not focused on. This is strange, because in many therapies, such as body therapy, and in some Gestalt techniques, you go after the implicit knowledge of the patient, but then you transfer it to the narrative explicit knowledge. My feeling is that Gestalt therapy knows about implicit knowledge and uses it, but it doesn't focalise on it theoretically, as it probably should. Maybe I'm wrong: we'll see.

Let me start with the distinction between implicit and explicit knowledge, which everybody knows, but which I want to make very clear.

Explicit knowledge is verbal, symbolic, and declarative. It's also what narration is made of: all interpretations are by definition explicit. Implicit

---

[1] This chapter is the transcription of a speech by the author in Siracusa, Italy, on January 18, 2002, for a seminar entitled "Creative Improvisation in Psychotherapy", which was organized by the Istituto di Gestalt, whose directors are Margherita Spagnuolo Lobb and Giovanni Salonia. Although the author has revised the text, the narrative style of this speech has been maintained. Transcribed by Stefania Benini.

[2] Members of the Boston Change Process Study Group include: N. Bruschweiler-Stern, A. Harrison, K. Lyons-Ruth, A. Morgan, J. Nahum, L. Sander, D. Stern, and E. Tronick.

[3] This refers to a seminar in Palermo, Italy, in January 2001 which, like the one in January 2002, was also organized by the Istituto di Gestalt.

knowledge is nonverbal. It is not symbolic, and it is not conscious, but not repressed: it simply has never come into consciousness. A couple of assumptions about implicit knowledge are very important, because we used to think – and I was taught – that implicit knowledge is mostly sensory-motor knowledge. The examples have always been things like the baby getting the thumb into the mouth or a child learning to ride a bicycle, etc. We now realize that implicit knowledge is much more than that: it includes affect, thoughts, anticipations, and "how to be with somebody" in all its senses. In fact, in the world that we all know and use in all of our relationships, I would say that 90% of knowledge is implicit. What do you do with your eyes when you talk to someone? How do you adjust your face to get exactly the right expression? And how do you read that on the other person's face? This is totally implicit: in fact, you can't even put it into words. When we talk about *transference* and *countertransference*, for instance, I believe that we are referring to largely implicit knowings of how to be with somebody who is an authority figure, an equal, or whatever they are.

We also used to think that implicit knowledge, with age and development, as Piaget says, progressively becomes explicit, because it becomes symbolized and talked about. According to this perspective, the development supposedly implies that implicit knowledge turns into explicit knowledge. This is not true for the most part. Some things do become explicit. But the majority of implicit knowledge remains implicit and, while the explicit knowledge expands, the implicit knowledge does the same: just more and more things are understood in that way. The other aspect we didn't realize about implicit knowledge is that we used to think it was less rich, less sophisticated, less elaborate, and less complicated than explicit knowledge – which isn't true. Implicit knowledge is extraordinarily rich and complicated. What you see children doing early on, such as "how they greet their mother after a reunion", "how should they feel about it", and "what should they think about it" are things they learn long before they can talk (at twelve months).

This is what I mean by the other side of the moon, because I'm am going to spend most of the time talking about implicitly knowing about things. You can see right away that my talking about implicit knowledge in psychotherapy with adults is a natural continuation of the work with babies. Because there everything is implicit, and so we've somehow become experts at looking at the implicit, since that's what you've got. I say this by way of introduction.

The other thing we're going to talk about is the relationship, but a special part of it, and I want to talk about the implicit knowledge of this special part of it, which is *intersubjectivity*.

I'll first describe a brief clinical example, in order to explain why understanding the implicit is so important. A colleague of mine, a psychoanalyst, was seeing a woman client on the couch, three times a week. They would talk about a lot of things, and every now and then the client would mention not knowing really what the therapist was doing back there. One morning, the client comes in and says, "You know, I'm sick of not seeing your face. I would like to see your face. I don't know what you're doing back there. You could be knitting, sleeping ... I don't know what." Now, the client didn't know she was going to do this. All of a sudden it popped up, and she said this, sat up, and turned around to look at the therapist. This had never happened in two years. She didn't plan to sit up, she just did sit up. You can say that that could have been handled in a lot of ways, or it could have been avoided, if you wanted to avoid it. But, in this case, we have this woman looking at the therapist, and the therapist looking at her, and there's a silence. And the tension rises. We call this a "now moment". What the therapist then did was a total improvisation – a very creative one – which is necessary at such times, which I'll talk about in a moment; I just want to complete this example, so all the background fits in. So the therapist, after a silence, looked at the client, slowly softened her face, and a very small smile started to come on her face, while the client was looking at her. Then the therapist said: "hello". More silence follows. Then the client laid back down. The therapeutic work is very different after this moment. It becomes much better and much deeper work. But the patient and the therapist never talked about this moment of looking at each other and about the latter saying "hello". Somehow, this moment had changed the relationship dramatically, without ever being talked about. It was only about a year and a half later that the client said: "You remember that time when I sat up and you said 'hello'. I think that was the first time I realized that you were open to me and on my side." And nothing more was said about it after that.

This is a rather simple example of how a piece of implicit knowledge was exchanged between these two women, expanding their shared intersubjective worlds. This is the kind of contact I'm most interested in, and it has many similarities with the contact Gestalt therapists talk about, but it also has some differences that I think we have to work through. That's going to be our "lovers' fight". In fact, in so many psychotherapy methods, these kinds of contact either move the therapy ahead or stop the therapy. Often they are not verbalized.

Now, let me elaborate on this *intersubjective contacting of people*. Here I think that my points of view and those of Gestalt therapists, in any case of this group, are very close. It's very clear now that human beings are constructed to read other people's minds, and not by waves or anything mysterious, but by "reading" their voice, their tone of voice, their postures, their gestures – in other words, all the ways they say things. Our nervous system is constructed to do that. One of the things it is best at is capturing what you imagine is the other person's experience. This is something we only do with other people. The conclusion (which I think we all agree about, because it's talking about what's between people) is that our minds are not so independent. Indeed, they are very *interdependent*. Our minds are not separate or isolated, and we are not the only owners of our own mind. The boundaries between two people, even a mother and a baby, are very clear, but are also very permeable; we live, and a baby develops, in an atmosphere where we are totally surrounded by other people's motives, desires, intentions, and feelings. Minds get created by virtue of being in constant interaction and dialogue with other minds, so that the whole idea of a "one-person psychology" ought not to exist, or at least it must be incomplete.

I would like to outline for you some evidence for this view of living in an *intersubjective matrix*:

The first piece of evidence is neuroscientific: so-called *mirror neurons* have been found in the brain, sitting right next to the motor neurons that make you act. So, if I reach for this glass, my motor neurons will fire, and the mirror neurons that are right next to them will fire, too. Now, as you watch me move my hand toward the glass, your mirror neurons will fire off in the exact same place as if *you* had done it. So your body is telling you in some way – we don't know exactly how – what it feels like for me to do this. Somehow, we are constructed to be inside of other people, if we pay attention, and participate in their experience. Also, if I make a lot of gestures, like the one I just made with my hand, your motor neurons will go off: they will discharge, so you know what I'm feeling when I do this. But if I again move my hand toward the glass, there's an intention, and you know it right away – before I touch the glass – that there's an intention. There is a part in the brain that has been identified that discharges as soon as you think there's an intention. If I just move my hand, but not go toward the glass, your motor-neurons will tell you what it feels like to be me – but that part of your brain will not fire off, and so you know that I did not have an interpretable intention. This means that the human brain is built so that it has a special way of detecting intentions on the other person's part.

Another thing we are born with that makes this intersubjective matrix are *adaptive oscillators,* which are really like little clocks in different muscles groups that can get into synchronization with something outside and can get reset all the time, so that they synchronize. If we didn't have adaptive oscillators, we could never kick a moving football. In other words, we have to synchronize our movements with the movements of somebody or something else. We see that all the time, but don't think about how hard it is. For instance, if you're washing the dishes and I'm drying them, and you hand me a dish, and then another one, you synchronize, and you do it totally smoothly, because both our adaptive oscillators have gone into synchronization. Think about it: even if you suddenly kiss somebody passionately, why is it that you don't break your front teeth? The answer is that it has to do with this very quick synchronization. It means that you know what the other person is feeling, because you have synchronized your whole body toward that. This is similar to what the mirror neurons do. The essential question is not why we participate in other people's experiences, but *how do we stop doing it?*

Let me tell you about some developmental evidences. Many people, including me, who work with babies before they can talk (Trevarthen, 1980; Trevarthen and Hubley, 1978; Meltzoff and Moore, 1977; Meltzoff and Gopnick, 1993; Meltzoff, 1995), speak of *primary intersubjectivity.* A baby is born with a capacity to read and to synchronize into other people's mental states. All of the literature on early imitation is like this: if you take a newborn, a three-day-old baby, and stick out your tongue, the baby will imitate you. The baby has to be in the right state, and he or she does it. It's not a reflex; we don't know how babies do it. The baby doesn't know that it's got a face and that it's taking a visual pattern on the face of the other person and

translating it into a motor pattern on itself. Babies have this intermodal capacity of being able to translate from one modality to another modality, which
make them sensitive to things such as the tone of voice, muscular movements
and so on. In this way, they can participate in another person's life.

For example, if you bring a baby before he can talk very well into a laboratory, and the experimenter lets some candy fall out of a glass several times,
like this, and then if the baby is sent home and returns the next day, and the
experimenter gives him the same object, he will do something similar: i.e.,
let the candy drop *into* the glass. In other words, the baby imitates not what
he saw, but what he assumed was the intention.

This also happens if you have, let's say, a dumbbell. The experimenter
shows the baby, like this, how to pull on the ends of the dumbbell, and he
doesn't succeed in detaching the two poles. Then the baby is brought back,
and the experimenter gives it to the baby. The baby will immediately try to
pull one off and, when he suceeds, smile. In the control experiment, there is
a robot that does this – and doesn't succeed – as the baby watches. When the
baby comes back, he won't try to pull the dumbbell pole off, because robots
don't have intentions for the baby: only people do.

The Norwegian psychologist, Stein Braten (1998), has talked about the
capacity for participating in another person's experience. He talks about
"other-centered participation", an acting or feeling from the other person's
orientation. This is a powerful thing, and it seems to be one of the most basic
aspects of being a human being with other human beings. It's a condition of
humanness, and it's one of the reasons why we talk about "theory of mind",
which is really this kind of intersubjectivity. It's one of the reasons, too, why
we say that autistic children have a failure of intersubjectivity, that they are
not interested in other people's minds and don't try, don't slip into other people's experience. If, for instance, you put the palms of your hands towards
me, like this – and I'm a baby – I'm going to imitate you, and I'll raise my
hands and hold them with the palms facing you. But if I hold them, then I'm
looking at the back of my hands. If I imitate you, why wouldn't I hold them
like this, with the palms facing me? Normal babies do not do that, but autistic children do: they hold their hands with the palms toward their chest, like
this.

The way we look at psychotherapy, and I think every method does this to
some extent, is that there are always two agendas: one is the content, which
is explicit and co-constructs the narrative; the other agenda is the intersubjective finding one another and the constantly expanding the intersubjective
sharing between the two people. This second agenda is largely implicit. I
will focus here only on the second agenda: how the intersubjective relationship gets put together between two people.

Fundamentally, I see this kind of intersubjective searching, improvising,
and co-creating between two people as a form of psycho-ethology. For instance, if you watch two dogs meet each other on the street, they do a very
interesting choreography of sniffing around, looking, and doing all these
movements to figure out what's going to happen between them. Sometime
it's a very delicate process – whether they will go in the direction of fighting

or playing together, with sexual or domination interests. This is how I see the intersubjective finding of one another in psychotherapy.

Pretend that our two dogs are people: that one of the dogs is the client, and the other dog is the therapist. Only they are tied to chairs, so they can't move. They are going to have to do everything the dogs do, but they will have to do it by mentalizing their actions. And this is where the implicit comes in, because they'll have to decide at every moment: "Am I interested in you? Do I like you? Do you like me? You are too far away – come closer. No, not that close; I'm not ready. Right now, don't do anything. Did you just hear what I said? But did you *really* hear? I wish you'd stop that." You see, all of these things are our two dogs with mentalizations, and nothing has to be spoken. It's done with words, but the implicit message involves what the two people are going to understand about how they are together.

Now I want to proceed with clinical examples.

We see a sort of cycle of moving towards contact and then moving away from contact; it's a slightly different cycle from the one that you use (Salonia, 1992; Spagnuolo Lobb, 1992, 2001), but it has a lot of similarities. We see the beginning part as what we call the *moving-along*. This *moving-along* is a fascinating process, because what it really amounts to is that the client says something, then the therapist really doesn't know what the two of them are going to say or do next, until the client actually says it. Then the client doesn't know what he is going to say, until the therapist has actually said what she is going to say. It's even worse than that. If I'm the therapist, I don't know what I am going to say until I say it. If the therapist knows what she is going to say too much in advance, or even before the client answers, then she is treating an abstraction or a theory and not treating a person.

This means that you've got two people who are constantly improvising together, and that's why we use the word *moving-along*. Not only are they improvising, but they are also co-creating where they are going to move. What one person says becomes the context that will determine in part what the other person says.

One very interesting feature about this improvisation is its enormous creativity. The reason it's so creative, is that the *moving-along* improvisation is very *sloppy*. You make, so to speak, mistakes all the time. You didn't quite understand that right, or you were thinking something while you said it, which gave it a different color. So there are constant derailments. And we see these derailments as an opportunity and not as an error. This is very true in mother-infant relationships. But it is also true in therapy relationships, because each error is an opportunity to learn a way to be together, to repair the error. With babies, we see that every time there is an error in this *moving-along* process, it is a chance for the baby to learn coping mechanisms, and for the mother, too. In psychotherapy situations, we see these errors or derailments as creative opportunities to take a slightly different path. This is why we call the process *sloppy*. And we have come to love the idea that it is sloppy, because that's what makes it creative.

In thinking about the improvisation, sloppiness, and creativity of this kind of process, we have found it very useful to consider *dynamic system theory* and *chaos theory*. It turns out that any system that is extremely complicated, with thousands of variables, all of a sudden, when it tries to organize itself, creates what we call *emergent properties*, which you can never fully explain. So when the woman client sat up from the couch and looked at the therapist, that was an *emergent property*, an emergent moment that was not completely predictable. One could predict from her, I assume, that one day she would want to know "are you open to me?", "are you on my side?", and "what do you do back there?" But you will never know which day and in what manner or form that will happen. In that sense, it's unpredictable. That's why you don't know what you're going to say until you say it.

To summarize: we have this *moving-along* process that we define in terms of relational moves where each person either says or does something, or they do it together. You string together these relational moves that would include a silence or onything else. While you can't predict what they are going to lead to, they do somehow rather help you get to a point where an *emergent property* can all of a sudden pop up. In that sense, they do lead somewhere, but not exactly. Then you suddenly have an *emergent property*, and the two people are thrown into a *now moment*. It doesn't matter what the method of treatment is. For instance, the "hello" and the "sitting up and looking at the therapist" was in a psychoanalytic treatment. But I've had the same thing happen to me in a psychotherapy, where we're sitting in chairs and the client says to me: "I'm sick of looking at your face; I don't want to see it anymore. I know what you're thinking; I'm going to turn my chair right around and look at the wall." And he turns around. And there's a silence. That's another *now moment*. What's interesting about these *now moments* is that the therapist doesn't know what to do and becomes anxious. The anxiety in both therapist and client mounts, and the therapist is, in a way, *désarçonné*. The first thing that one does if he doesn't have a way of accepting or handling this is to run back into technique and hide. There are many things you know, in either of those situations with the patient sitting up. You can say something that is technically correct, such as, "what are you feeling?" But, actually, that's a way of hiding from the contact. To have a *moment of meeting*, which is what the "hello" was, the therapist has to be spontaneous and authentic and say something that comes from him or herself. It has to be perfectly tuned to the situation, not to the theory, and it has to carry the signature of the therapist, so that it's personal experience. This permits the *moment of meeting*. It can be very simple, as when the therapist said "hello", or it can be a fairly complicated, much more dramatic one.

Here's another example from a case of Stephen A. Mitchell (2000, pp. 139–143). Mitchell had a client in psychotherapy who was a young and very intelligent and mean woman, who would give him hell. She would criticize him and tell him how bad he was. She made life difficult for him and, because she was so smart, she understood all his major faults and would get right into the fault, twist the knife, and make him feel awful. He tried everything a well-trained therapist would do to stop it. In fact, he was a very experienced therapist. One day, the client was being particularly difficult. She was really being bitchy, and then, all of a sudden, she stopped – which now signifies an *emergent moment* that is coming up, and I'll paraphrase what she said to Mitchell (p. 142): "If we were on the street right now, outside, and I wasn't your client, and this wasn't a psychotherapy session, and if I said to you what I just said to you, what would you tell me?" There was a silence – there's always a silence, here – and the therapist, Steve, said: "If we were out on the street? And this was not a therapy? And you just said all that to me? What would I say to you? I'd say 'go fuck yourself!'" That's a *moment of meeting*. There was a little silence, and then he added: "But I *am* your therapist and we *are* in therapy."

Right after that, once again, she calmed down and stopped going after him. And as with the "hello" client, this one, too, started to go much deeper and in another direction in her therapy; this exchange seemed really to shift the course. And here, too, they never talked about it. They never, never talked about that incident.

A variety of psychotherapy schools could criticize what he did: he let it go too long, didn't know how to stop it, was gratifying her by giving that kind of passionate response to her, and gave her control of the therapeutic situation by getting so excited. But, in fact, while you could make all these criticisms, it worked when nothing else had.

Usually, after these *moments of meeting*, we find what we call an *open space*, which is a sort of withdrawal. This word comes from baby experiments and baby observations. There is a kind of being alone but together, when some kind of assimilation occurs, which doesn't have to be verbalized. So we're still on the other side of the moon, here.

Now, I would like to put another issue on the table before starting with something else: that is, the importance of *here and now*. This is one of the places where I think Gestalt therapy has been really way ahead of other schools and where I'm in great agreement with it. But one of the things that has been fascinating me about *here and now* is that almost all therapies agree that things that happen in the here and now work more – they really take hold, and they make for better change and progress. We all agree. So I ask myself: *where is here* and *when is now*? And it turns out that the *when is now* is a very hard question to answer. We all agree, because I think that Gestalt therapy is very philosophically grounded in phenomenology: I've been wondering about many things here which I think may be of interest for us to discuss. I think we all agree that we only live directly *now*, subjectively. You are only alive now; there is no other time of living. If you have a memory, you're remembering it *now*. If you have an anticipation, you're having it *now*. There is no escape in this reality.

What is interesting, however, is that sometimes you need to have two times in order to have the experience. Take a memory – a very good example. One part of the memory is that you remember something that happened in the past and you can feel almost as if you're there but, at the same time, you have to know implicitly that you're in the *now*. It's the combination of being in the now and thinking about something in the past that makes you know that it's a memory, not a delusion, that you're not living in it but just remembering it. Thus, the act of memory requires that you know that it's happening now. But you don't know it intellectually – you know it implicitly. We actually have a lot of experiences that happen at the same time. Sometimes you feel like "well, I'm not completely in the present"; for instance, while I'm thinking of being here with you all, I'm thinking of what happened yesterday, or I'm thinking of what's going on in the other room. So it feels like you're only half in the present. But, in fact, you have not escaped from the present; you're just in two presents: this present and the present that you are experiencing next door or yesterday in the form of memory. It turns out that our experiences are mostly polyphonic and polyrhythmic. Then, there is another matter: what happens when all of a sudden there is a new present moment? What this feels like phenomenologically is what Merleau Ponty (1945) calls an *upsurge of a fresh present*, that you accept; you accept that all of a sudden there is this fresh present, and that's where you're living now.

Yet there's another problem with the present or the *now* of the here and now: *how long is the now?* How long is the present? Is it long enough for anything interesting to happen? If you use the vision of time that we use in the physical sciences, which is *chronòs* in ancient Greek, you will have a point of present that is extremely thin. It just moves along all the time, and it eats up the future as it moves, leaving the past in its wake. But it is itself just an instant; it's so small that nothing could happen in it. Yet, subjectively it feels like we're living in the present. This is a paradox that needs to be resolved.

Actually, some philosophers have solved this problem: I think that Husserl (1960, 1989) has been the most interesting, because he talks about a "three-part present". There is what he calls *the past of the present moment*, which is still present; *the instant of the present* that is passing; and *the future of the present moment*, which is also in the present. The whole thing is a *gestalt*, a whole. The best example for understanding this is found in music, because when you have a phrase of music, for example with six or seven notes in it, you hear the whole journey of the phrase across the notes, and that is what you seize in the present moment; it's all in the present, subjectively. You can't take a photograph of a musical phrase. Even the fact that it's written in notes doesn't matter; you don't hear it in notes but in phrases. The present moment actually is an *ensemble*; it's an aggregate of smaller units that make some kind of psychological sense and coherence. They make a *gestalt*.

This *gestalt* is very interesting, because it forms as it is happening. For instance, if we hear the first five notes of the seven-note phrase, we automatically create in our minds how it could end, which is influencing what you're hearing at this instant. In fact, if all of you hear the same five notes, and I ask you "how will it end?", you'll make a few implications of the first four notes, where you'll mostly agree on what are the possible endings. They are all just implications, not predictions. It's also very interesting that if I played the same music, which was Western traditional music and, instead of you, all of the people were Chinese who didn't know Western music, they would also be able to make implications that would be not very different from yours. During the present moment, the now, what happens is that the first three notes have not disappeared from the present: they do not go into memory, but rather they stay. The people who know the most about this are musicians and musicologists. In their interesting language, they talk about a phrase in music as where the crest of the present travels from the horizon of the past of the present moment to the horizon of the future of the present moment.

Till now, we've established that we have this very complicated *gestalt*, which is the *now*, and that we refer to it in therapy. Let's look at that carefully, since we are all talking about the here and the now.

Gestalt therapy frequently uses implicit knowledge, and the integration of the self is actually an implicit task or an implicit experience. The integration of the animal and the human souls is also an implicit knowledge. I can see that Gestalt therapy is very involved in implicit things, but I haven't seen a discussion about what *is* implicit knowledge. How is it different from other knowledge? What is its relationship to consciousness, how does implicit knowledge get into memory, and what kind of memory? These are what I call hard theoretical questions about implicit knowledge. We have been trying to think about those issues, and we don't have complete answers yet, of course, only small answers. This is what I mean when I say that I don't think that Gestalt therapy, or any psycotherapy method for that matter, has really tried to figure out what we mean by implicit knowledge: how it works and what makes it different. I think that one of the reasons why the Boston Change Process Study Group and I have been so interested in implicit knowledge, and how it is different from explicit, is that we have been forced by the reality of what a baby is to look at this.

As I said, it seems to me that Gestalt therapy works a lot with implicit knowledge (i.e., many techniques are not explicit), but – and this is a tricky comment – that its goal is to make the knowledge explicit. Here we have to cope with the big difference between *awareness* and *consciousness*. I just asked if *awareness* is a word in Italian, because, interestingly, there's no word for awareness in French, and since *conscience* is by definition verbal and symbolic, there's no way to be aware of something which isn't. I bring this up because you can be aware of things, but not conscious of them, and you can also be conscious of something and not be aware that you're conscious of it. I find the whole problem of consciousness is very much at the bottom of this and, as many of you may know, consciousness studies have become probably the single most exciting issue in modern cognitive psychology.

For instance, if you ask a client "what are you feeling?" or "where do you feel it?" or any kind of questions that helps him become aware of the feeling, then – once the client says what it is – it becomes conscious, or better, reflectively conscious: then the client knows that he is aware of it. Afterwards, you can take that consciouness and use the material to build up a narrative. But with implicit knowledge, it becomes conscious only with difficulty. What I'm suggesting is that you can make implicit knowledge conscious, but through a different mechanism: a two-person intersubjective mechanism. And there your implicit knowledge can become conscious. Let me try to explain it in the way I understand it.

Consciousness has always been a problem. Descartes had his model of consciousness, which you surely remember: everything you felt and sensed would come together in one place in the brain, which is what Damasio (1994) calls the *Cartesian theater*, like a theater where all comes together. In this case, however, you need somebody to watch the play. Modern scientists say that if there's somebody in your head watching what's going on in the theatre, then there has to be somebody inside of that person's head watching what's going on in his head, and so on.

This is what is called the error of Descartes. Descartes was very wrong; however, he was right in one regard: you need to have two different points of view on the same experience for it to become conscious: something you can experience, and then somebody to watch it from another place. And in all modern scientific theories of consciousness, when they speak in terms of brain circuits, they maintain that one has an experience, and that is one view, and then that experience has to be fed back into the brain in a different network. The second view is different from the first view. And the two together create consciousness. That's the explanation of consciousness within one person.

But there's another way to think about consciousness: to look at it as a social act: I have an experience, but I can intuit intersubjectively how the other person sees my experience. Now we have two views on my experience, and I acquire a different kind of consciousness, which I would call intersubjective consciousness. Therefore, consciousness doesn't have to be the work of my own brain; it can be the work of my brain with somebody else's brain. It's part of living in an intersubjective matrix, which makes an implicit experience become conscious, because it's public and it can be reflected on. But this way of becoming conscious is different from the usual one.

If we tell each other how the one perceives the other, we are creating a second level of truth, which is less good than the "animal level". Now, because you assume that the animal part is true, what each person has to do is to get another level of truth, which is implicit, in order to answer to the question: "To what extent is this person being sincere with words?" In this case, you get two layers of implicit knowledge.

As I mentioned earlier, the process of finding one another is sloppy, and words actually help the process of going other ways. But most psychotherapies pay attention to how it was put in words and what the words say. That's why I said to you at the very beginning: "I want to talk about the other side of the moon." I mean the side where I don't care what the words say. I am now exaggerating: of course they matter, but we know a lot about that. What we don't know about is the other side. I'm not trying to make comparisons and say one is more important than the other. I'm trying to say that they are complementary and very complicated sides, but we haven't paid enough attention to the implicit part.

In Gestalt therapy, you speak of figure/ground dynamics. I think that in therapy, this is exactly what happens: you get a change in figure and ground with regard to the implicit and explicit. We are so trained, and our culture is so verbal, that we privilege the verbal modality, and most of our therapies, including Gestalt therapy, grew out of the Freudian tradition, which says that if you can make the unconscious conscious, some good will be done. But you know, there is no reason to believe that this is true. One of the things that Freud found out very early on, was that if you could make the unconscious conscious, this didn't help. And that was when he and Ferenczi realized that it was the relationship that was most curative. Gestalt therapy, as I see it, comes out of the realization that making the unconscious conscious isn't really what makes the big change. But if it's the relationship, is it going to be *making what's unconscious about the relationship conscious?* Is that going to help? Yes, it helps, but there's this other part – which is what happens implicitly in the relationship – that becomes conscious differently and that may be more helpful. Again, I'm exaggerating, but this is why I say it's the other side of the moon.

You see, I find myself in a difficult position, because I still believe that talking about things really does help. But I get confused as to why it helps. And if it has to do with the relationship, then what is it about the relationship that makes it work? This is where I feel that it's the more "animal part" of the relationship that allows it to work. Here's an example to explain what I mean by the animal part. Suppose a patient says to you, "Have you given up hope on me? Do you really think I can change?" If you say: "I have not given up hope, and I do think you can change", it really doesn't matter *that* you say this, but *how* you say it. How you say it is an implicit piece of knowledge. This kind of situation arises all the time.

To answer Margherita Spagnuolo Lobb's question (Spagnuolo Lobb, 2001) about what is at the basis of creative improvisation, I find myself in agreement with her when she says that it is the self-regulatory processes of both the individual and the two of them, the dyad. Here we rely on the *dynamic systems theory*, because what self-organization means, especially intersubjectively, is that the amount of shared experience between two people keeps expanding and becoming more coherent. It's really the intersubjective field that grows and becomes more consistent and coherent. We agree on this concept, but I think that this is the way the *dynamic systems theory* and all of these new theories about organization support that idea.

An interesting question might be: "What happens when there is an inequality in either implicit or explicit knowledge?" For instance, when the age of the therapist and of the patient are very different, or when their cultures are very different? First of all, both people implicitly know that there's an age difference and a difference in experience: it's one of those situations where you're almost forced to make the implicit explicit, so the two of you can share this implicit knowledge. For instance, you say: "I've been in this situation too, you know, when I was a young therapist", or: "What is it like for you to work with somebody like me much younger than yourself?" What happens is that we may talk about it for some time; the implicit reality, which doesn't change, stays, but we have increased the intersubjective field, and now we both know that we're both involved with this question.

Let me give you a different example of the same problem.

I've treated a fair number of Black Americans, and usually at some point the moment arrives when they say to me, "You can't know my experience."

The only way I've found to answer that kind of question is: "I think you're probably right. The best we can do is that you try to explain it to me as best as you can, so that I can understand it as best as I can." And then I usually go back to the original contract and say: "Is that good enough for you? And if not, I'll find you a Black therapist." And I would do the same with somebody much older.

There are so many inequalities between the therapist and the client with regard to their knowledge – implicit and explicit – that we are brought back to the subject of the therapeutic treatment itself. For instance, one thing a therapist may ultimately say to a client is: "It's my experience that people who are neurotic are always better at doing their neuroses than people who don't have the same neuroses." One of the questions the therapist then has to ask her or him, and this is why it's not exactly technical, is something, such as: "You're better at your crazy patterns that involve me, than I am in not getting caught up in what you're doing. So tell me how you do it."

Let me just give one more example on inequality in either implicit or explicit knowledge.

When I was in New York, I had a client, a billionnaire, who was referred to me by someone very prestigious. Towards the end of the first session, he asked: "What is your fee?" And I answered: "A hundred dollars", or something like that. He replied: "A hundred dollars! That's all you make? You know, my friend who referred me to you – well, his therapist charges five hundred dollars." Now this is a man who has enormous knowledge, explicit and implicit, about money and what it does to people. And so he said to me: "Do you not believe in yourself? I don't want to go to somebody who doesn't value himself very highly, because I value myself very highly. And also I don't respect people who don't want to become richer. I don't understand that." I tried to explain that I have one fee for everybody, but he wasn't satisfied; rather, he was worried. So I said: "Okay, let's make a deal. How much do you make an hour?" It came to around five thousands dollars. So I set my fee there. He paid that for a few sessions. The point was made, and we went back to my usual fee, but with the issue of "could he work with me?" settled.

In Gestalt therapy, awareness is realized in the relationship between organism and environment: there is no awareness without the action, the moving of the organism toward the environment. What I say is slightly different: considering the acting of the organism toward its environment is not enough; a mutual recognition is needed for awareness to develop. Awareness is no longer an individual matter but a cultural one, a mutual sharing. Gestalt therapy might develop this aspect at a theoretical level.

These ideas excite me. I see intersubjectivity as a major human motivational system, like attachment, sex, and all of these things. I think that if you take it seriously as a major motivational system, then there are many things you come to expect: it has to help survival; it has to have a preemptive quality, so you have to do it; and, it has to organize your behavior to become intersubjective.

Let me just say another word about this relatively new concept – intersubjectivity. What I really mean by intersubjectivity is being able to say to you: "I know that you know that I know", or "I feel that you feel that I feel." That's ultimately what it is.

Returning now to a motivational system: if we didn't have this capacity I talked about, all the evidence for intersubjectivity, we could not survive as a species. We only survive in groups, families, or tribes, and intersubjectivity makes for great flexibility and adaptivity of group coordination. Thus, before somebody does something, you know what they are going to do, and you can coordinate with them. It also permits morality, because you only feel *coupable* or embarrassed if you know what somebody else thinks or sees when they watch you. Society would never have a moral system without intersubjectivity to keep it together. There are many aspects on this matter: if you didn't have intersubjectivity, you wouldn't talk. I would not talk to you, if I didn't believe that intersubjectively, you could paint the picture, the landscape in your mind, of what's in my mind. So, for all these reasons, it's at the base of the human condition. I once wondered: "Who would be a pure client to look at this with?" And I thought: Maybe, a prisoner who was in prison for life, and he was never going to get out, and he saw a psychologist once a week or once every two weeks; he could be a "pure client". They do talk to somebody, at least many of them do. I asked two people who have spent much time talking to prisoners: "Why do they talk to you? They get no benefits from it. If they get healthier, it doesn't matter, because they are not going to get out of prison sooner. What's the benefit?"

Both of them responded: "These prisoners talk sometimes, because if they can talk to somebody else about their experience, and if they think that somebody else can know what it is, they can stay in touch with themselves." These are the words that they used: *stay in touch with themselves*. And if they can't talk, they start to lose their identity; they can't touch their own experience. This is an interesting example. It's not a "pure client", of course, which doesn't exist. But from my point of view, the content of what they talk about doesn't seem to be as important as the process of talking. And the act of talking is the implicit relationship about talking, which is almost content-free.

Even in the situation where somebody has commited a sin or crime and goes to the priest for confession, there's a practical reason for going: they get exculpated. That's the explicit part. The implicit part is that the priest has validated their existence, so they're not alone in the cosmos with regard to their experience. They're back in touch with themselves. Well, sometimes I wonder which is the stronger motivation to go and confess?

The other way I think of intersubjectivity is as a complementary motivational system to *attachment*, because at the very core of attachment theory is the idea to have physical proximity and security. And you can be very attached to somebody without having any psychic intimacy with him or her. I see intersubjective motivation as a sort of modulating between, on the one hand, being completely alone in the whole cosmos and, on the other hand, being totally transparent, so that everybody can "read" you. And we all have to find in different contexts the right point, just the way we do with attachment. I think that what we do in all relationships is that we're constantly adjusting the relationship, we're adjusting the intersubjective field from minute to minute and second to second, because it's so important to know where you are relatively to somebody else.

This is part of the intersubjective matrix and of what you are self-regulating: you're regulating the relationship, organizing it, trying to make it more coherent and better, and you're also regulating yourself, your reality.

Another thing that I like about the implicit part of the relationship is that in the Western countries, especially in the developed Western countries, most of our relatively deep intersubjective contact and intimacy is in dyads or triads: in a family, a couple, or mother and child, etc. Also our therapies are done that way, so that you create this kind of psychic intimacy as well as attachment with the therapist. I think that in other societies, more tribal or traditional ones, you can do the same thing: have an implicit relationship by dancing together, or singing together, or moving together, or going through a ritual together.

References

Braten S (1998) Infant learning by altero-centric participation: The reverse of egocentric observation in autism. In: Braten A (ed) Intersubjective communication and emotion in early ontogeny. Cambridge Univ Press, Cambridge, pp. 105–124

Damasio A (1994) Decartes' error: Emotion, reason and the human brain. Putnam, New York

Husserl E (1960) Cartesian meditations (transl. Dorian Cairns). Martinus Nijohff, The Hague

Husserl E (1989) Ideas pertaining to a pure phenomenology and to a phenomenological philosophy. Second Book (transl. R. Rojcewicz & A. Schuwer). Kluwer Academic Publishers, Dordrecht

Meltzoff AN (1995) Understanding the intentions of others: Re-enactment of intended acts by eighteen-month-old children. Developmental Psychology 3: 838–850

Meltzoff AN, Gopnik A (1993) The role of imitation in understanding persons and developing a theory of mind. In: Baron-Cohen S, Tager-Flusberg H, Cohen DJ (eds) Understanding other minds: Perspectives from autism. Oxford Univ Press, New York, pp 335–366

Meltzoff AN, Moore MK (1977) Imitation of facial and manual gestures by human neonates. Science 198: 75–78

Merleau-Ponty M (1945) Phénoménologie de la perception. Librairie Gallimard, Paris

Mitchell SA (2000) Relationality: From attachment to intersubjectivity. Analytic Press, New Jersey

Salonia G (1992) Time and relation. Studies in Gestalt Therapy 1: 7–19

Spagnuolo Lobb M (1992) Specific support for each interruption of contact. Studies in Gestalt Therapy 1: 43–51

Spagnuolo Lobb M (2001) The theory of self in Gestalt therapy. A restatement of some aspects. Gestalt Review 4: 276–288

Trevarthen C (1980) The foundation of intersubjectivity: Development of interpersonal and cooperative understanding in infants. In: Olson D (ed) The social foundation of language and thought. Norton, New York, pp 316–342

Trevarthen C, Hubley P (1978) Secondary intersubjectivity: Confidence, confiding and acts of meaning in the first year. In: Lock A (ed) Action, gesture and symbol: The emergence of language. Academic Press, London

Therapeutic Meeting
as Improvisational Co-Creation

Margherita Spagnuolo Lobb

I. Introduction

In our times, it seems clear that psychotherapy, even Gestalt therapy, is not only a matter of supporting the patient's creativity, nor just a matter of being creative as psychotherapists. We think more in terms of co-creation, since our whole culture has acquired a new perspective on human nature, which takes the "relational"[1] and the "relative" as the basic hermeneutic code. If 50 years ago the New Age Movement supported personal growth as a way of emerging from the authoritarian model of the culture of that time, and therefore the concept of creativity was seen more in terms of personal development and freedom from cultural schemas, today, living in the post-modern era where no point of reference is secure or stable any longer, the concept of creativity has to be seen as a matter of the relationship, the only experienced phenomenon where a momentary truth can be found.

Basing myself on this premise, I will consider here the idea that therapeutic co-creation works on an improvisational basis: it cannot happen as a result of premeditated, known, schematic, and knowledgeable processes, but only when there is a person-to-person encounter, where the partners put their knowledge in the background and become instruments of the relationship itself. Improvisational co-creation demands that the partners are present and alive at the contact boundary: it is similar to the sophisticated ability of the jazz player who has all the musical knowledge in her blood and is able to be fresh, strong, contactful, and unique in her playing.

To look at therapeutic meeting as improvisational co-creation seems to be a most advanced – as well as difficult and divergent, but also universal and useful – concept in the theory of psychotherapeutic praxis.

This idea is supported by the most recent studies on psychotherapeutic change, conducted by researchers subscribing to Intersubjective Theory and

---

[1] I use the term "relational" here as a meta-concept for "contact". As a Gestalt therapist, I refer to relationship in its specific application to the experience of contact-with-drawal-from-contact.

especially by Daniel Stern and the Process of Change Study Group (1998a, b). On the other hand, Gestalt therapy has declared from its beginnings (Perls et al., 1994) the aim of attending in a clinical setting to that *quid* which makes spontaneity possible in the human experience of contacting the environment: in other words, those relational processes that lead to the fluid unfolding of the deliberateness of contact. The clinical genius of Frederick Perls who, even if not inclined to theoretical explanations, was certainly a master in this particular skill of co-creating new perceptual and relational patterns with the client, was by all accounts a live demonstration of that aim. Therefore, to look at the therapeutic encounter as a process that happens on an improvisational basis is already in our blood, and to draw support from colleagues who have arrived at remarkably similar results from a different perspective is the best validation of our theoretical basis. Gestalt therapy theory looks at co-creative processes from a physio-social point of view, and thus it refers to the organism/environment contact with an anthropological matrix of the Darwinian kind (Spagnuolo Lobb, 2001, pp. 277–282); Stern's group research, on the other hand, derives from the intersubjective tradition, therefore referring to what we might call "the present contact with the other's mind". I will try to demonstrate how certain basic concepts and developments in the Gestalt therapy approach to human nature and psychological treatment can contribute to Stern's courageous support of the "implicit relational knowledge" in psychotherapy.

I will present three aspects of the therapeutic meeting as improvisational co-creation: 1) improvisational co-creation as a typical characteristic of healthy relationships; 2) the dimension of time in therapeutic co-creation: the process of change and phases in the therapeutic meeting; 3) what makes change possible in therapeutic co-creation?

II. Improvisational Co-creation as a Typical Characteristic of Healthy Relationships

The day before her final examination in the fifth grade of elementary school, Laura, 10 years old, asks her father: "Dad, do I have to worry about the exams?" He answers: "No, Laura, you don't." Laura looks relieved: "Ah, okay!"

There is something in our daily relationships that makes them healing relationships. Most of the time we work well: our normality is our ability to not only understand the need of the other, but also to take the relationship one step further, to what we might call the satisfaction of our needs in a unique way, in an unrepeatable co-creation proper to that encounter.

The function of creative adjustment (a basic concept in this book) allows us to repair relational blocks and to correct our movements toward the other. The freer our senses are, the more we can openly perceive the field, the more we are able to adjust creatively. But even when our senses are numb or blocked (and they hallucinate a repetitive relational schema), we continue to adjust creatively to that difficult field.

A young girl says to her mother: "Mom, what a lot of beautiful things you have!" The mother replies: "You're beautiful, too!"

A borderline patient says to the therapist: "I will never be dependent on you any more!" The therapist warmly answers: "I feel moved by your dignity when you say so."

A special freedom from stereotyped perceptions is needed to be able to improvise, so that the selfing process in contact-making can unfold, basing itself fully on its id-functioning as well as on its personality-functioning and ego-functioning (Spagnuolo Lobb, 2001). The movement toward the other is harmonic and, like a dance, proceeds in small co-created steps.

Our founders (Perls et al., 1994) strongly asserted this perspective from the beginning. They were looking for a key to read the normality, the spontaneous regulation of the organism, of the healing relationship between wo/man and nature, and between wo/man and social group. How to build a theoretical model pertaining to the spontaneity of human nature, without devitalizing it in the process, but rather stating the principles of that *quid* which defines it: this was the dream, and also the epistemological risk, faced by the authors of *Gestalt Therapy* (ibid., p. 154). And it is also the risk that Stern et al. are running when they write: "(...) the micro-process of proceeding in a therapy session seems to occur in an improvisational mode in which the small steps needed to get to a goal are unpredictable (...)" (1998a, p. 300).

To look at normalities – instead of at deficiencies – constitutes a revolutionary change, not only as far as clinical praxis and development are concerned, but also for broader matters, such as the relationship between psychotherapy and politics, our anthropological perspective, and so on. To look at what one does as the best solution possible is the opposite of having in mind what one should do in order to make the world go better. One can speak of the positive in human nature and of unrevealed potentialities that can help human beings and social groups to live better, but this does not change the paradigm of "see-what-doesn't-work/do-what-makes-the world-work-better". Other humanistic psychotherapies have fallen into this epistemological trap, as well as many Gestalt therapists. To believe in what we call self-regulation of the organism/environment field means to look at our world through different lenses: we need not worry about what should be done, about seeing what does not work and building tools to repair the evil. Evil and good are part of the same whole: we can only stay with how they express themselves, without trying to change anything.

What led the research of the founders of Gestalt therapy was the need to revise psychoanalysis (the emergent psychotherapy model at that time) in a world which, after the Second World War, was drastically changed. What leads our research nowadays, in a world that has also drastically changed in the past 50 years (under the influence of a pervading process of globalization, which affects daily family life as well as terrorism), is the need to understand the healthy processes of our relationships. It is a new version of learning from nature, but this time it is a matter of learning about our being-with.

III. The Dimension of Time in Therapeutic Co-Creation:
The Process of Change and Phases in the Therapeutic Meeting

The experience of time has been researched in many ways, for instance in philosophical and psychotherapeutic terms. For those who look at experience from a phenomenological point of view, research on time is very exciting. Somehow, we do not do justice to the many meanings that the word "time" has when we use one term only. The ancient Greeks used at least four words to indicate time: time in general (*chronòs*); limited time, the hour (*ora*); the moment, the instant (*stigmi*); and *Kairòs*, the appropriate time, the doing-the-right-thing-in-the-right-moment, the being in time.

Daniel Stern (2003) has studied the chronological length of what is experienced as the present moment, and he considers it like a fractal (a form which is the same regardless of the scale we use); he researches how present moments connect with each other. Giovanni Salonia (1992; personal communication) replies that, in order to understand one moment, one has to refer to the whole length of the interaction: for instance, to understand a kiss between two partners, one has to consider the whole interaction, since it is very different if a kiss happens at the beginning, in the middle, or at the end of the entire interaction.

To stay closer to the concept of creative improvisation, we can think of the therapeutic encounter as a dance. When two people dance, they combine their movements in small steps. Each step is *per se* a co-creation, a play of the one who leads and the one who is led, of risking physical closeness and staying at a safe distance, of sharing the rhythm of the music. The whole dance moves from a start through a full involvement to an end. The small steps make the whole sequence, but to understand each step it is important to locate it in the phase of the sequence. In other words, a movement from one of the partners of pulling the other partner towards him- or herself, for instance, has a different meaning if acted at the beginning ("This dance is a way of staying closer to you"), in the middle ("This dance is involving us") or at the end ("I would not like to leave you", or "It has been nice to dance together").

The experience of time strongly determines the "intentional consciousness" of any small step in the dance as well as of any other experienced contact event where there has been an implicit or explicit agreement on the amount of time to be shared. In fact, among the many contacts we constantly make, only a few of them are particularly meaningful: they bring novelty to our perception and therefore make us grow. In this kind of contact, our experience of time interweaves with our contact-making (with the way we co-create the dance with the other), giving to every phase of this process a peculiar deliberateness. This reading, which might at first glance seem deterministic, in fact simply brings out an obviousness innate in ordinary human experiences: i.e., the fact that our organism prepares itself to develop every meaningful encounter in a *before*, a *during*, and an *after*, with a deliberateness that is functional to the carrying out of these phases. The therapeutic meeting is one of these meaningful contacts, where the amount of time to be shared is usually explicitly agreed upon.

In an ordinary healthy experience, as Perls et al. state:

"One is relaxed, there are many possible concerns, all accepted and all fairly vague – the self is a "weak gestalt." Then an interest assumes dominance and the forces spontaneously mobilize themselves, certain images brighten and motor responses are initiated. At this point, most often, there are also required certain deliberate exclusions and choices. (...) That is, deliberate limitations are imposed in the total functioning of the self, and the identification and alienation proceed according to these limits. (...) And finally, at the climax of excitement, the deliberateness is relaxed and the satisfaction is again spontaneous" (1994, p. 157).

It is precisely attention to the process that leads us to see the experience of contact as it develops, thus considering the time dimension. Although the description of the four phases of the experience of contact-withdrawal is very clear in *Gestalt Therapy*, the use of the concept of time is less so. Specifically, it is not clear whether these four phases express the *possible* development of the experience of contact, thus allowing space for the possibility that they will not be developed in every experience of contact, or whether the time dimension is to be understood in the Heideggerian sense, as a category which defines the sense of the relationship, so that every experience of contact, simply because it develops in time, involves a temporal experience, a sort of relational clock, which gives sense and meaning according to the temporal phase traversed. In other words, we should like to know whether the final contact (or any other phase in the process of contact) is a phase that in any case "takes place", in the sense that in that phase the contact is to be read with the meanings this phase implies, or whether it is a phase that takes place only if the relationship reaches a certain level of maturation. It seems to me that a sovereignty of the temporal dimension is implicit in a theory of the self that is fundamentally phenomenological and, in any case, this point remains undeveloped in the founding text; nor can we refer to later Gestalt literature, since sufficient attention has not been given to this aspect (Spagnuolo Lobb, 2001, pp. 285–286).[2]

If the fact that it is located in time modifies the experience of the self in contact, we may think of a different predisposition of the self to contact in the various phases. One consequence of this is that a particular perception or expression is located in a reference context that depends not on the intrinsic content, but on the teleological function of the phase in which it is inserted. The example I just gave of the different meanings of a pulling-toward movement during a dance is a good description of this. If we apply this matrix of relational meaning in the therapeutic process, i.e. during the therapy session, every sentence as well as any other communication the patient and the therapist utter take on meaning in the context of time.[3]

---

[2] In the group at the Gestalt Institute, which I direct with Giovanni Salonia, we have developed the time dimension of the experience of contact (Salonia, 1992; Spagnuolo Lobb et al., 1998), both because it seems to us hermeneutically correct, and because we have examined the validity of the clinical (Spagnuolo Lobb, 1997; Conte, 1999) and formative (Spagnuolo Lobb, 1992b) aspects.

[3] It is to Isadore From that we owe a primary development in temporal key of the theory of the process of contact. Although he left no written testimony on this matter, Isadore did leave his students a clear teaching on the phenomenological reading in the temporal key of the disturbance of contact in the therapist-patient relationship as it unfolds during the session (Müller, 1993).

Looking at an example from the patient's point of view, let us consider that she arrives for the first time for a session and immediately tells the therapist of the most intimate part of her problem. The therapist notices (and not necessarily makes it explicit) that the patient is avoiding the fore-contact with him. The anxiety that the patient experiences in the fore-contact phase of that situation does not allow her to develop the process of contact spontaneously, and so the self-function creates solutions which, through the loss of an ego-function, enable her not to feel anxiety.

The whole session is a process of contact-withdrawal from contact, which leads the partners to the contact boundary and which, after the fullness of the encounter, makes them withdraw.

We can see every session as a dance, and also the whole therapy as a dance. What happens in this dance? The patient comes to therapy with an intentional consciousness (of which he is more or less aware). The therapist attends to it – from her own deliberateness (of which she is usually aware). In dancing together, the therapist can "touch" where the patient's intentionality loses its spontaneity, therefore where his being-with, his contact-making carries anxiety and consequently becomes sterile and repetitive (in order to avoid that anxiety); on the other hand, the patient can "touch" how the therapist sees his process of being-with and intuits that the therapeutic meeting is a concrete chance to change his being-with and regain the spontaneity of his awareness (or of his intentional consciousness).

Let us take an example of the development of the co-creative therapeutic meeting. Just before and around the beginning of a new session, both the patient and the therapist activate themselves (fore-contacting phase). In this moment, excitements emerge, thus initiating the figure/ground process. There is a deliberateness in their experience, which starts and supports the process. There can be no excitation that is exclusively of the one or of the other; otherwise, there would be no novelty to be assimilated, and there would be neither self nor growth.

In fore-contacting, Perls et al. state: "The body is the ground, the appetite or environmental stimulus is the figure" (1994, p. 182). Shall we try to apply this description of the intentionalities of partners to an example of the experience of therapist and patient in session? The fore-contacting patient might think: "How will my therapist react to my recent change in the relationship with my husband?"; the fore-contacting therapist: "How did the patient develop what happened in the last session?" In the following phase, that of contacting, both therapist and patient expand their "selfing" toward the contact boundary between them, following the excitation, which in a first stage (orienting subphase) leads them to explore the other's presence in search of a set of possibilities to work through their initial wondering. For instance, the therapist's beard could remind the patient of her father's moral rigidity, thereby leading her to tell him the change with her husband in a cautious way. On the other hand, the restrained breathing of the patient alerts the therapist, who will pay particular attention to the patient's retroflections. It is exactly the wondering that now becomes the figure, while the initial need or desire is placed in the background. In a second sub-phase (manipulat-

ing subphase), therapist and patient "manipulate" the environment, choosing certain possibilities and rejecting others. For instance, the patient might choose to ask the therapist: "Have you always had a beard?" trying to understand whether for the therapist the beard is a momentary and not rigid choice, assuming from her experience that a man who has always had a beard, like her father, must have some moral rigidity in his blood. The therapist might choose to tell the truth and ask: "I haven't, and what is important for you in this aspect of my beard?" Therapist and patient "manipulate" the environment, "attacking" certain parts of the field and overcoming obstacles. Thus, the patient might actively grasp the possibility given to her by the therapist and risk explaining what her fear is about: "I feel changed with my husband and am afraid to tell you, because your beard reminds me of my father's rigidity." The therapist, on his part, might risk putting his person in his answer, instead of using pre-packed therapeutic tools (like using the empty chair technique: "Put your father on the empty chair and tell him about your change"); he realizes, for instance, that he feels surprised, and he decides to make it explicit: "I'm surprised and curious about this perception of yours." In a third phase, which is called *final contacting*, the final objective, the contact-making, is the figure, while the environment and the body are the ground. Both therapist and patient are occupied with their whole self in the spontaneous act of contacting the other, awareness[4] is at its height, the self is fully present at the contact boundary, and the whole ability to choose is relaxed, because there is nothing to choose at that moment, which must simply be fully lived. The partners prepare the ground for this very important moment of full-contacting or "healthy confluence", which might be lost. The patient might relax her fear and tell the therapist:

I had strange thoughts this last week, strange and exciting. I have never been like that. I have thought that I might be attracted by other men, and actually I looked at some handsome men with different eyes … and it seems to me that they were looking at me, too, in a way I had never experienced … All this is so exciting! On the other hand, I was nervous with my husband, I'm changing with him.

The therapist, who has just decided to make his feeling of curiosity explicit to the patient, might in this moment turn his personal involvement back (retroflecting) and, for instance, work on the patient's relationship with her husband. He feels that this methodologically correct intervention would take the very special atmosphere of that moment away from their meeting. If, on the contrary, he continues to risk being fully present as a person-therapist, he feels that there is a strong emotional involvement between them and has to take a decision on how to use it therapeutically. This is the phase that Stern et al. call the "now moment": "(…) now moments are like the ancient Greek concept of *Kairòs*, a unique moment of opportunity that must be seized, because your fate will turn on whether you seize it and how" (1998b, p. 911). This is the crucial moment in a therapeutic session, and meeting the

---

[4] Awareness is not consciousness; it is being awake, fully present at the contact boundary, with all the senses open (cf Salonia, 1986).

patient's need of contact is what makes the therapeutic meeting a successful one. The therapist has to decide whether and how much to relax his retro-flections and commit himself to an improvisational co-creation. He feels that the vibrancy that he experiences between them in that moment informs him that in the patient's words there must be some emotional intention ad-dressed to him. So he decides to leap into the void and asks: "Why are you telling me this? How am I involved in this change of yours toward men?" At this point, there is a brief and poignant silence; then the patient says:

> Maybe I felt that you were giving me permission during our last session, the permis-sion that I had always wanted from my father, to relax my sexual and sensual feelings to-ward you. I don't know how that happened exactly, maybe the way you looked at me when you told me that you liked the way I was dressed. There is another thing that hap-pened just last night and that I didn't have the courage to tell you: I had a dream last night, where you were hugging me, in such a sweet and warm and totally accepting way, that I felt a strong sexual pleasure in my whole body. And in telling you the dream, I still feel that wonderful sweetness in my body and feel peaceful and open to you.

The nourishing exchange, the contact with the novelty has happened. In Gestalt therapy, we say that the relational block, experienced as a block in the spontaneity of making contact with the therapist, has been dissolved, thanks to the support that the therapist gave at the right moment, when the ground had been properly prepared and their meeting was in the open mo-ment, when the patient was ready to experience another kind of contact, a more spontaneous one, and the therapist was ready to take the chance and support the energy, the excitement, of the patient addressed to the realiza-tion of full-contacting and withdrawal. In Gestalt therapy, this is the way the organism grows/changes through assimilation of the novelty brought by the other. For us, it is a matter of supporting the excitement which leads the pa-tient toward a spontaneous realization of his intentionality of contact; for Daniel Stern and his group (1998a, p. 300), it is a matter of both therapist and patient changing/expanding their "implicit relational knowledge", which is defined as a procedural knowledge of being-with, neither conscious nor un-conscious (not repressed). If, for them, the therapeutic change is measured by a change in the intersubjective relational knowledge of therapist and pa-tient, for us the change is measured by the regained spontaneity of the pa-tient-therapist contact-making. In both cases, we are speaking of a proce-dural competence which, as such, will apply to any other context of the patient's life.

In the last phase, *post-contacting*, the selfing activity diminishes, both therapist and patient withdraw from the contact boundary to allow the possi-bility of digesting the acquired novelty, in order to integrate it, all unaware, in the pre-existing structure of experiences. The process of assimilation is al-ways unaware and involuntary (as digestion is unaware and involuntary); it may become aware to the degree that there is a disturbance. It is the phase that Stern et al. call "an open space", where "the partners disengage from their specific meeting and *can be alone in the presence of the other*" (ibid., p. 307, emphasis added). This is a very beautiful description of the assimila-tion process.

The experience of time in all phases (not only in full-contacting or "now moments") of therapeutic co-creation can be defined as *Kairòs* (cf. Salonia, 1994), as the proper time, the being-in-time, the doing-the-right-thing-at-the-right-moment. Stern et al. (1998b, p. 915) describe well the other fates of the now moment when it is not seized therapeutically and does not end in a "moment of meeting": it can be missed, failed, repaired, "flagged", or endured. Their description and point of view is so much in line with Gestalt therapy theory that it might be even embarrassing for us to admit that they say better than we do what is in our – not in their – blood. "Now moments" (in our language, the "phase of full-contacting") happen anyway; it is a matter of the maturing of certain possibilities in the person's drive toward growth, in the relational time (*Kairòs*), in the momentary availability of the other; in other words, in the conditions of the field. *The response from the environment can support either the devitalized repetition of a previous relational pattern or the desired contacting.* The drive toward growth (deliberateness of contact) never disappears, not even in the most serious disturbances, like psychosis.

IV. What Makes Change Possible in Therapeutic Co-Creation?

What do we mean by therapeutic change? Each method provides an answer to this basic question, which is related to consistent anthropological, philosophical, and teleological principles. On the other hand, a change always occurs, and both therapist and patient are "called" to evaluate the change that they experience in psychotherapy. Sometimes, they think of certain changes in different terms. For instance, I have met therapists who speak positively of a change in the patient's life as a consequence of psychotherapy (such as, leaving a partner or starting a new relationship), which rather leads the patient into an increasingly depressive state. Hence, an interesting issue might be: "Who decides the value of a change and how?" Considering our relational perspective, we speak of change-in-the-therapeutic-relationship, which is theoretically explicable by every method and is perceived by both therapist and patient as a positive change, where previously blocked or undeveloped, implicit or explicit intentionalities are now exercised more freely.

In Gestalt therapy, we explain it theoretically in terms of re-gaining – or gaining – spontaneity in contact-making-and-withdrawal with the environment; in Intersubjective Theory, they speak of expanding the intersubjective knowledge, hence improving the relational abilities to manage the intersubjective space.

Now, how do we as therapists answer the question: "What made me really change in a therapeutic (or similar) relationship?"

And how do our patients answer the question: "What made you really change in your therapy?"

If I consider my own personal therapy, two qualities come to mind: the sense that what my therapist said or did (or not) provoked a deconstruction in what I expected (my habitual perceptive assessment); and the sense that what was happening was the right thing at the right moment, that is, that the same thing would have had a different effect at another moment.

Patients usually answer, first, that it is not so much the content of what the therapist said as the way she or he said it; second, it happens at certain moments when the therapist says something different from what the patient is expecting, and it is clear that the therapist is seeing in the patient something true, something that the patient has learned to hide in relationships or has forgotten.

We are speaking here of that change that is experienced during or after single sessions; the question is "how does each meeting create change?"

In an attempt to express in Gestalt therapy terms what brings about the change in psychotherapy, and with recourse to the studies of Stern et al. of the Process of Change Study Group, we may say that the unfolding of the self (selfing) of the therapist and of the patient during the session happens on the basis of the id and personality functions on the one hand, and of the ego function on the other.

The therapist actually works on two grounds: the method, that is, the theory which helps him to find his direction in his perceptions, like the map that helps us to find our way on a specific territory; and his own experience of personal growth and change. But the way he encounters the patient is *creative adjustment*, his dancing with the patient. This is done, for example, by using the patients' experiential linguistic categories, giving specific support for each interruption of contact (Spagnuolo Lobb, 1992a), addressing what is fascinating for him in the patient (Polster, 1987), and above all *risking* being-there in the relationship, while maintaining the boundaries imposed by his role as therapist.

On the other hand, the patient has an agenda when she goes to therapy, a more or less explicit demand of change. She also has habitual relational patterns, which consciously or unconsciously she will display in the session. But here, too, the manner in which she encounters the therapist is *creative adjustment*, and the *risk* that she runs, consciously or unconsciously, every time she finds herself faced with a habitual relational and perceptive modality, which may be deconstructed and which she wants to deconstruct, sometimes irrespective of the therapist's openness, precisely because she knows that she is in a therapeutic context. For Stern et al., in order for a "now moment" to be transformed into a "moment of meeting", it is required:

"(...) that each partner contributes something unique and authentic of his or herself as an individual in response to the 'now moment'. The response cannot be an application of technique nor an habitual therapeutic move. It must be created on the spot to fit the singularity of the unexpected situation, and it must carry the therapist's signature as coming from his own sensibility and experience, beyond technique and theory" (1998a, p. 306).

This "signature" of the therapist seems to me to be a masterly specification, a work of art by a master who conveys to us that, just as the baby recognizes the scent of its mother's nipple, so the patient recognizes what is intimately peculiar to the therapist; and it is only in an encounter that bears this mark, that the patient gives the therapist the power to teach him a new way of being-with.

A Clinical Example

At this point I will offer a clinical example of what I mean by "taking the risk", both on the therapist's and on the patient's side. One day, during a session, F. told me about something that had happened during a picnic lunch with her family (husband and two adolescent daughters) and a number of friends on the beach. One of her daughters was singing, while the other played on the keyboard. A man who was not part of the group, and whom the patient described as "peculiar", was listening a little way off. At the end of the performance, this man approached my patient and, inexplicably, said: "You must be the person responsible for all this." At that moment, the patient looked at me with a surprised expression, and I felt a powerful emotion; my eyes were wet, and I found it difficult to suppress this emotion.

The patient withdrew her gaze from mine and changed the subject, as though nothing had happened. She told me how clever the mother of one of her sisters-in-law was. At this point, I had to decide how to use my emotion: did it express a sensitivity linked to my own history, or was it an important element of a contact that she was avoiding with me? The examples quoted by Stern et al. (1998a) seem to stop at this point: they say that change in therapy comes about regardless of the verbalization of such episodes. In fact, there had already been a profound exchange – as profound as it was unexpected – between the two of us. But the method of Gestalt therapy focuses precisely on this kind of emotional experience; thus it was normal for me to take my own emotion into consideration. Besides, the field theory perspective, which is proper to Gestalt therapy, informed me that my emotion belonged to our field; therefore it was *both* my own sensitivity and her way to avoid contact-making. However, I wondered: if I suggested this kind of emotional contact to her, what advantage would there be for her? The answer is not provided in the fund of theoretical knowledge. This is what Stern et al. (1998a, b) call the "now moment", which can be compared to the very first phase of our "full contacting", in which there is a considerable element of risk, and a choice is imposed (in the sense that even not choosing anything is a choice). Stern et al. (2003) speak of a moment at which fate is ready to be fulfilled and is fulfilled in one sense or another. It is a moment at which our being in relationship decides our growth.

Thus, as a therapist, I was aware of the risks inherent in this moment: the risk of proposing my own emotion to the patient (and of inducing a misleading element), and the risk of letting the patient set in motion the usual relational modality. Of course, in this case, the main risk was that our encounter would not modify the patient's relational code, that it would remain based on the impossibility of being seen in her deep, hidden love for her daughters. I chose to share my emotion and said: "Did you notice that I was moved a moment ago when you told me about what happened on the beach?" She looked at me and said: "No, I didn't notice." But she started to watch me more carefully, almost as if she wanted to test her ability to accept the fact that I had been moved, only to withdraw from my gaze, almost as though she wanted to reconfirm the idea that it is impossible to "dance and sing" with another person. I asked her: "And how does it affect you to know that I was moved?"

At this point, F. took a deep breath and burst into tears; crying, she allowed her own feelings toward me to be released, in such a way that she experienced the feeling of being seen by me. By risking telling her how moved I had been, I had implicitly told her that I saw how, despite her having had to conceal her song, her love of life, in her birth family (the family environment was too hard-pressed by serious problems, such as migrations, finances, and the early loss of her father), she had "given" her daughters the chance to freely express their own song. Her telling me about this episode had made it possible for me to see all this and had allowed her to be accepted with warmth and complicity, rather than with hostility and concern. I said to her:

"I can see the great love you have for your daughters and how, although you are a very different sort of mother from what your mother was to you, you still hide your song of love for them. I can also see the chance you give me to see such an intimate part of you, which is your song of love for life."

Working through and verbalizing relational experiences (at an emotional, body, intellectual, and spiritual level) is part of Gestalt therapy's "normal" praxis.

I believe that this praxis must make a difference in the process of change.

V. Conclusion

We have seen how the concept of improvisational co-creation in psychotherapy, which forms the basis of the recent discoveries of Stern and of the Process of Change Study Group, perfectly coincides with the epistemological principles of the theory of Gestalt therapy. Furthermore, Gestalt therapy supplies a map, articulated in procedural terms, of the phases of the development of self in the episode of contact represented by the therapeutic session, which may constitute a contribution to the phases described by Stern and the Process of Change Study Group: above all, in order to understand the onset of the "now moment" during the "moving along" phase. In fact, the description of the phases of orientation and manipulation as active preparation for the moment of risk – when the patient gives the therapist the chance to "remake a relational history", and the therapist gives the patient the chance to stay at the contact boundary with a reciprocity made of the fullness of the senses – may explain the onset of the "now moment". Finally, we have conjectured that working therapeutically on "moments of meeting", recognizing them, and clarifying their connection with interruptions of the spontaneity of contact speed the process of change and make it more aware.

References

Conte V (1999) Work with a seriously disturbed patient in Gestalt therapy: The evolution of a therapeutic relationship. Studies in Gestalt Therapy 8: 154–161

Müller B (1993) Isadore From's contribution to the theory and practice of Gestalt therapy. Studies in Gestalt Therapy 2: 7–21

Perls FS, Hefferline R, Goodman P (1994) Gestalt therapy. Excitement and growth in the human personality. The Gestalt J Press, Highland, New York

Polster E (1987) Every person's life is worth a novel. Norton, New York

Salonia G (1986) La consapevolezza nella teoria e nella practica della psicoterapia della Gestalt. Quaderni di Gestalt 3: 125–146

Salonia G (1992) Time and relation. Relational deliberateness as hermeneutic horizon in Gestalt therapy. Studies in Gestalt Therapy 1: 7–19

Salonia G (1994) Kairòs. Direzione spirituale e animazione comunitaria. Editzioni Dehoniane, Bologna

Spagnuolo Lobb M (1992a) Specific support in the interruptions of contact. Studies in Gestalt Therapy 1: 43–51

Spagnuolo Lobb M (1992b) Training in Gestalt therapy. How the perspective of dental aggression changes the traditional concept of training. Studies in Gestalt Therapy 1: 21–29

Spagnuolo Lobb M (1997) Linee programmatiche di un modello gestaltico nelle comunità terapeutiche. Quaderni di Gestalt 24/25: 19–37

Spagnuolo Lobb M (2001) The Theory of Self in Gestalt Therapy. A Restatement of Some Aspects. Gestalt Review 4: 276–288

Spagnuolo Lobb M, Salonia G, Cavaleri P, Sichera A (1998) The experience of time as a dimension of the experience of contact-withdrawal. Australian Gestalt J 2: 29–37

Stern D (2003) The present moment. Norton, New York

Stern D, Bruschweiler-Stern N, Harrison A, Lyons-Ruth K, Morgan A, Nahum J, Sander L, Tronick E (1998a) The process of therapeutic change involving implicit knowledge: Some implications of developmental observations for adult psychotherapy. Infant Mental Health J 3: 300–308

Stern D, Bruschweiler-Stern N, Harrison A, Lyons-Ruth K, Morgan A, Nahum J, Sander L, Tronick E (1998b) Non-interpretive mechanisms in psychoanalytic therapy. The "something more" than interpretation. Int J Psycho-Anal. 79: 903–921

Creative Abilities and the Art of Living Well

Malcolm Parlett

I. Introduction

At a recent meeting of about twenty experienced Gestalt practitioners in Britain, someone asked the question: "What attracted us to Gestalt therapy?" The responses varied, but there was one recurring theme – that the Gestalt approach made sense in a real-life way. It was a philosophy and method to be lived, not just a theory to be talked about, and not merely a specialized approach to psychotherapy. Rather, it was suggestive of a way to be in the world that we had independently discovered to be richer, truer, and more satisfying for ourselves than other paths tried. It offered a means of cultivating "the art of living well".

This chapter takes off from the above idea namely, that living well is an art form. Life is not a science but an improvisation. The whole notion of creative adjustment, so central to Gestalt therapy theory, suggests having an adaptive and spontaneous response to living in this world. A Gestalt therapy exploration or therapy session is open-ended, experimental, and uniquely constructed – like a piece of art or sculpture, or a musical composition, poem, or dance. Epistemologically, Gestalt psychotherapists are engaged in an enterprise that is art and not medical science. Types of therapy that apply a fixed technique, or are couched in the deterministic language of science and technology, are antithetical to the Gestalt therapy tradition and fundamental ethos. The values of the approach are aesthetic and ethical – the same values with which artists contend.

This chapter investigates and plays with the metaphors of the artist, of developing artistry, and of living as an art form. These metaphors come as near as any description does to the heart and central purpose of Gestalt therapy, at least as many have developed it. There are multiple ways in which Gestalt ideas and methods overlap with the world of the arts and artists (not just painters, but poets and dancers, singers and sculptors, musicians and actors as well), so this analogy is apt.

The connection with the arts was there from the beginning. Paul Goodman, himself a published poet, drew many parallels between artistic creativity and living spontaneously[1]:

---

[1] Although this quotation comes from *Gestalt Therapy,* authored by F.S. Perls, R. Hefferline, and P. Goodman, it is well-known that Goodman wrote the section from which it has

"To the artist, of course, technique, style, is everything: he feels creativity as his natural excitement and his interest in the theme (...) the technique is *his* way of forming the real to be real; it occupies the foreground of his awareness, perception, manipulation. The style is himself, it is what he exhibits and communicates: style and not banal wishes of the day" (Perls et al.,1994, p.174, italics in original).

But it is Joseph Zinker, with his renowned 1977 book, *Creative Process in Gestalt Therapy*, who made the theme the most explicit: the Gestalt therapist needs to be a creative therapist, "with a rich personal background [who] celebrates life [and] another person's essence, beauty, goodness, capacities, and future possibilities [and is] inventive, experimental, [with] rich inner imagery, [and] a sense of grace, structure, order, and rhythm of life" (pp. 39–40). He continues to explore artistic themes in his latest book (Zinker, 2001).

I would like here to extend the parallels further – by reflecting on the development of Gestalt knowledge and skills as being rather like how an artist develops his abilities. Gestalt students do not go to a school for painting, sculpture, or dance, nor to a conservatory of music; but they, too, are undergoing an artistic education. They are acquiring ways of thinking, key notions, attitudes, and techniques and gaining access to a tradition – all the constituents of the Gestalt approach to living and practicing in creative ways. Every person, Zinker reminds us, has the capacity to be an artist. So I shall not be referring to Gestalt therapy training and trainees alone, but to all those studying the Gestalt philosophy and theory-in-practice – whether through training, personal development work, coaching, or therapy as a client or patient. Some psychotherapy patients may have little sense that they are receiving an education in an approach to living. They may be immured in the medical model view of themselves as receiving treatment for a specific complaint. But, hopefully, they soon transform their understanding to become more of an equal partner in supporting their therapy and "artistic development". For others – training to be psychotherapists, for instance – the educational journey is explicit, even to the point of their gaining a formal qualification at the end. Assessment, just as it does in schools of art, courts controversy: how can one measure artistic performance or therapeutic talent?

II. An Artistic Education

Gestalt students (trainees, clients, patients, participants in groups, etc.) are undergoing an education, whatever the precise contract and expectations. Although it is not always explicit, they are absorbing an approach to living and making sense of life and the world. Moreover, the education, once begun, is likely to be lifelong. To become an "artist of life" *via* the Gestalt tra-

---

been taken. It has become customary to acknowledge Paul Goodman's distinctive contribution, outlook, and voice and the fact that he was the primary author of this part of the book. In doing so, there is no disrespect to the other authors, particularly Frederick Perls, who initiated the book and brought in the other two authors to write the bulk of it.

dition is not a quick-fix acquisition of a bag of tricks, a fast route to success in conventional terms. Rather, it is a longer-term developmental process geared towards "opening doors", creating more options, extending the range of ways of living, and increasing the color, vividness, texture, and richness of one's existence. Along the way, blocks to living well are met and dismantled.

This dismantling, or recovery process, is critical. Staying with images from the arts for the moment, what is ill-formed, graceless, or no longer tuneful, or lacks color and vibrancy, or is played out in some half-hearted dance with another, become subjects of intense focus. They are attended to as points of inquiry, not out of an obsession with pathology, and not as an end in themselves, but because they stand in the way of fuller life and more abundant health. The educational journey is in part one of dealing with the blocks to creativity that weaken the full expression of the life-force and impede the spontaneous flow of living. What is unfinished, stale, too rule-governed, suppressed, or weakly fuelled by passion and interest, stands in the way of being present – as a creative artist, fruitfully engaging with the raw materials of contemporary existence, the "lifespace" and what fills it.

As an artistic education proceeds, people develop and learn and practice more in the mode and method of the particular art form or approach. They acquire skills and competencies. They become better able to do certain things, accomplish more, and do so with greater grace and ease. Their early attempts may be awkward and ill-formed, compared to what they may achieve later.

In short, they develop abilities. Of course, these are not just individual, personal attributes and skills that they acquire and then own, rather like personal pieces of psychological real-estate. What the abilities are, and how they are shaped, is also a function of what the school, group, or training program offers and prioritizes. The abilities learned are a product of the whole field in which they are presented and practiced. The extent to which students develop in specialized ways, has as much to do with the curriculum of the art school, the heritage, and the local traditions of teaching as it does with their individual learning styles.

III. Five Dimensions of Change and Development

In the remainder of the chapter I shall reflect on key abilities that are supported by, and intrinsic to, a Gestalt-style education (Parlett 2000). I suggest that they relate to the art of living well, flourishing as a human being, and living a full and satisfying life "with artistry". While they seem to describe well the kinds of developmental change that Gestalt students undergo, as a result of their education, they have a more general validity, too. Thus, artists of all kinds need to develop along these lines as well – as part of their own becoming – even if they never appear in an explicit curriculum.

The abilities I am referring to have been variously described in several ways. They can be regarded as five dimensions of creative adjustment (ibid., pp. 24–25) or (Parlett, 2003) as varieties of human strength (that are urgently needed in the world at large). I differentiate five of them and have named them as follows: (1) *responding*, (2) *interrelating*, (3) *self-recognizing*, (4) *embodying*, and (5) *experimenting*. As abilities called for in the art of living, I have argued (Parlett, 2000) that no Gestalt education can ignore them, and in my own experience of different training programs, they are not ignored but built into the training, even if they are not referred to by these names. They have not been part of the traditional presentation of the Gestalt approach, but that does not mean they have not been there – as high-level "meta-competencies" that are being imparted, practiced, demonstrated, and valued as important. I suggest in the first of the above publications, that the developmental shifts made by trainees and others in the course of their Gestalt training could be mapped in terms of the five abilities, or "if not these exactly, they have been acquiring some that are very similar indeed" (ibid., p. 25).

In the following sections I will now describe each of the above five abilities at some length. Continuing to follow the theme of the arts, I draw upon the life of the artist to exemplify each ability under discussion. There is no evidence that artists in general are different from the population at large in terms of their maturity, access to life competencies, or overall life satisfaction. But, inspired by Goodman and Zinker, I take the artist as a symbolic figure. The artist in mind is an idealization, almost an archetype.

A. Responding

The first of the abilities is *responding*. All the time, an artist is self-organizing. This is intrinsic to his being an artist. He organizes himself to paint the picture, compose the music, dance the dance, and write the verse. However, this process of self-expression, of creating and articulating, is never conducted in a vacuum. It is not a sealed-off and isolated operation, or separated in any way from the field of its emergence and expression. There is always a wider phenomenological field – full of what he or she will be experiencing as incentives and obstacles, matters of practicality, imagination, and problems to be overcome. In becoming an accomplished artist or performer, he learns that what lies as potential, possibility, or vision can only become actualized by *responding to the field that exists*.

Artistic work calls on different combinations of focus, commitment, imagination, and practice, according to context and practical circumstances. There are elements of risk-taking, taking advantages of opportunities, and being open to serendipity and chance. The artist needs to be ready to adapt and be responsive to conditions, while being prepared to intervene and direct events. At times, he will need to seek and call on support: creative, critical, and practical. There is a necessary appraisal of consequences of doing or not doing something. All these elements form part of what I am calling the ability to respond – i.e. self-organizing and self-managing within a field, singular in its configuration, and changing in its organization all the time.

Sometimes the responding is neither especially skillful, free, flowing nor accomplished. The artist may be experiencing apparently immovable difficulties, insufficient resources, inadequate facilities, or restrictive regulations. Or he may experience a sudden lack of confidence, a shift in interest, or a loss of energy. The original commitment seems for a time to weaken in the face of perceived impediments. He gets snagged. Patterns of self-protection developed in childhood may resurface in the face of some particular field conditions encountered today, flooding the present with the past. Given adverse field conditions, the self-organization may turn rapidly into self-*dis*organization.

The ability to respond is not a fixed and measurable attribute. It is highly field-dependent and variable according to circumstances. No individual's responses are ever exactly the same as another's. Each person's responding is a function of all that she or he has ever learned in the past and his or her habitual response patterns. The work of exploring fixed gestalten, or automatic configurations of the field, takes many different forms – meaning that an education in responding cannot be circumscribed in advance. Yet, the right context can help to cultivate, enhance, and strengthen the ability to respond. By contrast, some contexts – including, alas, many educational ones – can crush initiatives, reduce self-confidence, and create a "disabling field". In therapeutic work, a lot of artistry is required to create for the client and therapist working together a supportive yet challenging field of collaborative learning. To learn how to respond more intelligently and with greater confidence to challenges and difficulties requires the therapist to support the would-be artist, but not to the point where the artistry of the therapist becomes more figural than that of the client's. Nor, in any artist's journey, can anyone else do it for him: creative, skillful responding is ultimately self-learned.

Responding is the first ability. As readers will realize, from a Gestalt therapy theory point of view, it relates to issues of self-support and empowerment, to taking author-ity and response-ability for one's own life, and the existential nature of one's life choices. It is about supporting clear gestalt formation and completion, and achieving free-functioning – fluidity and flexibility within an ever-changing field. Alas, the field is often structured in ways that elicit automatic and habitual responses that are far from being artistic, so strengthening the capacity for creative self-organization in the field is a significant process in developing the artist's autonomy.

B. Interrelating

Interrelating is a second ability that almost all people have to a significant degree and yet can be enhanced. It is basic to life: from trivial transactions to sharing intimate life partnerships. The artist, like any human being, is a member of a social species, and her artistic talent has been cultivated in relationship. As an artist, she is also interrelating by communicating. Even if her work feels like a wholly private and personal process at times, the reality is never far away: the picture, poem, dance, or song is created in the context of others, and it is often for others as much as for herself. Whether performing in public, or showing the results of her work in public, she is engaging in an act of "communicating herself", speaking out in words, paint, sound, movement, or some other medium, to other human beings.

Human beings do not and can not exist alone. Artists are no different in this respect. They learn from others and are stimulated by what others create, do, and demonstrate. A painter notices another's technique. A photographer builds on a tradition of a favorite icon. A pianist listens over and over to a recording of a piece by a master. Inspiration often comes from others or is fired by somebody else's "solution". The ability to interrelate, to engage with other people productively, runs through the artistic life. Indeed, in an interconnected world, interrelating with others is obligatory, even for the would-be recluse. Notably, for instance, the artist will receive reactions and feedback – including appreciation and criticism laden with judgments and projections – and will develop over time a whole variety of ways of dealing with them. Other people are also important in that they compete for scarce resources. An underlying competitive ethos pervades most fields of the arts, and handling conflict and other complex relational issues in non-distracting ways can have a big effect on an artist's overall well-being.

Artistic work, too, is often collaborative. With film and theatre, the work is inherently interactive, a function of a number of people working as a team. But even with solo art – writing a novel, say, or playing the piano – the reality is generally that there are others involved – people who commission the work, as well as the audience, readers, or spectators, with whom the artist has to engage. An artist may not be a "natural" when it comes to interrelating: she may not be a people person, or be super-accomplished in skills, say, of negotiation. But, if the artistic enterprise is collective, relationships are important. And establishing a relationship with the receivers of the art may be of critical import.

Broadening our view to include the artistry of ordinary life, the ability to interrelate assumes still greater significance. Relating to our families, sexual partners, employers, friends, colleagues, neighbors, and fellow citizens involves a huge and important slice of human activity. Much of what happens between parties is a function of the field of the between, which is already set in place and which structures much of what takes place. The management of the "dance between" is an enterprise of skill and sensitivity, which the two (or more) parties may demonstrate to differing degrees. The process of identifying with individuals and groups – and thereby rendering others as "outsiders" – sets up tensions which can be destructive if not handled with understanding and compassion. Respect for the other, not least as a source of difference and creative stimulation, is not easily learned in a culture that is frequently polarized, where stereotyping is rampant, and where conflict is often mishandled.

In Gestalt therapy training and learning, the skills of interrelating are attended to throughout. As part of human functioning, how we relate to other people is basic, inevitable, and of universal import.[2]

---

[2] How we relate to animals, and more generally to the natural world, is also of critical relevance – a different branch of the interrelating ability that assumes added significance in today's world, with the urgent necessity to avoid further damage to the biosphere. This is discussed at greater length in Parlett, 2003.

Artists, like any other group, including Gestalt therapists and therapy clients and trainees, come to the tasks of engaging with others with varying degrees of skill. The ability to interrelate develops over a long time – a lifetime. Learning to meet, converse, argue, hang out together, collaborate, form friendships, become lovers, break up, fight, reconcile, ask for help, and so on, are all ways of interrelating that most people learn in the course of their social development. The very specialized study that Gestalt "art students" undertake is one that requires much practice and careful observation by others more skillful in spotting disturbances to contact or where the flow of engaged connection seems to falter or move backwards.

Even learning to listen, with all one's senses, and to give space to another to express him or herself, may sound easy but is known to be difficult for many beginning students. People's capacity to impose meanings rather than find meanings, or to be wedded to an agenda that is one-sided, or to change the subject when emotions rise, are all ways in which the delicate sinews of good contact can be easily bruised or strained. Practicing inclusion and learning to live the relationship (Yontef, 1993), or developing an intersubjective capacity to "enter another's world" with exquisite sensitivity, are developments of the interrelating ability to a very advanced level.

C. Self-Recognizing

The third ability identified, *self-recognizing*, is also at the heart of the artistic enterprise. Creative expression depends on finding within oneself the impulse, generating point, or compelling idea that fuels the work. There also needs to be a match, say, in an emerging picture or poem, between what is arriving in paint or words and what is imagined. Staying in touch with his emergent process, the artist is monitoring in a way that ideally is neither critical in some destructive, "topdog" way, nor so lax as to result in work or performance that falls below a satisfying level.

No artist – musical, visual, therapeutic or otherwise – can do without the ability to self-recognize. This ability – the hallmark of a conscious, learning, self-aware human being – has many levels and dimensions. For instance, a performer about to perform needs to be ready – centered, clearly focused, and grounded. Recognizing that he is *not* ready is a necessary first step in becoming so. He can take corrective action – a minute or two of meditative-type deep breathing perhaps, or reaching out for a reassuring hand. Likewise, an artist in the creative throes needs to know what is right for him and what he needs in order to continue to flow, to function at his most creative. These are essential questions to ask and to know the answers to. Recognizing when an idea or internal feeling is ripe, or needs to incubate longer in unexpressed form, is another essential observation of his creative process.

Of course, the kinds and degrees of self-recognizing are not constant, even for an experienced writer, actor, or painter. For instance, there will be times when he will be temporarily "lost in his world": he may need to become so engrossed that the boundary between him and what he is doing is temporarily dissolved. At such moments of full contact, his capacity (or will-ingness) to access and "report in to himself" on his state of being at that mo-ment may be minimal. While internal monitoring may be relaxed and by-passed, some quality control self-reviewing must still be taking place. And one suspects, in the most experienced practitioners, that it works at a level of just being in awareness without becoming a strong and intrusive new figure.

Self-recognizing is a general ability that, in Gestalt terms, accommodates many varieties of being aware. It includes having an accurate self-image, and knowing one's process. With more experience – of how one works best, for example – comes the added realization that awareness of such matters is worth acting upon. Realizing the value of greater awareness is another di-mension of self-recognizing. As Yontef (1993) describes, there are stages of development beginning with awareness and moving to "becoming aware of one's awareness process" and continuing up to having a profound "phenom-enological attitude" where, in the terms used here, a degree of self-recog-nizing is always present.

Artistic work draws upon both skill and inspiration, and self-recognizing provides an essential feedback loop. In the development of Gestalt students, self-recognizing takes many forms. Indeed, it becomes ubiquitous as a value and priority in the training. However, it needs to be differentiated from ego-tism, which can be thought of as self-"spectatoring" (Clarkson, 1989, p. 124) and which interrupts full involvement and living with spontaneity. Even more so, in many Western cultures, the influence of oppressive cultures has led to over-active self-critical thinking patterns. Self-recognizing can be con-fused for many with self-depreciation. Learning to spot such processes, in-trojected messages, and "shame binds" (Lee and Wheeler, 1996) – and to offset or disrupt them – is as important a project as any in becoming a confi-dent and creative artist of life.

D. Embodying

The fourth ability described, *embodying*, is central to all artistic activity. The arts are almost defined by embodying, in the sense that, through bodily movement and sensing, something – an idea, concept, story, theme – is brought into being, is expressed. And with all expression, the body is impli-cated. No artistic idea can come to fruition if it remains in the imagination. The painter living her picture, fully sensitive to it and to what she is paint-ing, is observing it constantly. The musician deeply involved in expressing the exact feeling of the piece is experiencing a sense of discomfort in her be-ing and body when it is not right. The sculptor stands back and senses in her hands the exact shape of what she wants to do next.

For many artists, the power of drawing upon more than purely mental skills is almost taken for granted. The arts are whole-body involving. In carving or sculpting, singing, calligraphy, dancing, piano playing, acting or drawing there is manifest physical activity, sensorimotor coordination of a high order that is crucial to the project at hand. Perhaps a part of poetry writ-

ing may be very private and "in the head", but it becomes much more alive –
and embodied – when spoken out loud. A major part of artistic activity,
broadly conceived, has a strong and direct physical aspect. The painter using her brush is extending her hand by other means; the saxophonist with
her fingers, breath, and lips, or the dancer with even a simple movement of
reaching out, are also using their entire bodies (more accurately, they are
being their bodies). The physical experience cannot be separated from the
whole expressive process.

Of course, all of life is lived in, through, and with the participation of the
whole body: an idea that is basic to the holistic philosophy of Gestalt therapy. To be embodied is to be living with one's whole being and not as a talking head. Everyday language informs us of the basic necessity to be embodied: knowing one's *heart's* desire or where one *stands* or something not
feeling *right in the gut*, are essential sources of human data that provide orientation to any artist. Our ordinary language is peppered with references to
body and physical process.

The Gestalt student learns to be interested not only in people's ways of
thinking and the content of their minds, but also in their physical reactions,
their "felt sense" (Gendlin, 1978), their experiences of emotional and physiological processes. She learns that powerful needs and energies – sexual,
angry, loving, grieving – are critical to human life and living fully. She learns
to listen to or sense the messages that come from deep in her body. She realizes that to be embodied means to be in touch with the physical and emotional manifestations of all experiencing. She progressively is able to understand teachings, such as those of the philosopher, Merleau-Ponty, when he
says: "My body is the vehicle of my *being-in-the-world*" (1967, p. 82). To develop a personal way of living that does full justice to the Gestalt approach,
and thus to live the art form, she has to comprehend, and know from the inside, what embodying is and how central it is for a deep appreciation of the
Gestalt approach.

For an artist to embody ideas (or ideals) is to live them with the whole of
her being – to breathe them, to walk the talk, and to give expression to them,
so that the whole body and being of a person is implicated. The creative process of the artist, the therapist, or the person just living in life entails this
kind of involvement of the whole being in their enterprise. To be embodied
also means living in fundamental harmony with oneself – in terms, for instance, of "organismic self-regulation". Recognizing and responding to rhythms
of tiredness and energy is part of this. Learning to be more embodied also
calls for being alive to the senses and learning to move with grace and fluidity (within an individual's physical limits).

There are numerous ways in which people are physically out of touch
with themselves. Some ignore signs of ill health, while others are obsessed
with their medical condition. Some force themselves to exercise when they
need rest, or over-eat, starve, or cut themselves. They may also fall prey to
any of number of physical addictions. To be "unembodied" means to be in
an inharmonious relationship with oneself – split, not in one's body but
thought-bound or out of touch (figuratively and often literally), desensitized

and emotionally damped down or emotionally "out of control". Or people may be narcissistically involved in the appearance of their body and may distort their lives in order to have a so-called perfect body. All of these conditions and states involve not living *in* (or *as*) their body, not being at ease physically, and being in a state of alienation that is not artistic in the wider sense that I have been using.

E. Experimenting

Artists of all kinds are *experimenting*. Of the five abilities discussed, this one, most of all, speaks to the essence of what we think of as the artistic experience. The creative artist lays claim to the right to experiment freely, to be unfettered by constraints of convention and precedent. The originality of expression, what Goodman (in the quote at the beginning of this chapter) calls the artist's technique or style "is himself", it is *his* way of forming the real to be real. It was one of the foremost principles of the founders of the Gestalt approach to offer support and challenge to a human being to free him- or herself, to make a life – to sculpt her existence or dance his particular dance of life. That there are constraints and costs in doing so, and often not-so-good consequences for others (like children), was not perhaps sufficiently considered. But the anarchistic, avant-garde, and rebellious impulse gave the approach a distinctive, life-affirming, and energetic boost that has fuelled Gestalt therapy throughout its history. And the image of the artist – with his or her integrity, courage, and willingness to fly in the face of other's expectations – captures this questing and unsettling quality as well as any. (That artists are also often pictured as troubled, socially alienated, and divided beings, is a reflection perhaps of over-emphasizing anarchistic and rebellious directions. Departing from the so-called natural order has attendant downsides. In reality, of course, many artists work regular hours, pay their taxes, and are contentedly married. This does not detract from the power of the image of the artist as an experimenter *par excellence*.)

Artists experiment in a multitude of ways – extending skills, altering formats, cutting corners, and playing with perspectives and presentation. An instrumentalist plays music in a new way; an actor portrays a character in a different guise; a painter tries out a novel technique in applying paint. Hallmarks of great artists include not only their originality – their seeing something from a new perspective that they communicate for others to see it (or hear it, or feel it) from a different angle, too – but also their readiness to take risks, make mistakes, and survive disappointments.

Experimenting calls for an exceptional degree of focus. There is an intensity of involvement and concentration as a change is made, the point at risk is surmounted, or a climactic moment reached and passed. Other considerations are put on hold: "during an intense experience of a work of art it is felt to be (…) the only possible work or at least the highest kind, and the experience of it inestimably valuable" (Goodman, in Perls et al., 1994, p. 199). The attitude of experimenting calls for being open to the unknown and finding what is offered in the present moment and in the field as it exists at the time of the experiment. Improvising, as in jazz or improv theatre, is pure experimenting. In other fields of activity it is "to fly by the seat of one's pants", or "to make it up as you go along". No experiment can ever be planned fully in advance, and readiness to improvise, with the artist working live and the situation "taking over," brings living in the NOW to a high point. It is not much of a leap to suggest that life itself can become an all-the-time experiment, with the here and now world of ongoing creative adjustment becoming the material out of which life is built. It is forever improvised, rather than rehearsed over and over in advance and, alas, usually to little or no avail, because the actuality is rarely what has been imagined.

The counter-forces to experimenting are when there is an automatic repetition, an addictive or compulsive pattern that is mindless, or other times when not being present leads to an uncreative solution, often by default. To experiment is not always to opt for the novel and untried. Discernment is called for, and the skillful experimenter is open to the possibility of doing something that is ultra-familiar, when it is consciously chosen. Experimenting is not about "constantly re-inventing the wheel"; nor is it a fixed pattern of always unsettling the *status quo* or always being a rebel. There are times when, after much flux and free flow, the artistic way might be to create "a rigid alternative".

Experimenting calls for a particular kind of courage and willingness to be fully alive, acting spontaneously and being open to departing from convention. At the same time, there is strength in reasserting what is stable, secure, and predictable. In a world in which much enforced change and disruption to people's lives occur in disabling ways, the capacity to experiment may need to be directed toward becoming more resilient in the face of the change or to reassert essentials that may be lost. Experimenting is as necessary in staying the same amid change as it is in promoting change and encouraging the different.

IV. Conclusion

The abilities I have briefly described are essential in all human living. They are abilities that everyone has and draws upon in the course of living a life. At the same time, they can also be cultivated – as key areas for development and strengthening. If given the right conditions of stimulation, opportunity, and support, they can become more pronounced, more generally available, to be drawn upon and utilized in the course of living, working, creating, and acting in the world. Equally, if conditions are unfavorable, or if the abilities are ignored and sidelined, they can fall out of use, or become atrophied or unavailable – with serious consequences both for the individuals and those around them.

The abilities, I suggest, are key dimensions of human development, as reflected in Gestalt therapy. They connect to (or are antidotes to) recurring, shared, human difficulties, well-known to be common departures from artistry in our society, sometimes to epidemic proportions. Examples of *responding* difficulties are in feeling hopeless, dis-empowered, and alienated. *Interrelating* is important because of the huge incidence of relationship difficulties and human beings' lack of sensitivity in handling differences of outlook between people. *Self-recognizing* relates to the confusion regarding direction, focus, sense of self, and how to live. *Embodying* stands as an alternative to desensitization and having disordered reactions to essential bodily functions (e.g., in relation to eating, sex, or sleep). And *experimenting* stands in opposition to operating "on automatic" or being addicted to something to the point that life options are decreased. All these human difficulties represent departures from artistry in contemporary living. They may be associated with behaviors and attitudes that derived from earlier creative adjustments, which at the time of their origination were indeed creative. However, similar behaviors, enacted in the present moment, are more likely to be obsolete and out of date, not related to present field conditions, and therefore not artistic.

In this chapter, I have taken seriously the image of the artist and the analogy of living life as an art form. They provide a framework for talking, describing, and making sense of developmental changes. The language of abilities is another way of doing this. I have intentionally woven these themes together here. Part of what Gestalt therapists have to do, if the essential strengths of our approach are to resonate with new readers and interest groups, is to recreate and articulate in new forms what define the essential tenets of our approach. In *responding* to the editors' invitation and organizing how I have been organizing myself to write this chapter, I have also been *experimenting*. I have wanted to be congruent with, or to *embody* the values of Gestalt therapy and to make good contact in *relating* to readers through my words and narrative. At the same time, I have wanted to remain conscious of what I have been proposing and doing (*self-recognizing*). In other words, the five abilities, or five dimensions of living artistically, have all come into play. In the process, I have done what every artist does – given the chapter my best shot, knowing that no work of art is ever fully complete.

References

Clarkson P (1989) Gestalt counselling in action. Sage Publications, London
Gendlin ET (1978) Focusing. Bantam Books, New York
Lee RG, Wheeler G (eds) (1996) The voice of shame. Jossey-Bass, San Francisco
Merleau-Ponty M (1967) The phenomenology of perception. Routledge and Kegan Paul, London
Parlett M (2000) Creative adjustment in the global field. British Gestalt J 9: 15–27
Parlett M (2003) Human strengths: Five abilities in an interconnected world. Raft Publications, Knighton
Perls F, Hefferline R, Goodman P (1994) Gestalt therapy: Excitement and growth in the human personality. The Gestalt J Press, Highland, New York
Yontef G (1993) Awareness, dialogue & process. The Gestalt J Press, Highland, New York
Zinker J (1977) Creative process in Gestalt therapy. Brunner/Mazel, New York
Zinker J (2001) Sketches: An anthology of essays, art, and poetry. GestaltPress/The Analytic Press, Hillsdale, New Jersey

"Tiger! Tiger! Burning Bright" – Aesthetic Values as Clinical Values in Gestalt Therapy

Daniel J. Bloom

> "'Beauty is truth, truth beauty', that is all
> Ye know on earth, and all Ye need to know."
> John Keats, Ode on a Grecian Urn

> "If you are in the now, you are creative, you are inventive."
> Frederick Perls (1969) Gestalt Therapy Verbatim, p.3

I. Introduction

The aesthetic is central to Gestalt therapy.[1] Its particular organization of sensation includes – without being limited to – the experience of beauty itself. This same aesthetic attitude that creates art and appreciates beauty accounts for life's harmonies and rhythms. Aesthetic qualities animate the life-work of an artist as well as the quotidian events of ordinary life. The theory and practice of Gestalt therapy is infused with these qualities. It is no accident that the first and most comprehensive elaboration of Gestalt therapy theory was written by Paul Goodman, whose efforts in creative literature (fiction and poetry) were as ambitious as his works in psychology and social theory. His collaboration with Frederick Perls is the coming together of European psychoanalysis, phenomenology, Gestalt psychology, and existentialism with the American pragmatism of William James, George Herbert Mead, and John Dewey (Richard Kitzler, "Three Lectures", article in preparation).

Creativity is intrinsic to Gestalt therapy's focus on novelty, excitement, and the finding, making, discovering, and inventing of contacting. It is the functioning of organism-environment.[2] Moreover, this focus links Gestalt therapy with biology since creativity factors centrally in natural selection. Gestalt ther-

---

[1] This chapter is a consummation of work initiated by the New York Institute for Gestalt Therapy and especially the original insight of Joe Lay, who coined the phrase "aesthetic criterion".

[2] I change the original "organism/environment" of Goodman to "organism-environment". Goodman's compound word punctuation is an either/or formulation, and this is inconsistent with his holistic theory.

apy takes the process of development from evolutionary biology, where development is a co-creative interaction among genes, organism, and other environment, enabling maximally successful adaptations to diverse conditions (Dewey, 1910, 1934, 1958; Oyama, 2000a, b; Lewontin, 2000). Through creativity, organisms invent diversity, which allows for natural selection among populations. Contact, which is the awareness process itself, is the *experience* of natural selection within the life-spans of aware organisms. Self is the artist of the human organism and, as the vital synthesis of contactings, it is experience of life itself. The aesthetic emerges from within sensible experience as the sight, sound, touch, and even smell of life. It divides the living from the dead.

This chapter will examine the centrality of aesthetics in Gestalt therapy's ideas of contact-boundary, contact, self, and creative-adjustment.[3] This convergence of aesthetic values with therapeutic values is one of Gestalt therapy's most unique attributes as a method of psychotherapy. This attitude in Gestalt therapy's clinical approach is its radical power.

II. Contact-Boundary, Contact, Self, Creative Adjustment: The Heart of Gestalt Therapy

A. Contact-Boundary

"Experience occurs at the boundary between organism and its environment, primarily the skin surface and the other organs of sensory and motor response. Experience is the function of this boundary, and psychologically what is real are the 'whole' configurations of this functioning, some meaning achieved, some action completed" (Perls F et al., 1951, p. 277).

With this often quoted passage from *Gestalt Therapy: Excitement and Growth in the Human Personality* (hereinafter referred to as PHG), Gestalt therapy attempts to settle one of the central questions in Western philosophy: the relationship of mind and matter.

A brief summary of this important philosophical concern may begin in the 17th century. René Descartes (1596–1650) approached the disparity between "inner" and "outer" experience by separating the mind from the external world: mind is essence (or consciousness) without extension (the spatial dimension of physical phenomena), while matter is extension without essence. John Locke (1632–1704) continued this distinction and further identified the primary and secondary qualities of objects, noting what he thought to be intrinsic qualities and those dependent on perception. To Locke, mind is a passive *tabula rasa*, a blank slate, whose content is entirely the result of sense perception. David Hume (1711–1776) approached the mind/body dualism and, with the sharp logic of his empiricism, severed any way of being certain that our senses could be a reliable indicator of the external world.

---

[3] I likewise change the original "creative adjustment" to "creative-adjustment". This compound word now conveys the wholeness of creative-adjustment. "Creative" is not an adjectival modifier of "adjustment", but is intrinsic to it.

Immanuel Kant (1724–1804) examined this dualism and considered the function of the human mind in great detail; he formulated the synthetic unity of apperception and suggested that human cognition functions by organizing knowledge into categories prior to any experience. Kant opened the way for Idealism, which dominated much of 19th- century thought; at its extreme, it ignored the role of experience. In the United States, drawing on European developments in philosophy and science, William James (1842–1910) appraised this formidable gap between cognition and the material world and re-grounded experience in sensation; he defined perception as the activity of the organism. Consciousness is no longer a "thing" separate from the perceived world, but a material and sensible process: the psychical is physical. James, George Herbert Mead (1863–1931), and Dewey (1859–1952) re-embedded human experience in biology and began to adapt Darwinian discoveries into human development (Mead,1936; Dewey, 1910). Perception is the activity of the aware organism's "passage" or process (Mead, 1934). Self is created by social acts; the "we" precedes the "I", and remains implicit in it. Life is effervescent with excitement, an *élan vital* (Henri Bergson, 1859–1941). Experiencing, moreover, is an aesthetic process of organism and environment in co-creative poise with grace, harmony, and rhythm (Dewey, 1934). Experience is extension impinging on essence.

Gestalt therapy is the psychotherapy that is called forth by this meeting of extension and essence; and at this junction (contact-boundary) are organism-environment, contact, self, and creative-adjustment. "Mind, body, and the external world" (PHG, p. 255) unite as wholes of experience in contacting. This is a creative interaction of organism-environment: this interaction creates experience while it is simultaneously further creating experience. The individual emerges from his or her social context or field, much as a sculptured human is formed from a block of marble. As a psychotherapy, Gestalt therapy looks to this process and evaluates it by reference to this emerging figure's experienced and observed attributes. Fixities, lack of grace, and dullness, for example, are evidence of interruptions in contacting, losses of ego functioning, and disturbances of self functioning that diminish creativity. It is the fluid process of assimilating the novel that sustains the organism and field (ibid., p. 234). This process presents with aesthetic[4] qualities. It is inherent to contact, self, and creative-adjustment.

B. Contact

Contact is the process by which a figure emerges from the organism-environment background (ibid., p. 231). Whenever the term "figure" is used in this chapter, it should be understood that it is a shortcut for saying "The process of the dynamic relationship of figure and ground". This "figure"

---

[4] Aesthethic. Etymology: German *ästhetisch,* from New Latin *aestheticus,* from Greek *aisthetikos* of sense perception, from *aisthanesthai* to perceive (Merriam-Webster Online Dictionary).

emerges through a process where sensations re-configure and become perceptions and, depending on the circumstances, reconfigure into further motivations and actions. Each minute-by-minute detail of contacting contains a developing aesthetic as a *felt* and *sensed* organizing of experience. The qualities of this aesthetic will be discussed below (III.C.). This is *creative* activity at the boundary of organism and environment. It is a fluid synthesis of organism and environment with a unity of sensory, motor, and affective elements. Where a creative artist manipulates the art medium into an artwork, anyone in ordinary contact manipulates and restructures organism-environment into meaningful wholes of experience (PHG, 1951; Dewey, 1934, 1958).

C. Self

Self is the structure built by the contingencies of organism-environment, assembled, as it were, for the function or teleological end of contacting (Spagnuolo Lobb, 2001). It is the nexus of organism-environment, and it is a synthetic unity with its own aesthetic. From the organism, self draws on interoceptions (e.g., thirst, hunger, pain) and proprioceptions (e.g., spatial orientation, somatic sensations); from the environment it draws on exteroceptions (e.g., touch, sight, hearing) and the raw material for physical needs. It is the artist of life (Bloom, 1997, "Self: Structuring/Functioning", unpublished manuscript). When circumstances require more deliberateness on the part of the organism to meet its needs, more self is created at the contact-boundary. It is co-created by the organism and environment at their meeting. In sleep, then, there is minimal self, whereas there is more self in any activity that requires concentration, imagination, deliberateness, or effort. Self is an ever-changing creatively developing function of organism-environment with the aesthetic qualities of contact: rhythm, grace, fluidity, vitality, harmony, vividness, cohesiveness. A list of these qualities could continue through the rich vocabulary that describes the ripeness of life. Within self are its partial structures that orient the organism, enable the environment to be manipulated, and facilitate novelty, yet provide continuity and support: id functioning, ego function, and personality function. For example, a person whose self functioning contains disturbances may approach eating with hesitations, self-recriminations, and disharmonious appetite leading to binging and/or anorexia. The aesthetic qualities of this self, then, would be quite different from the fluid organization of self in harmony with the opportunities and needs of organism-environment (see III.C., below).

D. Creative-Adjustment

The final concept to consider from the aesthetic perspective is creative-adjustment. This process equilibrates the tensions of organism-environment at the contact-boundary. A person experiences an urge or appetite and satisfies it. Or a person writes an article on the aesthetic in Gestalt therapy and spends many hours organizing ideas into words and rearranges text on the recalcitrant blank screen on his computer; starts and stops; stands and sits; and finishes the work with an exhale of relief. In both examples, either a simple or a complex result is achieved in their creatively-adjusting to different circumstantial constraints. This is contact creatively transforming the organism-environment field (PHG, p. 406). Overall, it is how the world is known and lived-in. If natural selection is the biological process that provokes species into creating solutions to challenges to its existence, then creative-adjustment is the means by which people overcome obstacles and adapt as successfully as possible to life's vagaries. Creative-adjustment means neither spontaneous discharge of animal impulses nor automatic resignation to demands of the field, but balances in between. Creativity without adjustment is superficial; adjustment without creativity is lifeless. Neurotic adjustment is an habitual imbalance in the equilibrium of creative-adjustment, leading to diminution of contact's vitality. The more creative solutions a person invents for any particular circumstance, the more adept a person is at the art of living. Perhaps the common experience that motivates people to seek psychotherapy is their sense that their choices are limited, that they are in a constriction-filled situation. It may be a dark mood that does not abate or a love relationship that persistently brings distress. Or it may be a sense that the tasks of the world demand responses that the person is unable to make. In each situation there is a limitation in the person's capacity to respond creatively: either to see fully the opportunities that are present or to fashion new possibilities from what is actually available. In each case the personal aesthetic of each person is an experience of imbalance, tension, and disharmony. It is artist's block.

III. Aesthetic Values as Clinical Values

A. Psychopathology and Qualities of Contacting

The Weltanschauung of Gestalt therapy is life as creative process. The aesthetic liveliness of contactful experience has describable attributes, which are indicators of the state of the organism-environment. Yet, there are formidable obstacles to a theory of psychopathology within Gestalt therapy. A therapy whose model for optimal functioning specifies the richness of creative responses must avoid a priori limitations to such responses. There are more things in heaven and earth than are dreamt of even in Gestalt therapy philosophy. A system of psychopathology is inherently perilous, since it invariably implies norms of emotional health and wellness subject to cultural bias and introjection. But, Gestalt therapy looks to the authority of the experienced field itself, rather than societal norms; it invites each person to evaluate his own experience with his own criteria. "Organismic self-regulation" is the wisdom inherent to contacting. "Natura sanat, non medicus", nature heals, not the physician (Goodman, 1977).

Rather than a psychopathology using psychodynamic formulations and character types, then, Gestalt therapy psychopathology is a "kind of art criticism". When PHG introduces character types, it notes that rather than being fixed forms they are more like genres in literature – more like the categories of farce and tragedy in Shakespearean drama (p. 449). Within these "character genres", there are many diverse possibilities and combinations, so that the very meaning of the genre is transformed in each unique whole: "In *applying* any typology (...) one experiences the absurdity that none of the types fits any particular person. (...) It is the nature of the creative – and in so far as the patient has any vitality he is creative – to make its own concrete uniqueness by reconciling apparent incompatibilities and altering their meaning" (ibid.). The therapy itself is simply to "help the patient develop his creative identity by his ordered passage from 'character' to 'character'" (ibid.): that is, from figure to figure, always created from the potentialities of the organism and the possibilities of the environment. "Most important of all," writes PHG, "the achievement of a strong [that is, vivid] gestalt is itself the cure, for the figure of contact is not a sign of, but is itself the creative integration of experience" (p. 232).

Gestalt diagnosis is an hypothesis about contact, containing an experiment that enables its own evaluation; diagnosis and therapy are identical. For example: "I notice that when you say the word 'mother,' your voice drops, and I lean forward in my chair. Would you say your sentence again and notice how it sounds to you? What do you experience?" The diagnosis is the "noticing that", which is itself the beginning of the experiment, the therapeutic intervention. As the experiment continues, it informs the developing diagnosis and enables further experiment. Thus, diagnosis becomes experiment, which then becomes further diagnosis, and so on, in a graceful rhythm of contact.

Sometimes PHG describes "good" and "bad" contact. This use may have derived from Gestalt psychology's use of the term "good gestalt", and has unfortunate connotations of either/or possibilities (see, also, III.D., below). Further, to speak of contact as "good" or "bad", "weak" or "strong", or most commonly, "in contact" and "out of contact" is merely to be descriptive, without advancing a useful mode for the evaluation of contacting. It is far better to evaluate contact with reference to finer distinctions, such as grace, fluidity, clarity, brightness, balance, and rhythm. These are aesthetic qualities to describe a creative process and can be employed with all the powers of their own aesthetic. To refer to an art work as "bad" does not open a discussion of its qualities; rather, it closes the door to any meaningful evaluation. However, to describe its aesthetic attributes is to engage with it creatively. If a person declares her experience of contact is "bad", she says very little about her experience. However, if she describes how cold are her fingers, how tight her lips, how constricted her breath, and how lifeless the spring day seems to her – a catalog of her aesthetic sensibilities – already she would be opening to a new experience. This would be Gestalt therapy.

When contact is fluid and flexible, when the emerging figure is bright and graceful, Gestalt therapy suggests there is little interruption in contacting and all is well in the world. However, where the emerging figures are dull, indistinct, or diffuse, and contacting is weak, there is reason to suspect trouble. This could be the result of deliberate inhibitions by someone aware of environmental restraints as, for instance, a person may suppress a spontaneous giggle at a funeral. Or it may be the result of unaware habitual interruptions that are the characteristics of neurotic functioning and which contain losses of ego functioning and disturbances of self functioning. The difference between neurosis and vitality is that when obstacles are encountered in the latter, there is continuing creativity and, in the former, there is confusion and lack of sensitivity (ibid., p. 465). Psychopathology, then, is a fluid concept based on experienced interruptions and flows in the stream of contacting.

B. Intrinsic vs. Comparative Evaluation

PHG distinguishes two modes for evaluating experience: intrinsic and comparative. In comparative evaluation, the qualities of gestalt forming are contrasted to some standard extrinsic to the act itself. But if what is being evaluated is the experience of contact, how can one compare one's own sense of grace, for example, with another's? This splits whole experiences into fragments and declares some abstraction to be a fixed standard. It is an irresistible invitation to competition and neurotic conflict. Rather, PHG proposes the intrinsic mode of evaluating, where the standard emerges in the on-going act itself (p. 288): by its "gestalt qualities" and by achievement of its end (the "end directedness of process"). An experience evaluates itself – affirms itself, as it were – by the authority of the attributes that emerge within it as a function of the organism-environment field.

Intrinsic evaluation looks to the qualities within the experience itself or "gestalt qualities". It is axiomatic that Gestalt therapy derives from Gestalt psychology. Paul Goodman, Fritz Perls, Laura Perls, and all those who followed them, described the Gestalt psychological principles they drew upon: "the relation of figure and background; the importance of interpreting the coherence or split of a figure in terms of the total context of the actual situation (...) the active organizing force of meaningful wholes" (ibid., p. 237). The whole is more than the sum of its parts. Parts can only be understood as they relate to other parts comprising the whole. There is a tendency for parts to organize into the simplest whole, which is a dynamic equilibration of the tensions of the field (*prägnanz*) Unfinished situations persist as tensions in the field. All these are important and useful aspects of Gestalt therapy. Nevertheless, the Gestalt psychologists refused to be associated with Gestalt therapy and quarreled with the application of their perceptual and cognitive hypotheses to personality, psychopathology, and psychotherapy (Henle, 1986). Furthermore, Gestalt therapy and Gestalt psychology are fundamentally different. Gestalt therapy is adamantly an holistic approach – the sensory-motor-affective unity of contacting is bedrock; Gestalt psychology, on the other hand, is dualistic. Gestalt psychology is based on the mind-body split of iso-

morphic parallelism – events in experience are structurally identical to but
separate from corresponding brain physiology (ibid.).

C. "Gestalt" Qualities or Aesthetic Criterion?

1. "Gestalt" Therapy?

If the above-mentioned "gestalt" qualities are also seen as aesthetic evaluations of figure forming, then this conflict with the Gestalt psychologists can
be side-stepped. Much of what Gestalt therapy drew from Gestalt psychology can also be carried by the work of James, Mead, and Dewey (Kitzler R,
"Three Lectures", unpublished manuscript). These social scientists and philosophers started their important work 50 years before the Gestalt psychologists and continued actively writing (on Dewey's part) through 1950, first as
a response to the challenges of modern science; indeed, much of the Gestalt
psychologists' work overlaps with their earlier insights. Laura Perls studied
with the Gestalt psychologists Max Wertheimer and Adhemar Gelb in Frankfurt. This is the *only direct* connection that is reported between the founders
of Gestalt therapy and Gestalt psychology. Yet Laura Perls objected to using
"Gestalt" as a name for her "new" modality, since she thought it had almost
nothing in common with Gestalt psychology (Barlow, 1981, p.37). In Rosenfeld's "An Oral History of Gestalt Therapy" (1978), L. Perls says: "Mainly
Gestalt is an *aesthetic concept*, but Köhler used it in connection with field
theory" (p. 26, emphasis added).

She would have chosen "existential psychotherapy", but this name was
already being used by others (Perls L, 1987). The founders wanted to grab
the public's attention. They chose the name "Gestalt therapy" to herald a
break from orthodox psychoanalysis. Moreover, Gestalt psychology still had
a revolutionary reputation at the time they used its name. It is unclear,
though, how widely read Fritz Perls or Paul Goodman were in Gestalt psychology. "The concept of the organism-as-a-whole," wrote F. Perls, "is the
center of the gestalt-psychological approach which is superseding the
mechanistic association psychology" (1948). Is this really the *center* of their
approach? In his first book, *Ego, Hunger and Aggression*, Perls hardly mentions Gestalt psychology at all; he gives more weight to a variety of other influences, such as Friedlaender's idea of "creative indifference" (Perls F,
1947). Fritz Perls often referred to his work with Kurt Goldstein in Germany:
"Goldstein broke with the rigid concept of the reflex arc. According to him,
both kinds of nerves, sensory and the motor, stretch from the organism to the
environment" (Perls F, 1948, p. 569). But in 1896, at least 20 years before
Goldstein, Dewey, of course, analyzed the reflex arc as a whole phenomenon
(Dewey, 1896). Goldstein was not a Gestalt psychologist. Although Goldstein
worked closely with Gelb and was certainly influenced by other Gestalt psychologists, he distinguished his own work from theirs (Goldstein, 1995). He
was a neuro-psychiatrist and referred to his work as organismic, not Gestalt.

The Gestalt psychology in Gestalt therapy comes filtered through Goldstein's organismic lens.

Paul Goodman studied for his doctoral degree at the University of Chicago when that institution had been a center for American pragmatism. Goodman directly credits James and Dewey as significantly influential sources for his own work (Goodman, 1972; Stoehr, 1994). The most affecting passages in all of Goodman are his lyrical descriptions of experience. By contrast, his applications of Gestalt psychology's ideas seem to lack conviction, as if they were by rote. The degree to which Gestalt therapy and American pragmatism are related is a topic whose richness deserves deeper study, and yet which falls outside the purview of this chapter. The nearly seamless flow of development from American pragmatism to the theory of Gestalt therapy warrants the assertion that they provide an adequate ground on which Gestalt therapy's intrinsic evaluation and aesthetic criterion may stand.

However, this is not a search for the "true" forbears of Gestalt therapy, so much as an examination of the broadest foundation from which Gestalt therapy developed. The intellectual river that brought forth Gestalt therapy has multiple overlapping tributaries. Gestalt therapy comes from the same European stream from which Gestalt psychology, Kurt Goldstein's theory of the organism, Edmund Husserl's phenomenology, Martin Heidegger's existentialism, and Hans-Georg Gadamer's hermeneutics flow. Indeed, the American pragmatists themselves were familiar with the Europeans Johann Fichte, Wilhelm Wundt, Ernst Mach, Franz Brentano, and Henri Bergson (Thayer, 1981; James, 1893).

2. Aesthetic Criterion and Pragmatism

John Dewey's writings on aesthetics, for example, show his influence on Gestalt therapy. Dewey examined the aesthetic experience as part of ordinary human experience and sought to recover the "continuity of esthetic experience with normal processes of living" (Dewey, 1934, p. 10). "Biological commonplaces" of experience "reach to the roots of the esthetic" (ibid., p. 14). The aesthetic of ordinary experience is the harmony and rhythm of all life and not only the domain of the artist (ibid., p. 16). An experience is aesthetic "in the degree in which organism and environment cooperate to institute an experience in which the two are so fully integrated that each disappears" (ibid., p. 249). This is, of course, contacting. Again, Dewey: "For only when an organism shares in the ordered relations of its environment does it secure the stability essential to loving. And when the participation comes after a phase of disruption and conflict, it bears within itself the germs of a consummation akin to the esthetic" (ibid., p. 18). "Order is not imposed from without," writes Dewey, "but is made out of the relations of harmonious interactions that energies bear to one another" (ibid., p. 14). Experience is understood by reason, imagination, and aesthetic perception (Dewey, 1958; Diggins, 1994, p. 319). In the interaction of organism and environment, there are "rhythmic beats of want and fulfillment, pulses of doing and being withheld from doing" (Dewey, 1934, p. 16). Here is organism-environment; here is contact and withdrawal in a flow of process with intrinsic aesthetic qualities.

Gestalt therapy looks to the observeable and experienceable interruptions in contact as evidence of neurotic functioning. At these moments, losses of ego functioning and disturbances of self functioning appear as disturbances in the flow of contact making and withdrawal (PHG; Isadore From, personal communication). Interruptions are synonymous with Dewey's aesthetic evaluation of "breaks in the harmony and rhythm" of organism-environment (1934). These interruptions are felt. They are sensed, or sensible, by the patient *and* the therapist. These are not hypotheses or abstractions – they are *sensed* actualities affecting the stream of contacting. This is the aesthetic criterion as a clinical value. It is not that this fluid experiential stream is equivalent to the inspired process that produces works of art. Obviously, not every experience is comparable to an artistic masterpiece. But ordinary experience and extraordinary creations share a common source: the creative impulse with the aesthetic qualities of harmony, rhythm, cohesion, vividness, and so on. A toddler, for example, is no ballerina when she stumbles and falters as she creatively-adjusts her maturing capacities to challenging environmental obstacles; but there is, nevertheless, a harmony and rhythm to her contacting (Frank, 2001).

D. Aesthetic Criterion as "Gestalt Ethics"

The aesthetic criterion provides a basis for psychotherapy, but does this provide a basis for other values? Can there be an ethics of Gestalt therapy? This question is being posed in contemporary Gestalt therapy literature (Wheeler, 1992; Lee, 2002). Since it also questions the efficacy of Gestalt therapy's intrinsic and aesthetic values, it is worthy of a reply. Psychotherapies are always dragged into the ethical arena. To the extent that they purport that there are values of normal and healthy functioning, it is inevitable that they would contribute to those who question the common good and wonder how best to behave toward one another. Certainly, psychoanalysis readily migrated into this, and with its emphasis on maturity, delay of gratification, oedipal rivalry, and adjustment to society, it became the principal modality supporting a culture of conformity and competition (Lichtenberg, 1969). Gestalt therapy began as a reply to psychoanalytic hegemony, but it was misused as a free-for-all ethos in the late 20th century (Bloom D, "A View from the Manhattan Skyline: Up-dating and Comparing Gestalt Therapy", submitted article) that is currently being reconsidered. A new "Gestalt ethics" is now proposed where figure and ground are reconnected and evaluation becomes an assessment of a person's relatedness to others (Wheeler, 1991, 1992; Lee, 2002; Yontef, 2001). There is nothing wrong in this reemphasis on core Gestalt therapy theory to correct previous misunderstanding. Yet, this impulse to assert a Gestalt ethics may turn Gestalt therapy's model of human functioning into a tool for comparative evaluation, if it locates ethical authority outside the process of figure forming, such as with an assessment of intersubjective relatedness.

Gestalt therapy attends to the forming of the figure, rather than the figure formed (PHG, p. 231). Content is thus of secondary import. Rather, what *is* crucial is the elasticity of how content is found and made. So long as this fluidity is maintained, discovery is supported and encouraged. This is Gestalt therapy's evaluation. Values can be wisdom's best fruits. Ethics as a mode for evaluating the formed figure is indispensable. It is a part of the social compact and assures civil safety. But ethics is not psychotherapy. A just society may be the foundation for optimum fulfillment; it may also be one of the conditions for increased fluidity in contact and one of its consequences. But this, like growth itself (ibid., p. 428), is a by-product of psychotherapy. Ethics is both a concern for just ends and a way to ensure its means. But ethical weather patterns are fickle; the climate for approved and condemned behaviors is always changing. The quest for a "preferred" or even a "just" figure impairs the free play of figure formation. Rather, the ethics of Gestalt therapy is intrinsic to the contact process: it is the self-justifying light of the emerging figure.

Moreover, the aesthetic criterion assures that valuation will be fluid and experiential and that it will be always changing as a function of a developing field. The aesthetic criterion is an ethical criterion only insofar as it is an alert to interruption in this process of human discovering, contacting. If this alert is sounded, Gestalt therapy proposes, there will indeed be a disruption in the relationship of figure to ground. But this is available as a *direct* experience, not as an opinion of the clinician evaluating from an abstract ethical construct. Further, this is an experience of the therapist that is offered to the patient as an experiment: "When you do 'A', I experience 'B'. What is your experience?" The moments of experience are always reciprocal, since they are of the contact-boundary. Clarity, grace, vividness, harmony, fluidity – these comprise the aesthetic ground for evaluating human vitality. This is Gestalt therapy's radical attribute:

"In its trials and conflicts the self is coming to be in *a way that did not exist before*. In contactful experience the 'I', alienating its safe structures, risks this leap and identifies with the growing self, gives it its services and knowledge, and at the moment of achievement stands out of the way" (ibid., p. 466, emphasis added).

Utopian dreams are woven into PHG. They are of an harmonious world flowing with natural grace. What if contactful experience, for example, culminates in murder? Brutality implies the treatment of another person as an object. This is evidence of an interruption in contact – a splitting-off of one aspect of a whole from an other, and an attempt to annihilate it (ibid., p. 340), probably through retroflection, projection, and egotism. This would be sensed and experienced in the qualities of the forming figure. But some acts, though passing muster when the aesthetic criterion is employed, may nevertheless be judged wrong and condemned. Society criminalizes objectionable behavior, yet sometimes later withdraws its sanction. For example, adultery was once a capital offense; it was once illegal to teach evolution, purchase contraceptives, or perform an abortion. The intrinsic evaluation of the aesthetic criterion does not beg this question, but lies outside it. It leaves the non-psychotherapeutic question of approved and condemned acts – comparative evaluations of the formed figure – to others.

IV. Clinical Aesthetic in Practice

Human vitality is its capacity to creatively-adjust to the contingencies of experience. The neurotic is the failed artist (Rank, 1932) for whom a lusterless neurosis takes the place of artistic achievement. Yet the creativity of the person is coiled and alive within the structure of any instance of contact interruption and is available in psychotherapy. A current symptom was a creative-adjustment to past contingencies that persists as a creative activity that maintains a fixed gestalt despite changed circumstances. In its finest distillation of theory and practice, Gestalt therapy focuses on a single moment in the stream of experience, and especially on its sensible aspects. Sensation is the portal of sight, sound, touch, taste, and smell from which the aesthetic criterion emerges. In this section, a moment is abstracted from context so as to elucidate this point: that within all process there is a creative pulse in creative-adjustment and that even within apparent neurotic fixities there are vital kernels of contact. The therapy is support of this creativity, so the interruptions of contacting may become aware. The powers of the person then may become engaged in finding and making, discovering, and inventing a new figure. The unaware now aware is assimilated.

A Clinical Example

Roger complains of dull headaches and lack of interest in life. He wonders if he is depressed. The therapist notices that Roger's face seems frozen and appears disconnected from the rest of him. He asks Roger to sense his face and attend to how his facial muscles change, how he is holding or releasing his expression. The therapist asks him to exaggerate and play with this contracting and releasing of his face. Roger appears to alternate among a variety of masks: frowning, open amazement, tight disapproval, and childlike awe:

"What do you notice, Roger?"
"Well, I feel excited and sort of out of breath. I seem to have gone all over the place."
They sit quietly as they attend to the rhythm of their breathing. Roger's face seems softer.
"Can you feel your face now?"
Tears well-up in his eyes. "I feel sad."
Roger begins to weep.
After a while, he looks to the therapist and says, "I forget how many of my friends are dead. I miss them." His face is flushed, and his eyes are warm.

Roger's fixed mask is his creative-adjustment to the magnitude of his losses. It holds his sadness and his joy within its tightness, crafted in the workshop of his personality to shield him from overwhelming grief. The interplay of grief, awe, anguish, and joy emerged when he experimented with this mask; but they were always there. How else could he have known that he lacked interest in life? These unaware feelings were held together in the muscular tension displayed by his facial mask. They were his dull headaches; the ache was their vitality constricted into pain. Most likely, other aspects of Roger, including his breathing pattern, carriage, and gait would offer the same announcement of interrupted contact through their lack of harmony or stiffness. The therapist chose what was most evident to him as he experienced Roger at that moment in that session. This choice was a creation of the therapist-patient field, which is the meeting of two apparently individual perspectives. The first experiment arose from the therapist's sense that Roger's facial expression was rigid and out of harmony with what he was saying. The experiment led to a release of excitement that became ground for the second experiment: "Can you feel your face now?" And this then led to Roger's awareness of his grief. The sequence of experiment-to-experience-to-further-experiment flowed with its own rhythm. In this example, the therapist's vitality reached out to the patient and enabled new figures to emerge, which included previously interrupted feelings.

Roger's frozen mask was a reaction formation, since it was how his intense feelings were maintained in unawareness. Instead of liveliness or sadness, he was fixed and frozen – as if feeling-less. This posture protected him from feelings that were once overwhelming and thus once an adequate and creative solution to that risk. The reaction formation masked the repression of the original impulse, permitting any anxiety occasioned by the emergence of the inhibited impulses to be avoided (PHG, p. 444). Such a creative-adjustment is a neurotic's form of art. Yet, unlike the work of a true artist, this creation served to drain vitality from Roger and, applying the aesthetic criterion, left him with dull, brittle, and diffuse figures – all of which he experienced.

V. Conclusion

"Tiger! Tiger! Burning bright
In the forests of the night
What immortal hand or eye
Could frame thy fearful symmetry?"
William Blake, *The Tiger*

Contacting, the aware life process, is the organism as artist shaping raw sensation into meaningful forms. It is the consummation of creation. This is nature alive. Figures and grounds develop and proceed with a rhythm and harmony specific to the organism-environment, their field of existence. These forms of experience glisten with intrinsic qualities, sound their own vitality, and declare their own authority through the aesthetic criterion.

Gestalt therapy understands human experience to be imbued with creative life and provides a method for the fullest expression of its vitality. Contact-boundary, contact, self, and creative-adjustment are constituents of this aesthetic method. By looking to the forming of experience itself and its intrinsic qualities, Gestalt therapy avoids the imposition of static values or prescriptions onto life. Its clinical values are aesthetic values; its attention is on sensible experience. Gestalt therapy holds fast to the notion that individual experience is a process unfolding within a fluid field. Its aesthetic qualities are attributes of human beings, who are finding and making their way through an evolving world. As William Blake expressed it, life burns brightly with "fearful symmetry". "Beauty is truth, truth beauty," John Keats so simply declared. The grace of the aesthetic is the harmony of contacting and the wisdom of the organism. This *is* all we know on earth and all we need to know.

References

Barlow AR (1981) Gestalt – Antecedent influence or historical accident. The Gestalt J 4(2): 35–54

Dewey J (1896) The reflex arc. Psychological Review 3: 357–370

Dewey J (1910) The influence of Darwin on philosophy. In: Dewey J, The influence of Darwin and philosophy and other essays. Henry Holt, New York, pp 1–19

Dewey J (1934) Art as experience. Perigree Books, New York

Dewey J (1958) Experience and nature. Dover Publications, New York

Diggins JP (1994) The promise of pragmatism. Univ of Chicago Press, Chicago

Frank, Ruella (2001) Body of awareness. Gestalt Press/Analytic Press, Hillsdale, New Jersey

Goldstein K (1995) The organism. Zone Books, New York

Goodman P (1972) Little prayers and finite experiences. Harper and Row, New York

Goodman P (1977) Nature heals. Free Life Editions, New York

Henle M (1986) Gestalt psychology and Gestalt therapy. In: Henle M, 1879 and all that, essays in the theory and history of psychology. Columbia Univ Press, New York, pp 22–35

James W (1893) The principles of psychology. Harvard Univ Press, Boston

James W (1904) Does consciousness exist. In: Kiklick B (ed) William James writings 1902–1910. Library of America, New York, pp 1141–1158

Lee R (2002) Ethics: A gestalt of values/the values of gestalt – a next step. Gestalt Review 6(1): 27–51

Lichtenberg P (1969) Psychoanalysis: Radical and conservative. Springer, New York

Lewontin R (2000) The triple helix. Harvard Univ Press, Boston

Mead GH (1934) Mind, self and society. Univ of Chicago Press, Chicago

Mead GH (1936) Movements of thought in the 19th century. Univ of Chicago Press, Chicago

Oyama S (2000a) Evolution's eye. Duke Univ Press, Durham London

Oyama S (2000b) Ontology of information. Duke Univ Press, Durham London

Perls F (1947) Ego, hunger and aggression. Random House, New York

Perls F (1948) Theory and technique of personality integration. American J of Psychotherapy 2(4): 565–586

Perls F (1969) Gestalt therapy verbatim. The Gestalt J Press, Highland, New York

Perls F, Hefflerline R, Goodman P (1951) Gestalt therapy: Excitement and growth in the human personality. Julian Press, New York

Perls L (1987) Interview with Gloria Natchez. Living Biographies, Derner Institute, Garden City, New York

Rank O (1932) Art and artist. W.W. Norton, New York London

Rosenfeld E (1978) An oral history of Gestalt therapy, part one: A conversation with Laura Perls. The Gestalt J 1(1): 8–31

Spagnuolo Lobb M (2001) From the epistemology of self to clinical specificity of Gestalt therapy. In: Robine JM (ed) Contact and relationship in a field perspective. L'exprimerie, Bordeaux, pp 49–78

Stoehr T (1994) Here now next. Jossey-Bass, San Francisco

Thayer HS (1981) Meaning and action. Hackett Publishing Company, Indianapolis

Wheeler G (1991) Gestalt reconsidered. GIC Press/Gardner Press, New York

Wheeler G (1992) Gestalt ethics. In: Nevis E (ed) Gestalt therapy perspectives and applications. GIC Press/Gardner Press, New York, pp 113–128

Yontef G (2001) Relational Gestalt therapy. In: Robine JM (ed) Contact and relationship in a field perspective. L'exprimerie, Bordeaux, pp 79–94

The Neuroscience of Creativity:
A Gestalt Perspective

Todd Burley

It is common to look for the roots of creativity in some aspect of the individual. We assume that the creative person must have a unique characteristic or characteristics unavailable to others. Usually these characteristics are sought in reductionist versions of personality theory, intellect and more recently, in some aspect of the neuroscience revolution. Unlike other theories of psychotherapy and personality, Gestalt theory takes the field as its basic unit of observation. By field, Gestaltists mean that the whole context or ecosystem of which the person and his or her neuropsychological system is a part or portion works as one, and that it is impossible and misleading to try to understand and observe a person "apart from" the field of which they are a portion. Paradoxically, the way we know the field or "about" the field is through a person's contact with other aspects of the field, which gives rise to awareness and, from a neurocognitive perspective, awareness (Damasio, 1999) and experience, or one's personal phenomenology. Thus the creative person's neurological and neuropsychological makeup, from a Gestalt perspective, is a part or portion of the field. Creativity is a field phenomenon and, as we shall see, neuroscience leads away from reductionistic explanations and clarifies the concept of creativity as a field phenomenon.

But first, what is neuroscience, and what does it have to contribute? Neuroscience and in particular cognitive neuroscience is the study of such higher functions as sensation, perception, language, purposive movement, spatial perception and organization, memory, emotion, planning, decision-making, learning, and assimilation or adaptation. All behavior, creative and otherwise, is in some manner, related to the brain. Whether one is riding a bicycle, composing a song, or gazing at a sunset, the underlying processes are guided and processed by the brain. Let us look at the brain: its basic structure and how it develops and functions to facilitate creative processes. The brain is fascinatingly organized with the brain stem working to regulate basic life functions and the energization (excitation) of the cortex. The sensory lobes are arranged in such a manner that the occipital lobe is responsible for receiving, analyzing, and assisting in storing visual information; the temporal lobes receive, process or analyze, and store auditory information;

and the parietal lobes receive, process or analyze, and store body information such as touch, temperature, pressure, movement, and position of various parts of the body. Each of these areas of the brain receives raw information that is relayed from the related sense organs, and this information must be analyzed so as to create meaning and understanding. For example, the occipital cortex receives a series of signals from the retina that indicate light, dark, color, movement, verticality, horizontality, and angle. Such information is not recognizable as a face. The information must be analyzed and processed in order for the person to perceive a recognizable face. An additional system works in unison with the sensory lobes and responds to thoughts and external stimuli. This is the limbic system, which is positioned between and deep within the two hemispheres and is associated with emotional reactions. This system is part of the brain normally associated with "feelings", and it functions to control arousal (excitement) as well as positive and aversive feelings that correspond to liking and wanting as well as disgust.

These four information "processors" work in constant coordination and communication in order to perform almost all cognitive/emotional functions. For example, simple arithmetical problems such as 1+1=2 are verbal problems, which can be performed by the left temporal lobe. However, as the addition problem becomes more complex (for example, adding columns of numbers), and the person has to "carry" numbers from one column to the other, the parietal lobes, where space is represented, are called into play. In still more complex mathematics, which becomes more abstract, the right parietal lobe is called upon to assist. Thus far, I have merely been describing "sensory" input into the brain and the manipulation of information that has a sensory basis such as reading, judging spatial relationships, imaging music, imagining a change in composition for a painting, or just recalling the name of a friend we are introducing to someone.

Guiding this complex system are the frontal lobes, which are responsible for expression and acting on the world rather than sensing the world. The frontal lobes create intentions, make plans, and verify that one's plans are indeed carried to fruition. In addition, the frontal lobes are responsible for movement – whether related to talking, dancing, hammering or other actions that carry out the person's plan to have an impact on the external world. The anterior areas of the frontal lobes are responsible for guiding one's thoughts to be able to visualize a mural, retrieve a particular sequence of notes from memory, or anticipate an angle for a sculpture, for example. Importantly, the frontal lobes also read the body state on a continual basis and thus form the information that Gestalt therapists often request of clients when asking "What are you feeling?" or "What are you aware of in your body?"

Just as no two persons have similarly functioning bodies or organ systems, no two persons have similarly functioning brains. For some people, it is very easy to think in terms of verbal (from the brain's perspective auditorily-based) metaphor, whereas for someone less auditorily oriented it may be easier to think in terms of movement, gesture, and other uses of space. For still others, visualizing is the central mode of thinking. Thus, overall, we have a sensory system, itself made up of three very different but interactive modalities (vision, audition, and the somato-sensory system); a system for planning, executing, and verifying behavior; and a system for giving emotional value, both positive and negative to any given object, thought, or other stimulus. While it is difficult to grasp the vast interconnected information and decision processing system involved here, it might help to imagine having a computer that processes information using five different information-processing systems each working on a different "operating system". The power is enormous. But then the amount of information that must be processed simply in everyday living is incredibly complex. Despite the tremendous capacity of today's robots and "artificial intelligence" systems, we are unable to come close to a system that could even cope with the daily tasks of a cave man who must plan his day based upon his needs as well as those of his immediate family. Decisions such as where to hunt, how not to be detected by game, how to judge time, how to keep track of where he is in the mental map of the territory that he has developed to understand the terrain, and how to get back home are part of a constant neurocognitive flow of the moment and day. These are simply a few of the thousands of mental processes and creative judgments that must be made if he and those he is responsible to are to survive. Each of these decisions requires a great store of experience and memory (witness what happens when someone with Alzheimer's disease loses so much memory that he or she cannot return to the home wandered away from just moments ago), and equally importantly, creativity. Many of the decisions we make daily, even simple decisions, require creativity. Clearly, creativity is a property of everyday life. Yet creativity is often mistakenly applied only to the artist who has created a new awareness or way of seeing the world; creativity cannot be limited in this way. There is enormous creativity, for example, in the Cuban auto mechanic, whose brain has found ways to keep automobiles that are forty to fifty years old, usefully functioning. At a less concrete level, there is creativity in the local priest who has found a way to help his local parishioners maintain self-respect in a situation where oppression seems to dehumanize one's worth. This processing is all generated in the interest of meeting organismic needs related to the ongoing adaptation to the environment. The brain must coordinate these organismically-based needs (whether for food or artistic expression) with its understanding of what is available in the self and in the environment. Thus the complexity of the neural system begins to appear as a minimal requirement. What we call cognition and creativity depends on large-scale processing and coordination of multiple distributed areas of the brain (Bressler, 2002). This is not the end of the complexity associated with the brain. Additional processing is associated with major biochemical systems as well as the programming that is inherent in development.

But how does creativity develop, and how is it created? In part, the development of creativity is parallel to and intertwined with the development of the brain, its structures, and its "programming" through its interaction with the person's physical and cognitive/emotional environment. The brain is not fully developed when we are born; nor is it adapted to the environment in which it must maintain itself, adapt, and thrive. Thus while the structure of a newborn child's brain is being formed over a period of about seven years, it is also being trained. In essence the child's brain is learning to perceive in unique and personal ways and to organize meaning. By age two, association areas are well formed within sensory areas and by age seven, association areas between sense modalities are also well formed. Association areas between sense modalities allow one to perceive and create meaning involving two senses such as audition and space. For example the question "Is the uncle's brother and the brother's uncle the same person?" relies both on the auditory and verbal meaning as well as the spatial relationships implied in the words "uncle" and "brother" as related to the family tree. During this period, the development of abilities, which begins at birth and probably prior to birth, is based upon interaction with the world around and specifically with the mother and father or other caretakers. The literature is quite clear in indicating that the quality of the environment and the ability to interact with it bear a direct relationship to a child's acquisition of sensory, perceptual, and manipulative abilities. It is also now quite clear that memory is active a few weeks after birth, if not before (Rovee Collier, 1996, 1997; Bauer et al., 1994; Bauer, 1996[1]) and that recall or memory lasts for at least two years and probably longer with regard to procedural memory, that is, the memory for how one does what one characteristically does (Tulving, 1985). Recent evidence (Quinn, 2002) indicates that infants at least as young as three or four months are already able to represent mentally a variety of categories at both a general level (for example, mammal, furniture) and a specific level (for example, cat, dog, chair, table). Adequate stimulation is required for the child's brain to be "programmed" effectively. The infant and child watch and listen to the available adults as they learn how to think and process information. In a sense, the parent is teaching the child how to think. These processes are building and programming the brain circuits needed for adaptation and creativity. As part of this process, neurotrophins are active in the construction of neural circuits and synapse selection. These neurotrophins also help maintain the viability of neurons and synaptic connection through continued practice and use (LeDoux, 2002).

Thus a child's environment interacts with his or her genetic and normal physiological capabilities in the development of the intellectual and creative capacities of that child's brain. Consequently, the quality and the content of early childhood experiences are of great importance. Thus when parents are not available to a child for significant periods of time, the selection of alternative caretakers becomes an issue of long-term importance. Indeed, parents should take great care to expose children to adequate and assimilable stimulation. Over-stimulation will tend to result in inability to concentrate and attend while under-stimulation will result in lagging development. Practicing skills changes the structure of the brain, its neural connections, and

---

[1] See also Burley TD, Freier MC (1999) "Character: Where it comes from and what to do about it." Paper presented at the 4th International Conference of the Association for the Advancement of Gestalt Therapy, New York.

the amount of cortical space relegated to the skill in question while skills that are not practiced are degraded over time (Recanzone, 2000). Of course plasticity does not stop with development. It is an ongoing process where one continues to be fascinated by novel possibilities and connections that form the basis of creativity. As Pfenninger (2001, p. 92) states:

"Creativity involves the vision or the determination of novel contexts between facts in our external or internal worlds – contexts that had not been recognized previously. This requires the association in the mind of diverse and apparently unrelated images and, thus, represents a higher level yet, of integrative capacity of the nervous system."

There are, of course, qualitative differences between people that are based upon genetics; but these by themselves are not crucial in nature in determining the difference between creative and less creative persons. Far more important is the nature of stimulation and development that every brain must undergo in order to responsibly and effectively learn and utilize the skills involved in simple everyday tasks. Consider, for example, the learning and creativity required in simply getting a spoon into one's mouth without jabbing and soiling one's face. Such seemingly simple tasks are indeed major accomplishments of learning and mastery as well as programming of the brain for the eventual performance of more complex skills such as ballet, masonry, surgery, or even sculpting. These experiences guide the creation of specific circuitry within the brain.

Damasio points out that creativity requires decision-making and emotional responsiveness. As he outlines his understanding of the process, cortical areas responsible for visual, auditory, and somatosensory (spatial) processing generate neural patterns associated with particular experiences or images such as a shape, a movement, a sound. A memory for such an item is actually "an extensive modification of the firing properties of numerous circuits in 'association cortices'", which he calls "dispositional representations" (Damasio, 2001, p. 66). Contrary to what is commonly thought, memory is not stored as an image but as a modification of the firing properties of neural networks. Thus memory is actually a process, and each "remembering" is a reconstruction; hence the poor reliability of memory. Such dispositional representations allow the person to bring back a face or a musical phrase without an external stimulus. This is not solely an intellectual process, but also an emotional one. The brain reacts emotionally to both internally generated as well as externally available stimuli. In a sense, the brain does not recognize the Western and Perlsian bifurcation of emotion and reason. In fact, it is the emotional reaction that makes possible an aesthetic response or experience and the processes of liking, disliking, rejection, and pleasure. Emotional responses to artistic representations, Damasio says, create a sense of pleasure, much of which is based upon bodily responses such as breathing, heart rates, and skin conductivity, all of which become associated with the perception of particular objects so that eventually the body is bypassed in the generation of the emotion in what he calls an "as-if body loop" (Damasio, 2001, p. 68). These responses allow decision-making and support for creative manipulations. Indeed, without the intertwining of cognition and emotion, humans do not seem to make decisions that are organismically adaptive or self-support-ive (Damasio, 1994).

It is important here to confront a myth that has often and over a period of many years appeared in the psychological and Gestalt literature (Burley, 1998). This unfortunate myth is the idea that the left hemisphere is linear (of-ten translated as less valuable), and the right hemisphere is creative and ar-tistic. It is hard to pinpoint where this error originated, but it is now part of "common knowledge". Possibly it came from a less than careful reading of Ornstein's (1972) *The Psychology of Consciousness*. Although Ornstein re-ported the literature accurately, others perhaps made some premature and unsupported interpretations. It is correct that at higher levels the right and left hemispheres process information differently, but those differences lie in the fact that the left hemisphere is more oriented toward auditory informa-tion, while the right hemisphere is oriented toward spatial information based upon somato-sensory data. The left hemisphere tends to take over tasks that are "over-learned", while the right hemisphere is oriented more toward the analysis of new and unfamiliar stimuli. In addition, the left hemisphere pro-cesses information more rapidly than the right. As a result of both this com-plexity and the programming process itself, a skill like reading moves around in the brain depending on one's reading skill and level. Young children begin by relying heavily on the right parietal lobe as they struggle to understand the differences between "b" and "d", while later, with more experience in making such discriminations, reliance on the right parietal areas are no longer neces-sary. Highly theoretical math skills tend to rely heavily on the right hemi-sphere. Creativity, of course, relies on the entire brain but draws more heavily on one or another portion depending on various aspects of the task. If one is writing a poem one might rely heavily on the auditory and word skills of the left temporal lobe for the words while at the same time relying on the as-pects of the right hemisphere for cadence, rhythm, and other qualities of sound. Sketching a landscape might depend heavily, but not exclusively, on visual experience organized by the right temporal/parietal areas. Fixing a car might depend heavily on the right hemisphere's sense of timing and the frontal lobe's sense of sequence. It is simply not true that the right hemi-sphere is more creative than the left. In fact, it clearly takes two hemispheres to create almost anything. Creativity is a function of the whole brain and its neural networks, not the function of a portion of the brain.

As can be seen from what has been argued thus far, the brain does not carry by itself an innate set of creative abilities. Rather, it is poised to interact with its environment and create a set of adaptive and creative abilities. There is a growing body of literature that regards creativity as something beyond the individual person, and thus regards it as a phenomenon of the interactions in the field. Nakamura and Csikszentmihalyi (2001, p. 337) ar-gue that:

"Creative contribution is jointly constituted by the interaction of three components of a system: (a) the innovating person; (b) the symbolic domain that the individual absorbs, works with, and contributes to; and (c) the social field of gatekeepers and practitioners who solicit, discourage, respond to, judge, and reward contributions."

Other creativity theorists such as Amabile (2001) – who emphasizes domain relevant skills, creativity relevant processes and love or motivation for the task – note that the social environment often plays a central role in the creativity of the individual.

Vygotsky (1978) implied and Luria (1973) stated explicitly that nothing is connected in the mind that is not first connected in the environment, thus taking a clear "field" perspective. The neural circuits that are necessary for creativity are the products of contact and the history of contacts that the organism makes. Creative persons have a great deal of experience, practice, and familiarity with the domain or medium within which they work. In a sense, creativity grows out of what cognitive psychologists call "expert systems". Such people spend a great deal of time getting to know the area of their interest. Indeed, they seem consumed by their interest and are willing to take the time and to discipline themselves to become so acquainted with their domain that they begin to see organizational patterns in places where others see nothing or see chaos. They are able to find a way to represent the patterns they perceive. In a study of the creative characteristics of Nobel Laureate Linus Pauling, Nakamura and Csikszentmihalyi (2001) note Pauling's unusual ability to present very complex ideas in a clear and simple manner. Experts also organize information in ways that allow them to include more information than the novice would be able to. This familiarity allows them to notice and recognize that which is novel. They are able to place the novel information in what cognitive psychologists call "working memory" (mediated by the frontal lobes) so that it is instantly and constantly available for comparison and inclusion in the task at hand. For example, a very creative and gifted therapist is able to absorb and recall a great deal of information about and from a particular patient. Out of a mass of disorganized information, the experienced and creative therapist is able to begin to discern patterns which he or she is then able to recall and relate to new information. Creativity does not require an unusual IQ (Gardner, 2001) or genius. Rather, the person needs enough experience with information in order to be able to see the patterns that emerge from confusion, to remember and connect seemingly disparate bits of information, and to recall it when the situation calls for it. Amabile (2001) notes that John Irving, a highly regarded American writer, was severely dyslexic and had to work hard to achieve and perfect his skills. He concludes:

"Rather than focusing single-mindedly on finding the most gifted children to accelerate or the most talented employees to hire, educators, policymakers, and managers might do well to create opportunities for learning effective work skills and environments that support active, deep engagement with challenging work – remembering that creativity depends not only on brilliance and wit but also on discipline and passionate desire" (p. 335).

Creative people have significant self-awareness to be able to recognize and notice their emotional responses to the information they are working with, so that they can make decisions and discriminations quickly and easily. They know what they like and what they dislike. Creative persons create, revise, discard, love, hate, and are sensitive to vague dissatisfactions that allow further revision, discarding, rethinking, and so on. In short, they are emotionally responsive and reactive in part because they are experienced and well-informed.

This self-awareness is crucial, because creativity requires the ability to detect novelty. This ability is also basic to orienting the organism's attention and awareness towards unusual environmental events in order to insure survival. The ability to detect novelty and the unusual is also crucial to the creative process, as noted by Pfenninger above (2001). Knight and Grabowecky (2000) have identified the dorsolateral aspects of the prefrontal cortex, the junction of the parietal and temporal lobes, the hippocampus, and the cingulated cortex as being involved in the detection of novelty as well as the production of novel behaviors. These areas are associated with memory, emotion, spatial-auditory stimulation, self-monitoring, and the sense of bodily status (Damasio, 1999). Novelty is associated with enhanced memory as well as learning. To detect novelty a person has to have a high level familiarity with the domain or material in which the novelty is embedded. For example, when one is introduced to a new area of art, it is difficult to ascertain the unusual and outstanding from the ordinary. Only after establishing a great deal of familiarity can one detect the unusual and distinctive. A high level of familiarity with a domain is one of the characteristics of individuals who exhibit creativity. They are often seen as, and are, experts in a particular field. Solso (1995) refers to the work of Glaser and Chi (1988) in identifying characteristics of experts: experts tend to excel primarily in a their chosen domain; experts perceive larger meaningful patterns of information or data than non-specialists; experts work at a greater speed than non-experts; experts seem to have superior long-term and short-term memories within their favored domain; experts perceive and organize issues at a deeper level of representation or organization than non-experts; experts take time to look at a problem from several perspectives; and lastly, experts seem to self-monitor their process as well as notice their errors and make appropriate corrections. Obviously, building neural networks that will function in these ways requires time, practice, and a great deal of familiarity and interaction between the neural system and the domain. Based on personal histories and observations, it takes an estimated ten years to build expertise in a relatively complex domain cluster.

I recently had the opportunity to visit the State Russian Museum at the Mikhailovsky Palace in St. Petersburg. A painting by K.A. Savitsky drew my attention because of the artist's ability to capture individual mood, feeling, humanness, and uncertainty, which is always an aspect of parting. The title of the painting is "To the War", and it depicts a large number of men boarding a train and parting from loved ones as they leave to take part in a war. After spending some time absorbing what, as a psychologist, I regarded as a remarkable ability to capture fleeting feelings in facial expressions, postures, and gestures, I turned around to find myself confronted with a large number of Savitsky's studies for the larger painting. Clearly recognizable were small tableaus of lovers, families, friends, and other groupings the artist had painted as fully finished pieces of art. Looking back at the full picture, one could see that the artist had changed a background here, the color of a scarf there, and a focused gaze to unfocused in the larger and finished painting. Suddenly, the thought, care, experimentation, consideration, and simply months of hard work that had preceded a finished masterpiece were clear. The mind and brain that created this painting were clearly possessing a great deal of life experience, thoughtful perception, practiced execution, decisions far too numerous to count, and a prodigious memory for glance, fear, and excitement. In a minor act of creativity of my own, I recognized what I had been trying to absorb in order to write this chapter: the life experience, the motor skill, the ability to control nuanced color, shape, and depth, the training, the repetition, and the manipulation of and experimentation with novelty. Beyond these, now, began to appear hints of the field aspects of this act of creation. Savitsky could not have executed this painting without years of immersion in relationships, feelings, visual observations, and the ability to plan and actively support his interest.

Another field aspect associated with creativity and its neural aspects is the frequently unacknowledged fact that creative acts are often a team effort. It was common for artists of the Renaissance to have a number of assistants and individuals whom they were mentoring work for them and at times take charge of aspects of a creative endeavor. Often artists are quite open regarding the fact that their work is the "result of a collaboration and the merge of several people's ideas and skills" (Chihuly, 2001, p. 20). Creative scientists, such as Nobel Prize winners Thomas Cech (2001), who demonstrated the catalytic function of RNA in cellular metabolism, and Linus Pauling (Nakamura and Csikszentmihalyi, 2001), who identified forces that hold matter together, both also worked as part of teams. Beyond the circle of helpers and collaborators that frequently surround creative persons, are the concepts and methods that arise as culture – whether popular, artistic, or scientific – evolves and makes new ideas and creations possible. Current historians, such as Barzun (2000), have noted that "new ideas" seldom originate with the person to whom credit is given. Rather, the new concepts are in the culture but not yet expressed in a manner that is notable. Freud, for example, has been credited as the discoverer of the unconscious, yet this concept was already in intellectual circles for many decades. Many Gestalt therapists are aware that the notion of dialogue and the presence of the therapist have been around at least since Perls, Hefferline, and Goodman (1951) and yet inter-subjectivity (Stolorow et al., 1994) and its attendant relational emphasis in therapy has been hailed by many as a new concept. Frequently, the efforts of many are attributed to one person who serves as the icon for a concept, and yet it is truly the beneficiary of the contributions of many others who have, at times, led the way, or done much of the labor and thinking that led to the final work.

It is said that after Einstein's death, his brain was preserved for autopsy and later study. The assumption was that at some point we would discover the secret of his creativity by looking at some structural aspect of his brain. It is now clear to many who study creativity, and to Gestalt theoreticians, that creativity is a field phenomenon. Neuroscience has brought us full circle.

The brain, its experiential awareness at the moment and over time, in the field with its rich abundance of stimulation as well as personal and impersonal relationships, are all needed to account for creativity.

References

Amabile TM (2001) Beyond talent: John Irving and the passionate craft of creativity. American Psychologist 56 (4): 333–336

Barzun J (2000) From dawn to decadence: 500 years of Western cultural life. HarperCollins, New York

Bauer P (1996) What do infants recall of their lives? Memory for specific events by one- to two-year olds. American Psychologist 51(1): 29–41

Bauer P, Hertsgaard L, Dow G (1994) After 8 months have passed: Long-term recall of events by 1- to 2-year-old children. Memory 2(4): 353–382

Bressler SL (2002) Understanding cognition through large-scale cortical networks. Current Directions in Psychological Science 11(2): 58–66

Burley TD (1998) Minds and brains for Gestalt therapists. Gestalt Review 2(2): 131–142

Burley TD (2002) A phenomenological theory of personality. In: Burley T (ed) GATLA reader. Gestalt Associates Training Los Angeles, Los Angeles, 29–42

Cech T (2001) Overturning the dogma: Catalytic DNA. In: Pfenninger KH, Shubik VR (eds) The origins of creativity. Oxford University Press, New York, 5–17

Chihuly D (2001) Form from fire. In: Pfenninger KH, Shubik VR (eds) The origins of creativity. Oxford University Press, New York, 19–30

Damasio AR (1994) Descartes' error: Emotion, reason, and the human brain. Grosset/Putnam, New York

Damasio AR (1999) The feeling of what happens: Body and emotion in the making of consciousness. Harcourt Brace and Company, New York

Damasio AR (2001) Some notes on brain, imagination and creativity. In: Pfenninger KH, Shubik VR (eds) The origins of creativity. Oxford Univ Press, New York, 59–68

Gardner H (2001) Creators: multiple intelligences. In: Pfenninger KH, Shubik VR (eds) The origins of creativity. Oxford Univ Press, New York, 117–144

Glaser R, Chi MTH (1988) Overview. In: Chi MTH, Glaser R, Farr MJ (eds) The nature of expertise. Erlbaum, Hillsdale, New Jersey, xv–xxviii

Knight RT, Grabowecky M (2000) Prefrontal cortex, time, and consciousness. In: Gazzaniga MS (ed) The new cognitive neurosciences. The MIT Press, Cambridge, Massachusetts, 1319–1339

LeDoux J (2002) Synaptic self: How our brains become who we are. Viking, New York

Luria AR (1973) The working brain: An introduction to neuropsychology. Basic Books, New York

Nakamura J, Csikszentmihalyi M (2001) Catalytic creativity: The Linus Pauling case. American Psychologist 56 (4): 337–341

Ornstein RE (1972) The psychology of consciousness. WH Freeman and Co., San Francisco

Perls F, Hefferline R, Goodman P (1951) Gestalt therapy: Excitement and growth in the human personality. Dell Publishing, New York

Pfenninger KH (2001) The evolving brain. In: Pfenninger KH, Shubik VR (eds) The origins of creativity. Oxford Univ Press, New York, 89–97

Quinn PC (2002) Category representation in young infants. Current Directions in Psychological Science 11 (2): 66–70

Recanzone GH (2000) Cerebral cortical plasticity: perception and skill acquisition. In: Gazzaniga MS (ed) The new cognitive neurosciences. MIT Press, Cambridge, Massachusetts, 237–247

Rovee-Collier C (1996) Shifting the focus from what to why. Infant Behavior and Development 19: 385–400

Rovee-Collier C (1997) Dissociations in infant memory: Rethinking the development of implicit and explicit memory. Psychological Review 104 (3): 467–498

Solso RL (1995) Cognitive psychology. Allyn and Bacon, Needham Heights, Massachusetts

Stolorow R, Atwood G, Brandschaft B (1994) The intersubjective perspective. Jason Aronson, Northvale, New Jersey

Tulving E (1985) How many memory systems are there? American Psychologist 40 (4): 385–398

Vygotsky LS (1978) Mind in society: The development of higher psychological processes. Harvard Univ Press, Cambridge, Mass

Part II
The Challenge of Defining
Creative Concepts

Therapy as an Aesthetic Issue: Creativity, Dreams, and Art in *Gestalt Therapy*

Antonio Sichera

I. Noun and Attribute: Creativity in *Gestalt Therapy*

The idea of creativity is central to *Gestalt Therapy*. Significantly, however, from a linguistic standpoint, it is not usually found in the form of a noun – "creativity", as such – but rather as an essential attribute of the experience of contact, which Perls and Goodman had already thought of immediately as "creative adjustment". In a word, *Gestalt Therapy* does not offer an abstract definition of creativity, of its *ousìa*[1], but understands it as a quality of the experience of the field, a property that cannot be isolated from the life context in which it is performed and made relevant. If the noun tends to block and harden, the attribute expands the elements of the discourse to that which, in each case, it is linked, connoting and orienting them in a new direction of meaning, which simultaneously accompanies and modifies them. Creativity is not defined in *Gestalt Therapy*; but it is implicitly stated that all that "happens" in the field, in relation to the contact, is in itself "creative", because without the creative contribution of the subjects involved there is no contact, no experience, no relationship.

Behind this choice lies the paradigmatic manner in which Gestalt theory understands the study of psychology. Perls and Goodman are not concerned with writing a chapter of cognitive psychology on creativity as an essential characteristic of human mental effort; rather they want to grasp the method according to which the process of experience, the concretization of the relationship, implies a *poiesis*, a "creation". What happens in the contact is that the organism and the environment "create" the very conditions of the meeting and grasp and make fruitful the possibilities given, rearranging them in a new gestalt, that "strong gestalt", which is itself contact (Perls et al., 1994, p. 8). It is not a matter of a mental restructuring of the cognitive field, but of a living mediation (we may recall Goodman's "middle mode"), a "fusion of horizons" (Gadamer, 1983; Salonia, 2000), which must *support* – in the ety-

---

[1] Essence, in ancient Greek [editors' note].

mological sense – the joy and effort of the word, the flavor, and even the imperceptible vibration of the emotion, the importance of gesture, the "animal" reality of the body of human organisms, of subjects in relationship, who by talking, hearing, touching, and looking at each other, construct the possibility of the encounter between themselves and the world. The word, gesture, emotion, and body are real, shared spaces in which organism and environment "come into contact", as actual living organs of creation of contact. In this perspective, creativity can only appear in the form of an adjective: in other words as an essential attribute of an act of the self, which implies research and conflict, passion and desire, construction of an intimate mutual understanding in word and body. It is words and living bodies that "re-create" themselves in the relationship and are modified to create at the boundary the invisible, real point of contact. This is why the self is "a creative contacting" (PHG[2], p. 24), an expression chosen by Goodman to bring out the intrinsic link between the creativity and creation of contact: the act of contacting itself.

But this is not all. It seems to me that the insistence of *Gestalt Therapy* on the adjectival form implies at bottom a view of human existence and its possibilities, which is not narcissistically delusional. Perls and Goodman do not sing the praises of creativity as a treasure to be found or a virtue to be exalted; they attribute it to the work of contact: what is creative for them is, in fact, at various times, the power, awareness, integration, and unification that are particular to the experience of contact. If the adjective expands and characterizes, it is equally true that the noun functions as a barrier, a limit. There is no such thing as creativity; there are only creative relationships and experiences. Hence, linguistically too, creativity does not appear except "in relationship" with the many aspects and the various actions of contact, of that creating, which is an intimate part of it.

In any case, the very concept of "creative adjustment" seems symbolically to show this intuition. In the original context in which the adjective creative appears in *Gestalt Therapy* – à propos the most recurrent definition of contact – creativity comes into play as a modification of a given reality, as a reformulating of situations, which must above all be submitted to: situations to which, in fact, one must adjust: "Creativity and adjustment are polar, they are mutually necessary" (ibid., p. 7). In contact, it is not a matter of fleeing from the reality in which one is immersed, or of building artificial paradises where a magical fusion can be hypothesized between the subjects involved in the field; it is instead a matter of remaking, re-creating the *positum* of existence, restoring meaning to it, and manipulating it with words and with the body. In this sense, contact is, for Perls and Goodman, "creative and dynamic" (ibid., p. 6), because the awareness that supports it is, at bottom, "a creative integration of the problem" (ibid., p. 8): the self, as "artist of life",

---

[2] In the text I use the abbreviation PHG for Perls F, Hefferline R, Goodman P (1994) Gestalt therapy: Excitement and growth in the human personality. Gestalt J Press, New York.

acts as an "integrator", which "plays the crucial role of finding and making the meanings that we grow by" (ibid., p. 11).

Hence creativity, in Gestalt therapy, is inextricably linked to the power of the self, which gives unity to experience, working unceasingly for creative adjustment. It is no mere chance that even when the self attacks and inhibits itself (an aggression, and even splitting, by which the symptom is generated), all it is doing, basically, is to act creatively, in the emergency conditions by which it is constrained, for the survival and minimal nourishing of the organism, for the construction of a field that is not wholly destructive. If this were not the case, it would not be possible to understand the emphasis in Gestalt therapy on the creativity of the symptom, on the "creative power" of the patient in therapy (ibid., p. 13), on the interpretation of "resistances and defenses" in the setting as fruit of "creative awareness (...) active expressions of vitality" (ibid., p. 25). On the other hand, therapeutic distress arises from "inhibiting the creative unification [and] the method of treatment is to come into closer and closer contact with the present crisis, until one identifies, risking the leap into the unknown, with the coming creative integration of the split" (ibid., p. 17). Thus therapy is the task of the self, which discovers and feels, in the dark painful areas, in danger and in difficulty, that space in which a "creative élan" (ibid, p. 26) is possible: what was not permitted to be done or felt, what had been blocked or, as it were, erased, if it is brought back into the light in the therapeutic relationship, is certainly a source of anguish, but also the perception of a new, disturbing flavor of existence. That "faith" in the generating background constituted by the setting actually enables the self to let itself go in the adventure, discovering new, yet old, territories: in making this leap in the dark, the patient knows, or rather feels, that the background – i.e., the relationship with the therapist – is upholding her; in this relationship she will certainly experience painful novelty, but she will also find the necessary support to make it her own.

Therapy is thus a vital space in which the creative power of the self is taken seriously, in the strongest, most intense manner. This is why it has an essentially aesthetic dimension: you cannot be a Gestalt therapist unless you have learned to admire the creating effort of the self and learned to discern it even despite the obstacles, the unease, the silences, the pointless or tedious gestures, the irritating or incongruous answers, the hallucinations and ravings of the patient. In a word, you cannot be a real therapist if you do not feel engaged, every time, by the beauty of the slow reflowing of the vital possibilities of the other, if you do not gaze in wonder at that profound repossession, that renewed belonging-to-oneself and to the world that therapy fundamentally is. As the relationship matures, this beauty becomes manifest, if therapist and patient take part in the adventure of "co-creating" the conditions of contact, an event which is not revealed by a test but, according to Perls and Goodman, appears and is imposed thanks to the signs of *aistesis*, the aesthetic sensation, first and foremost among which is grace.

II. Dreams as *mise en abîme*[3] of Therapy

But if all this is to come about, there must be a serene trust in the power of the self-in-relationship; its contributions in the field must be welcomed as real. And above all, the therapist must be convinced that what the patient does and says in the setting, all that the patient consciously performs, is not a kind of useless palimpsest, but represents the possible vitality of the self, the indication of the road to be taken if an effective relationship is to be constructed. Nothing can be created together if each does not give space to the creativity of the other, to the creative power of the self. In the framework of this fascinating connection between creativity, beauty, and therapy there is, for example, an important passage of *Gestalt Therapy*, which must be read, on the subject of working on dreams. This may serve to exemplify what has been said thus far as well as open up further interesting perspectives. In the course of dealing with the theme of free association, significantly in the chapter on verbalization and poetry, Perls and Goodman state:

"To begin with, the associations circle round a dream detail. Let us assume that the patient accepts the dream as his own, remembers and can say that he dreamt it rather than that a dream came to him. If now he can connect new words and thoughts with that act, there is a great enrichment of language. The dream speaks in the image-language of childhood; the advantage is not to recollect the infantile content, but to learn again something of the feeling and attitude of child speech, to recapture the mood of eidetic vision, and connect the verbal and pre-verbal. But from this point of view, the best exercise would perhaps be not free-association *from* the image and application of cold knowledge *to* the image, but just the contrary: careful literary and pictorial representation of it (surrealism)" (ibid., p. 108).

This is a text that demands careful consideration. Brief as it is, it seems to me to make an important breach in terms of working on dreams and on the importance of aesthetic creativity in therapy. As is known, in the classic theoretical model the dream is supposed to be a projection of parts of the self, parts which the patient must be helped, in the course of therapy, to repossess. Perls puts great stress on this element (which is decisive) in his therapeutic practice: the assumption of responsibility in the face of the dream. Much later, Isadore From was to put forward the proposal of integrating the classic idea: reading the "dreamed" dream during therapy as a form of retroflexion, and hence as a message about the relationship with the therapist, which the patient must be able to verbalize and in any case express in the setting. It does not, however, seem to me that there has been sufficient attention to a deeper study of the path traced, however apparently fleetingly, in this passage from *Gestalt Therapy*.

---

[3] The *mise en abime*, in the language of literary criticism, is the contraction of the sense and structure of a macrotext, e.g. a novel, within a scene from or fragment of that work. It is a rhetorical procedure which conceals in a textual microcosm what the macrocosm – the entire work – then develops on a broad scale. In my interpretation of *Gestalt Therapy*, the dream shared in therapy fulfills the function of the *mise en abime* in relation to the macrocosm of the therapeutic relationship, whose meaning and deep structure, albeit in hidden manner, it anticipates.

What is actually being said here? – that the most useful work on dreams would probably be their portrayal, in literary or pictorial form, by the dreamer. In other words, the "best exercise" in therapy is probably "letting the dream be" in complete autonomy, as a work of art, fruit of the extraordinary creative powers of childhood, which the patient must be able to experience fully and freely: as the artist, who creates and gives space to her or his own urge to *poiesis*, independently of all theoretical considerations and of all practical interests, simply for the enjoyment of creating, for the (perhaps effortful) pleasure of concentrating totally on an undertaking that makes her or him in the world in a form of absolute typicality, with the stamp of that artless audacity typical of children. While she portrays "herself", thanks to the mediation of language (whatever kind of language it may be), she re-creates herself and opens up a new unexplored world, one that is always, albeit implicitly, in search of the recognition of the other. A person who portrays herself, always, at bottom, communicates herself. In the background there is, for her, a communicating gaze.

But let us clarify these concepts. The first important aspect is indisputably the self-referential viewpoint of the dream, the affirmation of its existence independent of any further signification. It is as much as to say, in short, that the dream *is*. It presents itself to the dreamer, and hence also in therapy, charged with a *quantity* of being that makes it existent in itself, important in its form as dream: i.e., in its illogical language, in its violation of the most minimum principles of reality, in its disregarding, carelessly and unpredictably, the *empirìa*[4], giving life to a world which is "other". The creation of the dream is not to be instantly demolished, but welcomed. Into it flows and is manifested the legendary energy, the original infantile creative strength of the subject, who makes a myth of his own existence, dramatizing it and restoring it shaped in a language that refers to the hellish and heavenly forces, the ancestral nature that abolishes the boundaries between life and death, between being born and coming to an end, in a universe permeated by magic and Hermeticism. In the remembered, narrated, and portrayed dream the aesthetic resources of the self are shown to a high degree. When it is able to narrate and rework the dream, portraying it in the forms of poetry and the visual arts, without constraining it in the web of syntax and ordinary prose, the self transfigures its subjective experiences, the history of the dreamer, transporting it into the atmosphere of myth, in the sense of the fictitious foundation of existence, profound interpretation of the decisive points of life.

But what, in more precise terms, does it mean to portray a dream? It is not a matter of dramatizing it, of making it into a theatrical play, nor of freely associating to it other words or images, but of reviving its imaginative structure in appropriate language, making it the stuff of poetry, the generative fire of a creative energy that belongs to it. Clearly it makes no sense, here, to set up sterile contrasts or facile dichotomies. We are face to face with an

---

[4] Experience, in ancient Greek [editors' note].

epistemological question, an axiology that gives primacy to representation over interpretation and, at most, includes it. In a word, as always in *Gestalt Therapy*, but absolutely radically, it is a matter of taking "the dynamic structure of experience not as a clue to some unconscious unknown or a symptom, but as the important thing itself" (ibid., p. 14). The portrayal of the dream, in the presence of and together with the therapist, puts the dream itself into the circuit of the relationship, in the development of the present experience between an I and a Thou. The dream is not, then, to be thought of as the content *produced* by the subject's unconscious, nor by the collective imagination, but as a pure aesthetic form to be listened to and developed together.

This means enjoying it together, benefiting from the oneiric *eidos* as an enchanted universe, enthralling and moving as is any image in art, any word that tends toward poetry. But it also means making the dream portrayed in the therapeutic relationship "play", recovering, in a different sense, From's intuition: the dream not as relational message, but as the aesthetic portrayal of the therapeutic relationship. In the dream, the patient, before and perhaps more than *talking* implicitly to the therapist as a result of retroflexion, attempts to construct the script of the relationship, reproduces it and – involving the therapist in the aesthetic emotion – projects forward the actual course of the therapy. Before being the fruit of an avoidance of contact, the dream, if respected in its aesthetic essence, is probably the possible portrayal of the contact itself, the conformation of an opportunity for encounter, the celebration and drama of the desire for the other.

III. Therapy and Poetry: The View of Art in *Gestalt Therapy*

If the dream represents the most intensely and markedly aesthetic phase of the therapist-patient relationship, nevertheless it is no mere chance that Perls and Goodman cast the whole of therapy under the name of art, inasmuch as they transfer it to the metaphor of poetry. There is, in *Gestalt Therapy*, contiguity between poetry and therapeutic work, and a few brief reflections on this analogy may enable us to confirm and deepen our thoughts on dreams as well as cast further light on the Gestalt view of art. Given the obvious limitations of space, I shall confine myself to two items of reflection.

First, what is aesthetic *poiesis* in *Gestalt Therapy*? It is essentially a way in which the poet "solves his own problems". In the language of Goodman, this means that although art has to do with (and in some cases arises from) psychic disturbance, in other words the blocking of the spontaneous flow of contact, it is not the case – as Freud thought – that it simply testifies to a wound. In portraying his suffering, his desire for contact, the poet "solves" his own problem, in the sense that he anticipates and, at the aesthetic level, on the linguistic plane, fulfills the lost contact. The corporeal and existential depth of his professing himself, in whatever form it may come about, looks anguish in the face and solves it creatively, though on a plane of existence other than the day-to-day (but which, we must remember, for the poet represents the essential part of his very identity). Now, if this poetry can be assimilated to therapy, if the therapeutic process can reconstruct the creative flow of poetry in the actual relationship, the portrayal of the dream acts as a symbol of the Gestalt therapy aesthetic. As a poet, recreating the dream, the patient anticipates the solution of the problem, foreshadowing the possible contact, opening the relationship with the therapist to the decisive fulfillment of the contact and marking its paths by means of the creative unification of art.

Secondly, the parallelism between poetry and therapy rest, in *Gestalt Therapy*, on a linguistic-type basis. This is partly because poetry is *par excellence* self-referential language, the greatest alternative to any instrumental use of words: the meaning dwelling in the poetic word is announced *in* the song and not beyond or by means of it (Heidegger, 1994; Gadamer, 1990). But this is not all. For Perls and Goodman, the miracle of poetry lies in the revitalization of everyday language, so often disfigured and debased, we may add, by the elephantine instrumental use made of even the simplest and finest words. In this context, therapy may be thought of as a long journey toward poetry, a path along which the worn-out words of the patient, afflicted by the worm of verbalization, recovers light and warmth within the therapeutic relationship, thus becoming, for the disturbed individual, "good" words with which to speak, to narrate himself. The therapist is not called on to give her own words to the patient, nor to make of the patient's utterances and *lexis* a content to be investigated or modified through interpretation. It is not a question of remaking language, nor of unearthing a hidden meaning, but of giving it new form, restoring its lost freshness thanks to the hazardous but crucial warp and weft of the therapeutic dialogue.

As in dream, so in the whole course of therapy, the question is therefore one of *form*: *how* to make the patient's own words resonate anew, how to bring to the world, in a new integration, his gestures, movements, breathing. All therapy is at bottom an aesthetic matter, a problem of beauty, in the sense in which Plato wrote of it in the *Symposium*. In the dream, or rather in its portrayal, which as such respects its linguistic self-referentiality, the self performs the function of annunciation of the word "good", that word which would win back the body.

References

Perls F, Hefferline R, Goodman P (1994) Gestalt therapy: Excitement and growth in the human personality. The Gestalt J Press, Highland, New York
Gadamer HG (1983) Verità e metodo (Italian translation). Bompiani, Milano
Gadamer HG (1990) Interpretazioni di poeti (1). Marietti, Genova
Heidegger M (1994) La poesia di Hölderlin. Adelphi, Milano
Salonia G (2000) Tempo e relazione. In: Spagnuolo Lobb M (ed) Psicoterapia della Gestalt. Ermeneutica e clinica. Franco Angeli, Milano, pp 65–85

Creativity as Gestalt Therapy

Richard Kitzler

I. In the Beginning

In the beginning there was always art – and creativity. And there were always the artists and creators. Drama and dance, music and composers, painters and poets were all there: as patients, but many also as nascent practitioners of Gestalt therapy. And there was a reason central to the theory and practice: Gestalt therapy was and is still not an adjustive therapy, and its practitioners and clients thought of themselves as creative artists, making and doing in the world with their tools, materials, and gifts. And they were there, active in their roles in aesthetic/social/professional creativity. For us, it was all of a piece.

II. The Scene

Let me take you to the scene at the Perls' brownstone on West 76th Street in the fall of 1949. In Frederick Perls' upstairs front office, as one lay upon the couch in clouds of cigarette smoke and heard in the background music from Lore Perls' Bechstein piano, he could see on the far wall on each side of the entrance door, two paintings. They were somewhat interesting, fairly well executed and replete with the classical symbols of psychoanalysis. Both were painted by Perls himself and can now be seen on the illustrated cover of his autobiography, *In and Out the Garbage Pail* (1969), which itself is crammed with his poetry, some of it quite good and some frequently doggerel. The picture to the left had a hurtling subway train bursting toward the viewer, and at the upper right, a profile view of Sigmund Freud, copied from the autographed photo that hung in Perls' office. At the right of the door was a picture of what appeared to me a fetal-like comet, if there is such a thing. They were clearly Perls' attempts to handle creatively the themes of life and death, but also (as I now think) to rework his own history as well as his and Lore's revision of psychoanalysis in the oral aggression of *Ego, Hunger and Aggression* (1942). For this "sin", he had to leave the International Psychoanalytic Association.

III. Enter Paul Goodman

Awaiting the chime to signal my hour to ascend the stairs for my session, I was joined on the waiting bench by a twitching, unkempt, pipe-smoking creature, who muttered into his pipe, shed showers of tobacco ashes on his shirt front, and had the merriest of eyes I have ever seen on a human being. This was Paul Goodman, awaiting his session with Lore Perls. We didn't talk. I suppose at that time he had written only about thirty books, articles, plays, and poetry and was living "on the wages of a sharecropper", as he frequently said. His collaboration with F. Perls on *Gestalt Therapy: Excitement and Growth in the Human Personality* (1951) had yet to be published.

On the other hand, Goodman's philosophy, or rather psychology of art – though he frequently cited his influences as William James and John Dewey – rested on Otto Rank, whose book he cited as "beyond praise". (That reference has been attributed to F. Perls; it is a mistake.) This psychology found its way into *Gestalt Therapy*, especially in the chapter "Verbalizing and Poetry". The psychology of art and creativity is not to be found in the symbolic meanings the artist uses (as in Freud's writings on Leonardo and Moses and monotheism), but in the activity, the handling of the materials as the work is created. In a sense, the product is an intended consequence of the activity, but not its psychology. It is not the creative unveiling of the contents of the unconscious in its symbols, but a very active doing-and-making with its novelty and surprises.

IV. Dream Work

The crucial connection here to psychotherapy is obvious; but, let me give an example in the dream work that was truly astonishing. When presented with a dream, the usual way was to ask: "What do you associate to it?" This produced some interesting material, ultimately making explicit what the dream meant to the dreamer. If such meaning was self-generated, we would have an important (I believe finally also essential) interpretation. Gestalt therapy stood the relation on its head: it was not the meaning that was crucial, but what the dreamer did with the dream in the session – that is, in the experiment. The emphasis was on the *how* of the dream, the work of it, where it was going (by itself!): its colors or chiaroscuro, movement, sounds, and its novelties. Above all, its novelties, that which had not appeared in the dream itself, but which generated themselves within the structure as it revealed itself.

The dream was seen as a creative work of art, in which the dreamer was the creator/artist, the dramatist and demiurge, the sculptor and the Carrara marble. And with this work came the integration and aesthetic sense of *Io facit*. And so the interpretation was found-and-made, discovered-and-invented, the activities of the working ego: a temporary, self-generated, and partial structure of the self.

At this stage, the patient becomes his own art critic, and the meaning rests on the question: "Did I, in this therapeutic work, convey clearly and figurally the center of emotion around which my dream became itself?" If the answer is adequately affirmative, then, as Lore Perls said, patients are free to make their own interpretations.

And this was not an individual activity, i.e., the work of the patient/therapist field. The Perls' always brought their patients into their social field, and one became part of a larger society. And there was a level of support and cooperation that interpenetrated the usual isolations and rivalries of family, though not without the rumblings and tremblers that always accompany the transferences of volcanic family geology. But eruptions were few and usually produced more fire than heat.

V. Dance as Co-Creation

In the early 1950s, on their own initiatives, the Perls' combined therapy groups found a dancer who had fled the rigidities of Martha Graham and was developing his own choreography. About twelve of us went to his and his wife's studio and worked hard at elementary movement. At the end of the first session, to the sound of tambourine and drum beat, we danced across the studio floor, in unison, contacting the environment that is our bodies in the co-creation of real dance.

That creative act remains in my memory as the great intrinsic self-actualizing work of my therapy. Moreover, it remains an affirmation and a point of ground-on-which-to-stand whenever doubt and despair begin peeping out from their fortress of extrinsic evaluation and its foreign standards: That! That there! We and I made that great moment, and it stands free and breathing and unshakable.

The dance sessions lasted for weeks. Even very conservative Isadore From came to some of them. Our teacher went on to become part of a troupe that taught dance to children in minority neighborhoods. Now there's self-affirming work! And the political and social-change component of Gestalt therapy. And so the creativity of change and of dynamisms inherent in it for self and social development spreads, and one's existence makes a difference.

VI. The First Gestalt Therapy Professional Group

The early fifties' professional group was itself a creative integration that supported brilliant and very strong personalities. "Outcasts," Elliot Shapiro called us. There were educators, psychologists, psychiatrists, artists, and social workers (respectively, Shapiro, Lore, a husband and wife team, myself, F. Perls, Paul Weisz, Paul Goodman, and Sylvia Conrad from South Africa). In those days, the state of professional psychology and psychiatry was such that one did not speak in the workplace of Gestalt therapy if one wanted to keep his job. That ordinary prudence made the group even more coherent, the battles stronger, and the theorizing brilliant. The group met regularly; Paul Goodman once said in the group that it was wise to have an elevating experience once a week. The group was the nucleus of what was incorporated, in late 1952, as The New York Institute for Gestalt Therapy.

VII. Political Implications of Gestalt Therapy

This was long pre-Vietnam, and Goodman was to become editor of *Liberation*, a pacifist journal. In 1945, he had already written *The May Pamphlet or Reflections on Drawing the Line*, an anti-war and anti-draft document to help concerned people discover what they could do in the movement, rather than have expectations or demands on themselves that they were unable to meet: then resignation in despair. For example, one could sign a petition; another could participate in a march; another could lead the march; yet another could run for office. Still others could paint a picture or write a poem. It was classic of Goodman's "tinkering" approach: here a little and there a little, as it is also in good psychotherapy. Paul Weisz said in the professional group: "We work on the uppermost surface, millimeter by millimeter." Sometimes he called it "working overneath".

Paradoxically, an exception to the political activism, taken for granted as part of the personal/social/political gestalt that was the New York Institute, was Frederick Perls himself. He would have nothing to do with it. He had seen such "horrible things" (Lore Perls' locution), soldiering in World War I; he had also seen the chaos and desolation of postwar Germany, including early on the rise of Nazism, which persuaded him that nothing works politically and that violence and wars were inevitable. He seemed quite cynical about this and would greet any initiative with scathing sarcasm. "World-changers" and "do-gooders" were the least of his epithets. He did not dare to hope anymore, and he was bitter. He could roll his lower lip down in disdain, curl his upper lip in contempt, and affect an air of imperial distance as he gazed on the canaille of political activism. It seemed to me an example of Paul Goodman's adage: "The therapist greets the manipulation with patience in the framework of a larger impatience."

VIII. Drawing the Line: A Boundary Phenomenon

The operant test for what one could choose to do rested not on the activity sui generis, but where it rested on a scale: i.e., the direction in which one clearly wanted to go, versus the direction one clearly did not want to go; this from the zero point of doing nothing. Thus *any* action in the desired direction was "drawing the line" beyond which one could not go. In one stroke, all the angst and metaphysical calculations disappeared in the simple act of drawing the line.

My point above is an example from politics to personality and is made and illustrates cleanly the political and personal concern for social change that was in fact possible. Actually, I made a direct application of the "test" from *Drawing the Line* in therapy, where obsessive/compulsive features were dominant. We could always draw the line somewhere and from there make an approach to the bottomless despair and loneliness (depression?) "overneath", which could otherwise be intractable.

One will see the variation on Descartes' method of doubting, which led to the *cogito* beyond which he could not doubt and which established a separate consciousness, interacting with the body by way of the pineal gland. Ultimately, it all rested on faith in God, the lack of which in personal alienation was the problem in the first place. The pre-cursors (in *Drawing the Line*) to an existential psychotherapy without its Romantic Heideggerian bells and whistles need not be spelled out.

IX. Human Creativity and Social Constraint

Again: The making-and-doing, the discovering-and-inventing in the present emergency of the experiment in psychotherapy, arising out of human creativity and social constraint, and resulting in a genuine work of art as it formed itself (in this case, the dream) informed the politics and guided social action practically. The good was not sacrificed for the best. Gestalt therapy practitioners preached what they practiced, and if it was a little underground, so much the better. Lore Perls had it right: real psychotherapy is always somewhat subversive of the existing order. In this she rested on the authority of the grand First Amendment of the United States Constitution:

> Congress shall make no law respecting an establishment of religion, or prohibiting the free exercise thereof; or abridging the freedom of speech, or of the press; or the right of the people peaceably to assemble, and to petition the Government for a redress of grievances.

So we draw the line: "We draw the line in their conditions; we proceed on our conditions" (Goodman, 1962, p. 28).

X. An Example in Practice: The Living Theater

The "Living Theater" of Judith Malina and Julian Beck, which became so famous years later, especially in Europe, where it was known as the "Living", is a case history. It was avant-garde, yet firmly grounded in the traditions of the theater, standing on which it strove to bring the audience into the play itself. Intensely pacifist and anti-war, it not only presented theater aggressively, promoting those values, but also participated in every public event as a strike for peace, such as peace marches, workers' rights and, paradoxically, the necessity for everyone's voice to be heard as a testament to one's natural right in noncoerced behavior. Again, an example of creativity from the beginning: a gestalt of strongly felt opinion, articulated in a social context, which is politics, and founded on an enduring aesthetic in western civilization: that miracle, drama.

They were proud of their intellectuality, but they were careful to keep one foot in the swim of things, so as to avoid the powerlessness of complete isolation. This was "ordinary prudence" (one of Goodman's pet locutions) and an example of "drawing the line in their conditions".

These were dreary conditions. It was the time of yet another Red scare in America. It was very much the situation the Perls' thought they had left behind in Germany. Communists were "under every bed". It was the era of congressional investigations, blacklists, purges, and the famous: "I have in my hand a list of two hundred and five [people] that were known to the Secretary of State as being members of the Communist Party and who nevertheless are still working and shaping the policy of the State Department"(Joseph McCarthy's speech at Wheeling, West Virginia, 9 February 1950). It boiled down to one black lady who dished out food in the cafeteria. It took courage and "a certain foolish optimism" to remind people of that First Amendment to the Constitution of this country and that Senator McCarthy was a liar and probably a thief.

But my small community had little to worry about. The Grand Inquisitors were after much bigger fish. Where were the votes in persecuting a collection of screwballs that no one gave a damn about or had even heard of in the first place? And so it proved. The bubble burst when the witch hunters took on the United States Army and, by implication, President Eisenhower himself, a product of it. And the Army destroyed McCarthy in the famous 1954 televised hearings, as Special Counsel Joseph N. Welch asked the Senator: "Have you no sense of decency sir, at long last? Have you left no sense of decency?" Imagine, a demagogue done in by "decency" in the mouth of a Boston aristocrat!

I did not at the time understand that this was a replay of the Red scares and anti-immigrant Palmer raids of the late 1920s. The academics in the United States, who had studied in turn-of-the-century Europe, especially Germany, had brought over not only their idealist philosophy, but also Social Democrat politics, and they thought to create a grass-roots movement within labor and the great urban centers: Chicago and New York. It was the time of the settlement houses, beginning social work, public health and housing policy, child labor agitation, and labor strife. Among those active in these programs were, of course, John Dewey, so often cited by Paul Goodman as a major influence, and George Herbert Mead, never to my knowledge so cited, but whose writings so uncannily forecast Goodman's.

Chancellor Hutchins forced Mead out of his chair of philosophy at the University of Chicago. Mead had been there over forty years. President Nicholas Murray Butler at Columbia University forced out John Reed (*Ten Days that Shook the World* [1919]) and Charles Beard (*An Economic Interpretation of the Constitution of the United States* [1913]). John Dewey left the University of Chicago for Teachers College in New York (an affiliate of Columbia University) in 1904, where with his philosophy reputation secure he was untouchable.

So "drawing the line", to return to the example, and drawing it even to us small fry, took courage and perhaps a relentless disbelief in the ordinary dangers of pointing out the Emperor's lack of clothes.

A dreary, yet comical and intensely meant action will make my meaning clear. The police, breaking up a peace demonstration in Times Square, arrested Julian and Judith. Julian was literally thrown into the police wagon. His shoulder was broken. Judith, arrested and put in front of the judge, was extremely nervous when the judge asked her if "she had ever been in Bellevue?" (Bellevue was then the mental ward in Bellevue Hospital; in the judge's reference, the equivalent of Bedlam in London.) Judith's reply was a classic of anxiety, embarrassment, and amazing naiveté: "No, have you?"

The next afternoon, in my office at Columbia University Health Center, I got a phone call (from Paul?), which described Judith's plight and terrors and total incapacity to function in the hospital mental ward. I walked through our secretary's office to my colleague, Allison Montague, the University psychiatrist, who had been senior resident at Bellevue. He knew the night psychiatric supervisor, and he intervened. Judith was sprung, I believe, the following morning, considerably shaken; I don't know if the wiser.

Appositely, after the publication of Gestalt Therapy in 1951, Goodman always maintained that the theory section – his section – provided the theoretical basis for the development of the counter-culture of the sixties and the human potential movement. But, as he became an elder of that culture and with the student strikes and so forth of the period, he realized that it was all counter and no culture, and he became bitterly disillusioned. Then his mantra became: "They don't know enough to come in out of the rain!"

XI. Gestalt Therapy and Gestalt Psychology

Although Paul Goodman tried to establish a psychotherapy upon the base of Gestalt psychology, particularly "the whole is more than the sum of its parts", and "the completion of unfinished tasks" with the corollary in a theory of "dominance" of unfinished need until completed in "contact" with a formal four-step theory of contact, it was very little discussed as being fundamental in the professional group. (Indeed, I now feel that Köhler and Mary Henle, professor of psychology at the Graduate Faculty of the New School for Social Research, had it right. There was no place for therapy in Gestalt psychology, in spite of Goodman's famous letter to Köhler that Gestalt therapy was a "development within Gestalt psychology".)

XII. The New York Institute Emerges
from the Professional Group

Earlier, I said that the professional group preached what they practiced; they certainly did not practice what they preached. These were giants of very strong opinion, who really believed in creative conflict: strong medicine for strong people. And they were not easily dissuaded from an opinion. There was very little, if any, group sense. But what stunned every newcomer was – as the great Episcopalian hymn – "the strife is o'er, the battle done, the victory of life is won, the song of triumph has begun. Alleluia". And that after-wards, the combatants wandered about making dinner arrangements, clari-fying points, apologizing (but not for the content), and restoring the civility of process. To an outsider, it was so fierce that conditions had occurred under which no one would ever speak to another again. Thus, to modify "there was no group sense", as we now understand a more dilated notion of group, there *was* intense collegiality.

They understood that their relationship was founded, that battles cleared the air, and that hurt feelings were okay but had to be made clear. "How did you feel when you said that?" was the ultimate mantra, uniting the state-ment with its ground, where all awareness made sense. This tradition car-ried over to the Institute.

However, the progress toward a genuinely social understanding of pro-cess and development had to await new members, versed in the beginnings of large/small group interaction, group culture, training groups practice, and street culture. When they did come in, they came in hesitatingly, but swing-ing with both fists. But this was a development of the late 1960s and early 1970s, and we are here focussed on the beginnings of the theory, that by keeping the roots watered and refreshed, we could make the leaves and branches sturdy, lively, colorful, beautiful, and into an aesthetic in which one could breathe.

XIII. The Republic of Letters

In what will perhaps become a long aside, I would like to give another *his-toire* that more clearly exhibits the learning, creativity, activity, free-wheel-ing adaptation, and wise eclecticism that was the gestalt that called itself The New York Institute for Gestalt Therapy.

The New York Institute celebrated its fiftieth anniversary last year. In 1952, the first offerings of the Institute included Paul Goodman's work-shop "On Writer's Block" – as perhaps paraphrased: "How to work with monumental despair and collapse as the typewriter stares at you, daring you to push a single key." This can be cosmic, and anyone who has not experienced it is an imbecile. Many are the gnashings and grindings and, alas, resignations from the field, vowing, "never to write another paper in their lives!" I say "alas", because that paper and those words and those ideas and those mistakes and those idiocies are then lost to us forever. Only in the Fechnerian all-consciousness is the part of the tissue of our ex-perience retained forever in the universe. Is this a consolation that doesn't console?

Goodman did not experience writer's block and frequently said so. He said he could write anywhere, he said, even on the subway. And, of course, he was eager to help those who had not, as he had, published at age twelve and who were beset to paralysis with the problem. But, as he considered himself a man of letters, it is likely he felt placed in a long line of writers; he did not feel isolated or orphaned by the empty face of a blank sheet of paper.

On the surface, he was an adept at making the thing his own, and he could proceed merrily in his work, seemingly without the gust for utter originality that cripples so many of us, but reveling in the joy of a benevolent literary eclecticism that liberated his Creator Spirit.

XIV. A Man of Letters

For example: that a person could write even on the subway has a notable provenance. In Boswell's famous *Life of Samuel Johnson*, we have: "A man may write at any time, if he will set himself doggedly to it" (entry March 1750). Now, memory tells me that Johnson further said that the sentiment was from Christopher Smart. (Smart was committed to Bedlam, i.e., Bellevue in the example from Judith Malina, because he insisted on kneeling and praying in public, and because he did not love "clean linen". Johnson said it was better to pray than not and, as for clean linen [modern underwear], he himself had no passion for it.)

You will remember Paul Goodman's pique that he was forced to live on the wages of a sharecropper. Johnson weighed in on that one, too: "No man but a blockhead ever wrote, except for money" (ibid., entry 5 April 1776). Goodman chose to be an artist, a creative writer, and he therefore chose the income that the literature he was able to do – without, as he said to us, "vomiting in the crowd" – was willing to pay.

Now I think I am sure that Paul knew all this and was thus placed in that long line of classical literature, which perhaps comforted him when he was writing on the subway. This is manifest in *Five Years. Thoughts During a Useless Time, 1955–60*, where he says that he is quite clear as to the provenance of this phrase, that sentence, the other locution, or another sentiment. But unlike a pedant like me, he was not above massaging here, tweaking there, suppressing another place, and shamelessly paraphrasing without attribution to make the thing his own. The learning goes into the "fertile void" and comes out again on the page, re-wrought, unencumbered, *practically* his original.

The matter is one of the experience of inclusion and exclusion or, to put it another way: how to maintain one's originality in the minority, while maintaining the majority against which to be original in the first place! It is a variation on one who would "rather be head man in Rome than second head man in Italy". It is sometimes said "a big fish in a small pond." I think this last was Perls' solution: he simply ignored anything to the contrary and went on being "original".

But for someone like Goodman, who maintained that the minority is an essential part of the majority and occupies therefore the moral position in the total – since it, the minority, is the compass point for the total and locates its concerns and problems – it is essential to remain in the minority, even perhaps in order to function at all. This is hard. As the solution to the problem, its pros and cons, would come to form in the conflict, the gadfly becomes aware that he will, as Goodman said: "Be isolated [again] in the know."

Often in the professional group, just as the creative solution to the dis-agreement was getting clear in its lineaments, and we were all about to be able to breathe again, I could see (I was looking for it) the red light of lunacy and deviltry in those flashing eyes and the anticipatory licking of his chops, as Goodman was preparing to upset the apple cart; and, I braced myself. And so it proved, when everybody then ganged up on him. He was vindi-cated! And loved. And thus able again to use his full powers.

An example of swirling arguments is the controversy in those days of *self* and *ego*. Everyone agreed that this was the weakest point in psychoanalytic theory, and the controversy in *Gestalt Therapy* is treated largely within Chapter 11, "Criticism that Makes the Self Otiose." The philosophy behind it is the Kantian synthesizer that somehow takes the experience and makes it available to the self. In ordinary language, the experience becomes phe-nomenon. But the synthesizer stands in-between and has nothing else to do with the experience. Goodman utterly rejected that, yet he continued to maintain the synthetic unity of apperception. And ultimately, in *Five Years*, he declared that he was a Kantian.

XV. Reflections

(Re-reading the above, in the reference to Christopher Smart as the origin of "writing anywhere" if one just sticks to it, I realized that my memory con-flated two items, both of which Goodman appropriated: 1) "Writing any-where" and 2) As I recall, he wrote: "Life should be like a good poem: have a beginning, middle and an end, and make a good point." Johnson attrib-uted the second item to Smart. I interject this insight to give you, the reader, entrée to a process that we may perhaps call my creativity; further, it relieves me of the tedium of searching out and correcting within the Rules [which must be obeyed under the penalty of death] of the Holy Grail of Reference, which is a complete pain in the ass.)

XVI. Postscript

I have attempted to locate in time, place, and event the crucial notion of cre-ativity in Gestalt therapy and its developing theory. In so doing, I have empha-sized its global character containing as a concept not only its usual aesthetic, but also its force as a social and political Anschauung. I have assumed "per-sonal" as product of the former. If this outlook is accurate, then I believe that rather than a synonym for "awareness", as it is used in Gestalt therapy (and where it is central), we have a unifying concept where awareness is a part.

Then the notion that mere awareness is curative fills itself out and makes more sensible and coherent that something new has entered the experience, and this is a movement of growth. The something new in the experience of contact is the creative fore-promise fulfilled in the adjusting, the creativity in that process called life.

References

Goodman P (1962) The may pamphlet or reflections on drawing the line. Random House, New York

Goodman P (1966) Five years. Thoughts during a useless time, 1955–1960. Brussel and Brussel, New York

Perls FS (1942) Ego, hunger and aggression. Knox Publ. Co., South Africa

Perls FS (1969) In and out the garbage pail. Real People Press, Moab, Utah

Perls F, Hefferline R, Goodman P (1951) Gestalt therapy: Excitement and growth in the human personality. Julian Press, New York

The Weighty World of Nothingness:
Salomo Friedlaender's "Creative Indifference"*

Ludwig Frambach

Any serious discussion on creativity and Gestalt therapy must include the name Salomo Friedlaender. Indeed, Friedlaender should be given special recognition; not only is he one of Gestalt therapy's main theorists, but also his relation to the theme of creativity is already clearly alluded to in the title of his principal work: *Creative Indifference* (1918). Yet, Friedlaender is hardly known in Gestalt therapy circles (especially to non-German speakers), even though Fritz Perls explicitly referred to Friedlaender's central importance in his own approach:

> "For a long period of my own life I belonged to those who, though interested, could not derive any benefit from the study of academic philosophy and psychology, until I came across the writings of Sigmund Freud, who was then still completely outside academic science, and S. Friedlaender's philosophy of *Creative Indifference*" (Perls, 1969, p. 13).

Perls, in his first book, *Ego, Hunger and Aggression* (1969), writes unambiguously about these men whose intellectual impetuses decisively affected his thinking: Sigmund Freud was one of the most prominent intellectuals of the twentieth century, and the significance of his psychoanalytic theory as a source of Gestalt therapy has since been properly appreciated (Bocian, 1994, 1995a, b); Salomo Friedlaender's importance for Gestalt therapy, on the other hand, has until now barely been noticed, let alone acknowledged and appreciated.[1]

---

* Translated from the German by Nancy Amendt-Lyon.
[1] Felix Branger (1981) was the first person to carefully consider Friedlaender in a Gestalt therapeutic context; unfortunately, however, this article ("Schöpferische Indifferenz – Salomo Friedlaender. Eine geistesgeschichtliche Einordnung einer Quelle der Gestalttherapie" [Graduierungsarbeit am Fritz Perls Institut, Düsseldorf]) has never been published. Branger throws light on Friedlaender's biographical and intellectual background and relates him to Perls' understanding of process. Hilarion Petzold's depiction of Gestalt therapy (1984), based on Branger, calls attention to the fundamental importance of Friedlaender for the principles of the Gestalt approach. Heik Portele (1992, pp. 91–103) compares *Creative Indifference* to Perls' concept of the "fertile void" and points out the connection to constructivist concepts and Buddhistic spirituality. My own understanding of Friedlaender's significance for Gestalt therapy in the context of a book on Gestalt therapy are found in *Zen and Christian spirituality* (1994) as well as in "Salomo Friedlaender/

Even Perls (like many others) would get Friedlaender's name wrong, although he highly respected him both as a person and as a writer/philosopher: "As a personality, he was the first man in whose presence I felt humble, bowing in veneration. There was no room for my chronic arrogance" (1972, p. 75). In his autobiography, Perls describes this personal relationship to the first of his three gurus[2]: "His philosophical work *Creative Indifference* had a tremendous impact on me" (ibid., pp. 74–75). This *tremendous impact* is evident in *Ego, Hunger and Aggression*. Perls, here, proposes a revision of psychoanalysis in three points. Before even addressing the connections to Gestalt psychology and his concept of the organism, Perls first argues the need "to apply differential thinking, based on S. Friedlaender's *Creative Indifference*" (1969, p. 14). Creative indifference and polar differentiation – Friedlaender's basic philosophical subject – are in fact the starting points for Perls' therapy theory reflections. In my opinion, they comprise the central, structuring theme of his Gestalt therapeutic approach and can be traced to his fundamental therapeutic concepts, particularly to his "five-layer theory of personality", to which I will return. Perls adhered faithfully to the basic course of Friedlaender's philosophy up until the end, publicly and explicitly declaring his allegiance: "The orientation of the creative indifference is lucid to me. I have nothing to add to the first chapter of *Ego, Hunger and Aggression*" (1972, p. 76).

I. Who was Salomo Friedlaender?[3]

His full name was, in fact, Salomo Friedlaender/Mynona. For, besides the philosopher Salomo Friedlaender, there was Mynona, the author of widely read, wacky, grotesque stories (an innovative literary form that he coined).[4] Mynona, the German word for "anonymous" written backwards, was the pseudonym he chose to represent his alter ego, or in his words: "I am a serious philosopher and a humorist all rolled into one" (Friedlaender, 1982b, p. 35). Others called him "the Chaplin of philosophy" and "a German Voltaire" (Harden, in Huder, 1972, p. 14). He was a scintillating, independent, and intellectual figure whom one could not describe with conventional clichés. Friedlaender felt more at ease in creative, bohemian, artistic, and intellectual circles than in groups of conventional academics. He was also largely

---

Mynona" (1996a). I have also addressed aspects of Friedlaender's thoughts in other articles (see 1995, 1996b, c). Lore Perls and Paul Goodman, the other founders of Gestalt therapy, never explicitly named Friedlaender in their publications.

[2] Selig, an architect and sculptor at Esalen Institute, was the second. Mitzie, a white cat, was the third (Perls, 1972, pp. 70–71).

[3] Lisbeth Exner's (1996) published dissertation in German philology gives us the most detailed information on the life and work of Friedlaender; Cardoff (1988) offers a valuable philosophical perspective; Kuxdorf (1990a) presents Friedlaender as "the commentator of an epoch".

[4] I quote Friedlaender's works by using the following abbreviations: F = Friedlaender; M = Mynona; F/K = S. Friedlaender/Mynona – A. Kubin, Correspondence.

ignored by his fellow philosophers, to whom he referred (see Exner, 1996, p. 244), exemplifying his talent for puns, as the Akademlichen [translator's note(tn): roughly translated as "acadumbics", a contraction of Akademiker (academics) and dämlich (stupid, dumb)].

Friedlaender's Autobiographical Sketch (1936), part of which has been published (M, 1965, pp. 203–233), begins with: "Let the little children come to their senses", a parody on the New Testament (Mark 10, 14). He considers his life story as "recovering his senses", as a tale of internal, intellectual development and discovery. Externals, such as dates and places, are of no interest to him: "My theme is always just the EGO", he wrote when he was at an advanced age (Friedlaender, 1982b, p. 205). This EGO, however, was not to be understood in the current and habitual psychological manner. For Friedlaender, based on a deep and comprehensive philosophical perspective, the EGO was a human being's – or the world's, for that matter – spiritually individual and essential center. Thus, philosophy was "the autobiography of the world" (Friedlaender, 1911, p. 6), the self-description of the spiritual, creative principle of the world.

Despite Friedlaender's disinterest in externals, some highlights of his path through life should be briefly mentioned: Salomo Friedlaender was born on May 4, 1871, as the first of five children to Jewish parents in Gollantsch, in the province of Poznan.[5] As a boy, Salomo was extremely introverted: "There was always philosophizing and fantasizing going on in me, yet I wasn't able to express myself freely and easily" (M, 1965, p. 206). A mediocre pupil, he was sent to boarding school. "Saly", as he was called at school, was the "philosophical neighbor at the desk to the left" of Ernst Barlach, who later became a sculptor and playwright (Barlach, 1977, p. 37). After his late graduation from high school, Friedlaender began, at his father's urging, to study medicine. But he himself was interested in philosophy, which he began to study in 1896, whereupon his father disinherited him.

One particular philosopher fascinated him: "For the first time in my life, Schopenhauer's work united me with a genius of high philosophical breeding, and I succumbed to him helplessly and passionately" (M, 1965, p. 218). In addition to his philosophical urges, Friedlaender experienced strong sexual longing. He felt torn between the two: "My mind despised life, but my body loved it" (ibid., p. 220). His life style as "being at the same time oddly both an ascetic and a debauchee" (ibid.) led him into a deep, existential crisis:

"From within the debauchee, who was I, came the enraptured, dark voice of moral demands – initially as Schopenhauer's negation of life. I felt pressured to make a decision. I began to sink progressively into ruminations about the world and life. I was losing the ability to understand myself. There were two diametrically opposed extremes of [my] will's direction. Out of the tension between these opposites, I saw a formula flash up; I knew hardly anything about its history and, thus, ignored the fact that it was an age-old formula. In school I stumbled across the polarity formula by way of certain chapters on physics, in particular Schopenhauer's color theory which, in turn, also led me to Goethe's.

---

[5] At that time, Poznan (Posen) was part of Germany; after World War I, the province was returned to Poland.

I had savored the pole of embracing life all too drastically. In order to make a decision, I was thus compelled to experience the opposite pole. In the course of these internal experiments, in which I was over and above directed by ascetic intentions, I completely forgot about eating and drinking, and I experienced fantastic ecstasies. These raptures contained visions of polar life, in the center of which my undecided ego, increasingly radiant, sprang up between all the poles of life, between the yes and no of one's will. I drew up a philosophy that I entitled 'From lively indifference to world polarity'" (ibid., pp. 222–223).

At the age of 25, then, in 1896, Friedlaender had thus found his theme – indifference and polar differentiation. He would subsequently let his mind encircle it, deepen his thoughts about it, and allow these thoughts to mature. In 1902, he received his doctorate, having written a dissertation on Schopenhauer and Kant. Nietzsche, too, began to fascinate him: "His critique of the ascetic ideal [made him] into a skeptical free spirit" (ibid., p. 224).

From 1905, he became increasingly industrious, writing books on Julius Robert Mayer and his polar law of equivalence (1905), on logic and psychology (1907), and an edition each on Schopenhauer's and Jean Paul's selected works, with commentaries (1907). In 1911, he wrote *Friedrich Nietzsche. An Intellectual Biography*. In the same year, he married Lise Schwinghoff. Two years later their son was born.

In 1918, *Creative Indifference*, the book that developed his own basic philosophical understanding, was finally published. Many received the book with interest, some even with enthusiasm, especially in Expressionist circles. But the *Akademlichen* ignored it. In his foreword to the book's second edition in 1926, Friedlaender confessed his mentors: Immanuel Kant and Ernst Marcus (1856–1928). Thanks to Marcus, whom he referred to as the "Krupp of logic" (due to Marcus' residence in Essen), the principal – as it were "Copernican" – significance of Kant for the history of thought, he realized, was that "Kant is just another name for intelligence, and Marcus focuses this intelligence" (Friedlaender, 1926, p. 9).

"Creative Indifference", his own philosophical approach, was neither superfluous nor questioned as a result but, rather, aligned within a new framework. And Friedlaender authored texts that expressed his new orientation (1924/25). Motivated by his philosophical convictions, he swung Harlequin's wooden sword against "the Eminences" of intellectual modernity (Friedlaender, 1982b, p. 99), since they ignored Kant's revolution of the critical way of thinking and, thereby, not only failed to achieve freedom, but also supported the rise of barbarity. He bestowed upon Remarque, Bloch, Benn, Thomas Mann, Tucholsky, Sartre, and others the "possibly most trenchant and pertinent polemic in modern German literature" (Geerken, in: M, 1980, Vol 2, p. 292).

Besides being a philosopher, Friedlaender was also a creative man of letters. Mynona, the word juggler and alphabet anarchist, turned things upside down and switched perspectives to a "carnival of logic" (Friedlaender, 1913). Friedlaender/Mynona are received enthusiastically by literary critics, among them Tucholsky. In "The Trappist Strike", for example, the strictly ascetic order of monks, who have taken vows of silence, turn into a brawling mob of drunkards (M, 1922). He invented such words as *Trauringkampf* [tn:

literally, *wedding ring fight*, an allusion to boxing matches in the ring] and *Zionanie* [tn: a contraction of the words Zionism and onanism], which were offensive and irreverent, especially toward venerable authorities. The number of his readers who wanted to hear public lectures – command performances – of his grotesque stories grew.

From 1906, he lived in Berlin, where he was a well-known figure in the bohemian scene, which was an exceptionally colorful circle of artists and writers. They met in Café of the West, nicknamed Café Megalomania. He was closely associated with the Dadaists, yet he was always critically independent. Alfred Kubin, Else Lasker-Schüler, Walter Benjamin, Martin Buber, and Gustav Landauer belonged to his circle of friends and acquaintances. In addition to stories as *The Creator* (1920) and *Graue Magie. Ein Berliner Nachschlüsselroman* (1922) [tn: Friedlaender's ironically titled novel *Grey Magic: A Berlin Imitation Identity Novel*], his works of lyric poetry are comprehensive (Kuxdorf 1990b).

Mynona the satirist cannot be separated from Friedlaender the philosopher. They are complementary, polar to one another: "As a polarist, this philosopher carries his buffoon in his bosom. He christened him Mynona and, with his *Eulenspiegeleien*, he frightened the world of Philistines" (Rukser, in Friedlaender, 1982b, p. 210); Mynona, the "soul-fumigator [who] must impregnate this world here that envelops us with sulphur, in order to cleanse it [and to check] how close or far away one's soul is from a genuine one" (M, in Kapfer and Lindenmeyer, 1993, p. 82).

Friedlaender had to flee in 1933. His satirical criticism of the "swastika greenhorns" allowed him only one exit – exile. He took his wife and son with him to Paris. There he became increasingly isolated and seriously ill, which paradoxically permitted him to survive the German occupation: he was too ill to be transported to a concentration camp. Meanwhile, he wrote. During his years in exile, he composed what he considered to be his most important philosophical works.[6] On September 9, 1946, Salomo Friedlaender died; his funeral, in Paris' Pantin Cemetery, was paid for by charity.

II. Philosophy

The basic philosophical insight (dating from 1896) that Friedlaender developed in his later writings is one of pure simplicity and, because of this, not easily understood at all: "The most general characteristic of any possible phenomenon is the distinction that can go to extremes" (Friedlaender, 1926, p. xv). In order for a phenomenon to be perceptible and appreciable, it must stand for an opposite of something else; it must be different from some other thing. This distinction or difference constitutes, in the most elementary way,

---

[6] All of his unpublished works are stored in the German Literature Archives in Marbach (= DLA) and in the Friedlaender/Mynona Archives of Hartmut Geerken (= FMAG) in Herrsching, Germany. Since 1972, a collection of Friedlaender/Mynona works can be found at the Academy of Arts, Berlin.

the figures of the world, the forms of phenomena (see Spencer-Brown, 1979). The elementary principle of creation that structures this distinction of phenomena is that of polarities, the original opposite: "Even the most complicated relativity can be disentangled into correlative pairs" (Friedlaender, 1926, p. 41). Going consequentially to the root of relative reality can be explained by polar relations [*tn*: mutual relations]: such as, plus and minus, in and out, large and small, high and deep, near and far, repel and attract, giving and receiving, etc.: "Polarity is Ariadne's thread in the world's labyrinth" (ibid., p. 333). In fact, the polar structure of reality is evident in all fields of science, especially basic to physics, for example, in the complementarity of particles and waves in quantum theory (Bohr/Heisenberg), in antimatter, or even in the double helix of the genetic code of DNA which, by the way, corresponds exactly to the structure of the Chinese book of oracles *I-Ging* (Schönberger, 1981). Friedlaender defines poles as "oppositively (symmetrically) homogenous" (Friedlaender, 1926, p. 20). It appears, in this polar opposition, as a phenomenon whose identity, unity, and totality cannot be perceived, because it cannot be distinguished. For instance, it is always *relatively* light in distinguishing comparison to the polar opposite of dark. The unity and identity of light and dark cannot be differentiated. The unity of polar differentiation, as it were, is its very *middle point*, its *indifference*. Friedlaender's philosophy focuses precisely on this indifferent middle point:

"From time immemorial, when dealing with polarities, more attention has been paid to the poles than to the indifference. Yet in this indifference lies the real secret, the creative will, the polarizing one itself, which objectively is absolutely nothing. However, without indifference there would be no world" (ibid., p. 337).

A. The Creative Naught of Indifference

This indifference is the creative, central dimension of reality or, to be more precise, the "immension of all dimensions" (ibid., p. 341). This is where Friedlaender's thinking indefatigably revolves and of which he attempts to make us conscious by presenting new variations on the theme. Here we are at the original source, in the center of all creativity. The main problem, however, is that one is dealing with something undifferentiated or undistinguishable, which can be understood, negatively, as naught: "A mistake in reasoning and life prevails: one confuses the naught of plus and minus with the minus. (...) Precisely the naught of the difference is its creator, the reality of all realities. (...) Precisely the objective naught is the subjective heart of the world" (ibid., pp. 18, 4).

We confuse the effects with the doer, forget the really creative indifference in the obviously dominant differences, and thus we don't recognize the "subjective heart of the world". According to Friedlaender, that which is objective is the polar-differentiated *external*, the entire variety of distinguishable apparitions in the phenomenal world. The subject, however, is the creatively indifferent internal part, the center, the being, the "weighty world of nothingness" (ibid., p. 30): "The naught of the world is the center of the world" (ibid., p. 19).

In order to point out the lively center of the naught of creative indifference in differentiated multiplicity, Friedlaender uses a variety of terms: *ego* (later on he frequently uses *ego-heliocenter*), *self, being, subject, individual, identity, person, mind, soul, absoluteness, ∞, insistence, will, freedom* and so forth. He is reluctant to let himself be bound to definite words or labels. Rather, he attempts to circumscribe that which is ultimately indescribable in his creative, multi-perspective manner.

B. Liberating Indifferentiation

"The heart, properly integrated, properly divest of all differences, is the heart of the world" (ibid., p. 51).

The existential fulfillment of the philosophy of polar indifference consists in the indifferentiation of one's own awareness, in a renunciation, a releasing of all differentiated contents of awareness, until an indifferent clarity of the mind can be achieved, one deemed to be the deepest source of authentic creativity. In this way, humans become centered, find their own center, capable of integrating everything, find their heart, which cannot consist in something that is differentiated but, rather, in that rationally intangible naught on which the entire diversity of all possible phenomena is based: "One's own heart, our innermost part, will not rest until it is all in all" (ibid., p. 50). But a really fundamental separation is necessary in order to achieve a liberating understanding of the ego, the self, and the true identity: "You have to know who you are" (ibid., p. 58). The path that Friedlaender indicates is the indifferentiation of the internal part of the subject, the "evacuation of the self from differences" (ibid., p. 391). Or, in other words, the dis-identification from that with which one "pseudo-identifies"(ibid., p. 458). If someone is in any way still identified with something differentiated or external, to which feelings and thoughts also belong, then he failed to find himself, because "at first, indifference is the naked soul, the human soul. The psychological differences relate to the soul as clothes relate to limbs" (ibid., p. 352).

A complete separation, even from the most subtly differentiated identifications, is necessary to be liberated from the center of one's real "own being", because the "idea of identity can not be experienced intimately enough. (...) Only the self, in which all differences are destroyed, is the genuine self" (ibid., pp. 60, 99). In constantly new variations, Friedlaender's philosophy revolves around this central aspect of one's own existence, as well as around everything else that exists, an aspect that, due to its transcendence, finally evades differentiated understanding: "The creating self is without form" (ibid., p. 458); it cannot be cognitively perceived with our distinguishing intellect (Frambach, 1996a).

Friedlaender, however, warns us about getting lost in indifference. The point is not about withdrawal from the world, but about active, creative production of the world, beginning in its intellectual, creative center. In this context, he speaks of *Indo-Americanism*: "The East presses for a culture of indifference, the West for one of difference; I want to be West-Eastern, Indo-American. I reject a culture of mere indifference just as much as a culture of mere difference; both are seductive fictions" (F/K, 1986, p. 57).

Real "creative" indifference strives for creative development: "Being ∞ is not enough; one should also *become* it (in a polarized way)" (ibid., p. 18). The creative art of life that arises from the indifferent center, consists principally in a balance of polar opposites, in an *equilibration*. It is important not to be absorbed one-sidedly and distortedly by one of the respective poles, but to center oneself within the creative center of the poles and, like a bird, to move both of them as if they were wings. An unprejudiced "readiness to like both" (Friedlaender, 1926, p. 340), an even-temperedness, characterizes a person who is centered in his or her indifferent center, according to the basic rule of the "weighty world of nothingness": "It prohibits nothing in particular, just the lack of balance between polar specifics" (ibid., p. 30). Concretely, rage and gentleness, for example, should not be isolated from each other as mutually exclusive contradictions, but should be experienced as a polarly differentiated unit of opposites [*tn*: mutually related] by being flexibly centered in their indifferent center. Thus, one can remain "elastically identical" (ibid., p. 82), and react freely and appropriately, either angrily or with gentleness, to the demands of the situation from a "totality of experience" (ibid., p. 33). The experience of time is also influenced by this centering. The poles of the past and future refer exactly to their center, the now of the present, and balance an individual in an "indifferent, central presence of mind" (F/K, 1986, p. 210). Creative indifference "provides for the *magnetism of the extremes*" (Friedlaender, 1926, p. 32) by relating the poles to each other harmoniously by way of their indistinguishable center. Friedlaender considers his philosophy to be instructions for an *"orthopedics of life"* that is still out of joint (F/K, 1986, p. 210). He intends to bend our perspective fundamentally, from the very beginning, back into its polar-regulating center: "The basis of things is therefore not their lower position, but their central, middle position; things are polar. 'Below' is the center of the polar 'above'" (Friedlaender, 1926, p. 24).

Friedlaender is concerned with "FUNDAMENTAL truth" (Friedlaender, 1982b, p. 144, upper case in the original); therefore, he is also an elementary logician. For him, logic is to the intellect what the skeleton is to the body (F/K, 1986, p. 171): support, structure, and thus principle. He is not a rationalistic, formal logician but, rather, aligned with the translogical, intuitive source of all logic in creative indifference. The goal of his logical reasoning clearly surpasses a narrowing, rationalistic perspective: "To be able to think about the concept of God so that it fits into our world and our lives is the first and ultimate task of applied logic. The world is either divine or incorporeal!" (Friedlaender, 1907a, p. 75).

Thus we have explicitly reached the spiritual and religious dimension to which Friedlaender always relates in his philosophical exploration of reality, and which is quite fundamentally connected to the topic of creativity. Even though he didn't exclusively identify with any one single religion or confession, he had a constructively critical way of showing that the philosophically clarifying permeation of religious themes mattered to him: "If the ego just believes piously, then it castrates itself on the brain, and becomes a 'brainless'" heart (F/K, 1986, p. 205). Having been influenced by Nietzsche, he had a critical attitude toward the real hypostases of Christianity; but he valued mysticism, particularly Meister Eckhart: "Eckehardt [sic] enchants me; he is the divine free spirit in nearly the purest sense" (ibid., p. 35). He knew very little about Buddhism and Taoism, although their fundamental ideas exhibit an astonishing similarity to his philosophy. In the broad sense of the word, Friedlaender is a kind of philosophical mystic, and his insight into the creative indifferentiation of an individual's center is an accurate view, from a Western philosophical perspective, of the central theme of authentic spirituality, the liberating fundamental behavior in the core of identity.

According to Friedlaender, philosophizing cannot be taught in an *Akademliche* and aloof manner, but must be a radical confrontation with the foundations of one's own existence. He is neither concerned with the broad knowledge of many things, nor with a confrontation with a philosophical tradition, so that he hardly seriously considers other thinkers – except Schopenhauer, Nietzsche, and Kant. By contrast, he is interested in existentially and mentally profound penetration through supposed certainties and truisms till the really sustaining certainties are reached. In his central intellectual insights, he has the liberating feeling that he is directly one with the creative, formative principles of life: "My philosophy is no longer philosophy; on the contrary, it is life itself" (ibid., p. 11).

III. Friedlaender's Philosophy and Gestalt Therapy

Friedlaender's basic concepts, indifference and polar differentiation, become operative in Fritz Perls' writings in the form of various writings, as seen in terms such as *middle, center, zero-point, naught, void, pre-difference, equilibrium, balance, centering, opposites, poles*, and *polarization*. An examination of these terms reveals the basic structure of Friedlaender's philosophy.

In the revisional concept of psychoanalysis in his first book, Perls called Friedlaender's polar philosophy "differential thinking" and considered it to be a "mental precision tool" (Perls, 1969, p. 16), since it can find the point of "predifference", as he also refers to creative indifference, as well as the zero-point, the center from which balancing equilibrium is possible and

"we could find a point from which the observer could gain the most comprehensive and undistorted view. (...) By remaining alert in the centre, we can acquire a creative ability of seeing both sides of an occurrence and completing an incomplete half. By avoiding a one-sided outlook we gain a much deeper insight into the structure and function of the organism" (ibid., pp. 14–15).

The center is a "magical" word for Friedlaender (F/K, 1986, p. 220); likewise, for Perls, "to center one's existence" (Perls, 1972, p. 31), or centering, is the most basic goal of therapy, because we "acquire a creative ability of seeing both sides of an occurrence", as Perls mentions above. A Gestalt therapy example is the characteristic "present-centeredness" (Naranjo, 1979): "The present is the ever-moving zero-point of the opposites past and future" (Perls, 1969, p. 95).

The next two points in Perls' revision – the integration of the Gestalt psychological perspective and his concept of the organism – are also clearly influenced by Friedlaender's philosophy (Petzold, 1984, p. 11). He takes on the basic figure/background concept of Gestalt psychology. Accordingly, perception differentiates principally into an unclear, diffuse background and a precise figure that is not *in* but *as* the foreground. This is the fundamental principle of our differential perception: the recognition of distinctive forms. Thus, it is not hard to comprehend *fore*ground and *back*ground as the poles of a polarity, just as we perceive *before* and *behind*. They are structurally analogous to Friedlaender's polar differentiation. Now, what would be the analogy to creative indifference? Neither in Gestalt psychology nor in Gestalt theory can a clear parallel be found. If we tackle the question logically (language-wise), then the answer must be: the ground (Frambach, 1994, p. 55). Polar differentiation into foreground and background has its indifference in the ground. The ground is not to be mistaken for the background. The latter is diffuse, yet the ground is indifferent. The ground is not a perceivable, differentiated phenomenon. It is that which is differentiated, the creative center and source of all differentiation. Perls discussed the content of that which can be understood as the indifferent ground in terms of "nothingness" and the "fertile void": "My first philosophical encounter with nothingness was the naught, in the form of zero. I found it under the name of *creative indifference* through Sigmund [sic] Friedlander" (Perls, 1972, p. 70).

The main meaning of nothingness for Perls – "*nothing* equals *real*" (Perls, 1971b, p. 62) – to which he often refers in the context of Buddhism and Taoism – is essentially derived from Friedlaender, to whom he interestingly enough ascribes Freud's first name. Although he wasn't completely aware of it – otherwise he would have developed an explicit analogy between indifference and ground – I am convinced that the implicit structural analogy between the figure/background concept and Friedlaender's way of thinking in polarities was cause for Perls to be fascinated by Gestalt psychology. Here he could again deal with Friedlaender's elementary theme, now transposed into new concepts and in another intellectual context.

This theme can also be distinctly heard in the third point of Perls' revision, the chapter entitled "The Organism and its Balance" (1969, p. 31). In his concept of the organism, in which he refers particularly to the works of Goldstein, Smuts, and Reich, the main subject concerns *homeostasis* and *organismic self-regulation*. The plus-and-minus-functions of physical metabolism are transposed as polar-regulatory principles onto "mental metabolism" (ibid., pp. 122–27). The human being as an "organism", according to Perls a metaphor for the unity of body, soul, and mind in the context of the field of one's world, is homeostatically self-regulated in its entirety by a lively, complex balancing process.

Friedlaender's polar approach to thinking can also be found in the theoretical part of *Gestalt Therapy* (Perls et al., 1951), in which Paul Goodman elaborated Perls' concepts, although there is no specific reference to Fried-laender. In my opinion, the most significant concepts within this context are the *self* and *middle mode*: "Self is spontaneous, middle in mode" (ibid., p. 376); it integrates the poles of activity and passivity, both willing and done to; through the "creative impartiality" (ibid.) of their indifference and center, it opens the basis for spontaneous, free feeling, thinking, and doing.

IV. The Five-Layer Model of Neurosis

Fritz Perls' theoretical foundations of Gestalt therapy in the first chapter of *Ego, Hunger and Aggression* demonstrate the decisive structural influence of Friedlaender's polar thinking. From this stems an appropriate, psycho-*log-ically* stringent interpretation of the five-layer theory of neurosis (Frambach, 1994, pp. 83–114), which was elaborated on vaguely by Perls and, with few exceptions (Staemmler and Bock, 1987, 1991[7]), was only superficially ac-knowledged. The *phoney layer* of roles and games is the point of departure for Perls. Neurotic bondage is principally comprised of a *fixation* to certain aspects of identity that have taken over the foreground of awareness. Other, expropriated aspects of the personality have been more or less permanently repressed into the shadow of the background, behind the scenes of the stage of life. In the *phobic layer*, one becomes increasingly aware not only of these avoided impulses, but also of the anxiety, the phobic attitude that led to the avoidance and maintains it. Then, a modification takes place, and aware-ness becomes more differentiated, since the psyche has not-yet-experienced oppositely-poled aspects, and now needs are what have the chance, at least partially and for a limited time, to be experienced and take shape. For in-stance, an aggression that was permanently suppressed into the back-ground comes into the foreground, which is otherwise constantly occupied by an artificial and almost chronic friendliness. The conflict of the *e-motion*, the *motion out of*, and the suppressing opposite motion of anxiety, thicken into a *diffusion*, which Perls called the "impasse". In this "bottleneck", this dead-end or blockade [tn: impasse refers to a dead-end, whereas the Ger-man word *Engpaß* literally means bottleneck or narrow pass], the old struc-ture of the previous foreground identification-fixation dissolves into diffuse disorder. If one is able to endure this terrifying phase, then a *vacuum* en-sues, which Perls named the *death layer*, the "fertile void", or "implosion". No polar differentiation into foreground and background takes place here. Rather, their creative center, the ground, the nothingness of creative indif-

---

[7] Frank Staemmler and Werner Bock presented a differentiated interpretation of the five-layer model (1987, revised edition 1991). I differ in my interpretation, especially of the fourth layer, which I have developed with reference to Friedlaender's polar philoso-phy and in comparison to transformative processes of spirituality (Zen and Christian mys-ticism). This is, in my opinion, an experience characteristic of the creative indifference in Friedlaender's sense, as the experience of the ground. Staemmler/Bock do not deal with Friedlaender any further in their interpretation.

ference can be experienced. What threatened us as a "terrible" (*furchtbar*) void, as a loss, turns out to be a "fertile" (*fruchtbar*) one. After the initial one-sided, imbalanced identification, the individual finds his or her way back to the middle mode, out of which the self can proceed freely and spontaneously. This occurs also in the immediately successive phase, which Perls calls "explosion". A mental aspect that was previously in the background, such as aggression or sadness, can now unrestrainedly develop in the foreground and thereby close an "unfinished situation", an "open gestalt". A previously rejected aspect of the psyche is *integrated* into the realm of responsibility of the personality as the balancing polarity, together with the already accepted psychological opposite pole. The stages fixation, differentiation, diffusion, vacuum, and integration of the five-layer model, which are experienced in infinitely varied individual intensities, duration, repetition, etc., result in a fitting course of development, if Friedlaender's philosophy of polar indifference is used as a framework of interpretation, particularly if fore- and background are seen as polar differentiation and the ground as indifference. Although Perls never explicitly developed these connections, there are clear indications in his writings:

"The basic philosophy of Gestalt therapy is that of nature – differentiation and integration. Differentiation by itself leads to polarities. As dualitites these polarities will easily fight and paralyze one another. By integrating opposite traits we make the person whole again. For instance, weakness and bullying integrate as silent firmness" (Perls, in Stevens, 1977, p. 7).

Perls' basically polar outlook on the dynamics of the psyche thus come to the fore. The aim is to integrate dualities, or one-sided identifications with actually equal psychic poles, into balanced polarities. In other words, we are striving to find the center, the "middle mode" of the self, the ground of the "creative indifference", from which the creative, situatively appropriate polar differentiations can result. A mentally "disturbed" personality, one which has lost its mental balance, can be compared to a seesaw, whose balancing center has been displaced because the person has been too one-sidedly and predominantly identified with only one pole of a mental pair of opposites, such as joy and sadness. In this way, the inner balance is tilted and a lopsided position ensues, in which a person can only maintain an upright position by the strenuous work of employing compensatory neurotic mechanisms. The actually existentially "weightier" pole, from which the person pulled away, because of some anxieties, sinks under the level of awareness, in the shadow of the background, and the "lighter" pole becomes pseudo-dominant in the foreground. Someone who is truly "predominantly" sad "tends" to compensate by showing off a gleeful facade. The healing path basically involves the "process of *centering*, the reconciliation of opposites so that they no longer waste energy in useless struggle with each other, but can join in productive combination and interplay" (Perls, in Fagan and Shepherd, 1971, p. 19). This reconciliation comes to pass by finding the center, the creative indifference, which produces the "magnetism of the extremes" (Friedlaender, 1926, p. 32) that integrates the conflicting dualities into complementary polarities. If one applies Friedlaender's polar way of thinking consequently, then we can assume that the psyche, as every other phenomenon, is essentially polar, paired, and complementarily structured. No single, isolated mental phenomena exist. On the contrary, we can assume units of opposites as, for example, liking and disliking, joy and sadness, prevailing and yielding, and so on.

Polarity is of fundamental importance for understanding the psyche. Polarity is more or less clearly exhibited in all approaches stemming from psychoanalysis (Jung, Adler, Reich, Szondi et al.). The polar perspective taken by Perls is unmistakably traceable to Friedlaender who, besides the principle of polar differentiation, also conveyed to him the main importance of integrating indifference. Friedlaender's philosophy of polar indifference influenced the theoretical inputs of Gestalt therapy initially and decisively with this subject and, accordingly, it is considered to be its fundamental philosophical background.[8] From this viewpoint, it is the goal of the Gestalt therapeutic process to lead increasingly from the one-sided fixation to that which is in the foreground to the ground, from the periphery to the middle and center, by way of integrating rigid dualities into flexible polarities. Due to the necessarily condensed representation of the interrelationships, I would like to propose an appropriate definition within the framework of the history of influences: Fritz Perls' Gestalt therapy is the psychotherapeutic realization of Salomo Friedlaender's philosophy of polar indifference on the basis of Sigmund Freud's psychoanalysis, mainly expressed and defined by the central concepts of Gestalt theory and Gestalt psychology, and determined by the holistic "organismic" conception of Man (Goldstein, Reich, Smuts). In addition, a multitude of further sources from philosophy, psychology, art, and religion played an influential role, with special emphasis given to the aspects of dialogical encounter (Buber) and phenomenology.

V. Conclusion

What Friedlaender, this outstanding representative of the German-Jewish cultural avant-garde during the first decades of the twentieth century (Kiefer, 1986), called "creative indifference" from his philosophical perspective is the basic creative dimension of human existence. A phase of indifference, fertile void, or nothingness must be experienced, no matter if we are considering creativity in the sense of artistic activity, in the sense of new realizations and insights in the scientific field, or in the sense of psychotherapeutic or spiritual processes. In a certain way, every really creative act is a *creatio ex nihilo*, a creation out of nothingness. If we can let go of the famil-

---

[8] Claudio Naranjo communicated to me personally, that he has long supposed that a particular philosophy must have been behind the brand of Gestalt therapy he came to know through Fritz Perls. Once he became more familiar with Friedlaender's (German-language) original texts, he realized that he had found this specific philosophical source of Gestalt therapy.

iar, which is more or less associated with uncertainty and anxiety, then we necessarily enter a stage of indifference, from which new differentiations and new creations can result. We thereby experience ourselves in this creative "middle mode", between activity and passivity, in the role of the active doer as well as in the role of the passive recipient who is given an insight, an idea, etc. Friedlaender, who was regarded as the "philosopher of Expressionism" (Taylor, 1990), philosophically explored this fundamentally creative act of human existence with his teachings of "creative indifference", and he thus made it accessible to consciousness in a novel way. With his "nose" for fundamental intellectual concepts, Fritz Perls (Frambach 1996b) recognized the far-reaching practical potency of Friedlaender's philosophy and realized it on a psychotherapeutic level. Beginning with the elementary themes of polar differentiation and the center of creative indifference, we can more deeply comprehend many principles of the Gestalt approach, especially the polar foreground/background-differentiation, which is complemented by understanding the indifferent ground. This ground of "creative indifference" is the source and strength of the spirit through which creative development takes place. It is the "weighty world of nothingness".

References

Barlach E (1977) Ein selbsterzähltes Leben. Heyne, München
Bocian B (1994/1995a, b) Gestalttherapie und Psychoanalyse I/II/III. Gestalttherapie 1994/
    2: 12–36; 1995/1: 61–83; 1995/2: 69–83
Cardorff P (1988) Friedlaender (Mynona) zur Einführung. Junius, Hamburg
Exner L (1996) Fasching als Logik. Über Salomo Friedlaender/Mynona. Bellville, München
Frambach L (1994) Identität und Befreiung in Gestalttherapie, Zen und christlicher Spiritualität. Via Nova, Petersberg
Frambach L (1995) Gestalttherapie und Spiritualität. Transpersonale Psychologie und Psychotherapie 2: 22–39
Frambach L (1996a) Salomo Friedlaender/Mynona. Ausgrabung einer fast vergessenen Quelle der Gestalttherapie. Gestalttherapie 1: 5–25
Frambach L (1996b): Von der Unfähigkeit des Intellekts das Absolute zu erkennen oder der Wettlauf zwischen Hase und Igel. Transpersonale Psychologie u. Psychotherapie 1: 51–65
Frambach L (1996c) Die Ursprünge der Gestalttherapie. Gestaltkritik 2: 40–47
Friedlaender S (1905) Julius Robert Mayer. Theodor Thomas, Leipzig
Friedlaender S (1907a) Logik. Die Lehre vom Denken. H Hillger, Berlin
Friedlaender S (1907b) Psychologie. Die Lehre von der Seele. H Hillger, Berlin
Friedlaender S (1908) Durch blaue Schleier. Gedichte. AR Meyer, Berlin
Friedlaender S (1911) Friedrich Nietzsche. Eine intellektuale Biographie. GJ Göschen, Leipzig
Friedlaender S (1918) Schöpferische Indifferenz. Georg Müller, München
Friedlaender S (1924) Kant für Kinder. Fragelehrbuch zum sittlichen Unterricht. Steegemann, Hannover
Friedlaender S (1926) Schöpferische Indifferenz. 2. um ein Vorw. vermehrte Aufl. E Reinhardt, München
Friedlaender S (1978) Katechismus der Magie. Reprint von Friedlaender (1925) mit Kommentar von M Schönberger: Das magische Prinzip der Natur. Aurum, Freiburg i. Br.

Friedlaender S (1982a) Aus den philosophischen Tagebüchern/Moral und Politik. Merkur 7: 679–683

Friedlaender S (1982b) Briefe aus dem Exil. H Geerken (ed) v. Hase & Koehler, Mainz

Friedlaender/Mynona S, Kubin A (1986) Briefwechsel. Geerken H, Hauff S (eds) edition neue texte, Wien

Huder W (1972) Salomo Friedlaender/Mynona 1871–1946. Akademie der Künste Berlin, 5. Mai bis 4. Juni 1972. Ausstellungskatalog. Berlin

Kapfer H, Lindenmeyer C (eds) (1993) Maßnahmen des Verschwindens. – Salomo Friedlaender/Mynona, Anselm Ruest, Heinz-Ludwig Friedlaender im französischen Exil. Ausstellung und Hörspiele von Hartmut Geerken. Redaktion: S Hauff. München

Kiefer KH (1986) Avantgarde – Weltkrieg – Exil. Materialien zu Carl Einstein und Salomo Friedlaender/Mynona. Peter Lang, Frankfurt a.M

Kuxdorf M (1990a) Der Schriftsteller Salomo Friedlaender/Mynona: Kommentator einer Epoche. Peter Lang Frankfurt a.M

Kuxdorf M (1990b) Die Lyrik Salomo Friedlaender/Mynonas: Traum, Parodie und Weltverbesserung. Peter Lang, Frankfurt a.M

Mynona (1913) Rosa die schöne Schutzmannsfrau. Verlag der Weißen Bücher, Leipzig

Mynona (1914) Für Hunde und andere Menschen. Der Sturm, Berlin

Mynona (1919) Die Bank der Spötter. Ein Unroman. Kurt Wolff, München Leipzig

Mynona (1920) Der Schöpfer. Phantasie. Kurt Wolff, München

Mynona (1922) Trappistenstreik und andere Grotesken. Walter Heinrich, Freiburg/Baden

Mynona (1965) Rosa die schöne Schutzmannsfrau und andere Grotesken. Otten E (ed) Arche, Zürich

Mynona (1980) Prosa. Bd. 1 & 2. Geerken (ed) edition text+kritik, München

Mynona (1988) Das Eisenbahnglück oder der Anti-Freud. Junius, Hamburg

Mynona (1989) Graue Magie. Ein Berliner Nachschlüsselroman. Fannei & Walz, Berlin

Naranjo C (1979) Zentrierung im Jetzt. Integrative Therapie 3: 165–191

Perls FS (1969) Ego, hunger and aggression. The beginning of Gestalt therapy. Vintage/Random House, New York

Perls FS (1971a) Four lectures. In: Fagan J, Shepherd IL (1971) Gestalt therapy now. Theory/techniques/applications. Harper Colophon, New York, pp 14–38

Perls FS (1971b) Gestalt therapy verbatim. Bantam, New York

Perls FS (1972) In and out the garbage pail. Bantam, New York

Perls FS (1966) Gestalt therapy and human potentialities. In: Stevens JO (ed)(1977) gestalt is. Bantam, New York, pp 1–8

Perls FS, Hefferline R, Goodman P (1951) Gestalt therapy: Excitement and growth in the human personality. Dell, New York

Petzold H (1984) Die Gestalttherapie von Fritz Perls, Lore Perls und Paul Goodman. Integrative Therapie 1–2: 5–72

Portele G H (1992) Der Mensch ist kein Wägelchen. Ed Humanistische Psychologie, Köln

Schlegel L (1982) Die Psychodynamik der Polarität in der Psychologie von Jung. In: Eicke D (ed) Tiefenpsychologie. Bd 4. Beltz, Weinheim, pp 265–276

Schönberger M (1981) Vergborgener Schlüssel zum Leben. Weltformel I-GING im genetischen Code. Scherz, Bern

Spencer-Brown G (1979) Laws of form. EP Dutton, New York

Staemmler FM, Bock W (1987) Neuentwurf der Gestalttherapie. Pfeiffer, München

Staemmler FM, Bock W (1990) Ganzheitliche Veränderung in der Gestalttherapie. Pfeiffer, München

Taylor S (1990) Left-wing Nietzscheans. The politics of German expressionism 1910–1920. de Gruyter, Berlin

The Influence of Otto Rank's Concept of Creative Will on Gestalt Therapy*

Bertram Müller

Consideration of Otto Rank's ideas merits inclusion in a book on art and creativity in Gestalt therapy. Indeed, the assertion by Perls et al. (1951) that Rank's theoretical magnum opus, *Art and Artist*, is "beyond praise" (p. 395) is just one of many positive references to his works. In this regard, then, it appears all the more astonishing that in the further development of Gestalt therapy, precisely the contribution of this "great master" in research on the creative personality, creative life, and artistic creation as well as the use of such findings for the understanding and relief of mental suffering has as yet not been more intensively consulted. Certainly Isadore From, a founding teacher of Gestalt therapy, and Taylor Stoehr, Paul Goodman's biographer, considered Rank's writings for the development of Gestalt therapy as – if not more – important as the theories by Gestalt psychologists (Müller, 1993). Yet, an examination of the broader development of Gestalt therapy and practice suggests, unfortunately, that proper recognition of Rank has yet not taken place. Therefore, due to the scant number of theoretical publications by the most varied of Gestalt therapy authors on the subject of creativity in psychotherapy, I concur with Nancy Amendt-Lyon's charge, that in spite of a few inspirational contributions on Gestalt therapy, as yet no conclusive theory of creativity in Gestalt therapy exists (Amendt-Lyon, 1999). Rank can provide crucial insight, and thus this chapter will partially readdress this shortcoming, restricting itself to the development and influence of Rank's concept of creative will on Gestalt therapy.

More unnoticed than any one of Rank's psychological writings is his literary legacy to art, artistic creation, and the artistic personality. Precisely these fundamental works on the creative acts of human beings can contribute in essential ways to both better understanding and use of creative as well as psychologically blocked processes in psychotherapy and art creation.

Especially in his post-Freudian writings (from 1925 on), Rank posed central questions as regards the human creative urge, artistic creation, and de-

---

* Translated from the German by Laurie R. Cohen.

velopment of the artistic personality, ethics, and aesthetics (Rank, 1968), such as: *Where* does the human "urge to create" originate? *What* is needed to develop it? In which different ways and epochs is this creative urge expressed? What is its function for the individual and for society? How does it contribute to an explanation of the development and the functioning of the human personality? What is it that urges a person to create an artistic work rather than to simply enjoy life? What spurs one person to perform superhuman feats in order to become famous and possibly even eternal, while another, in seclusion, seeks wisdom, individual happiness, and even eternal bliss? For Rank, the answers to these questions are not only important for a deeper understanding of the creative process of the artist, but also for human psychology in general.

Creative motives, Rank argued, particularly in his discussions with Freud, do not arise from innate, sublimated drives, and they are not satisfyingly explained by socialization, since much of what is human and creative occurs either without or against natural instincts and against all actual past experiences. Only the creative interacting with the world around, with all its realities, illusions, and ideologies, is able to explain the specific inner dynamism through which the creative work is born. Thus unlike Freud, though similar to Perls et al. (1951), Rank emphasized the strength of the creative will, which is more or less at work within each individual in the task and process of assimilating past and present experience.

The reason Rank scrutinized the creative personality and the process of creation is because he perceived particularly in creative individuals, and especially artists, an example of an independent personality, independent from others – the collective, as he calls it – that is both ready to accept support socially from the collective and (through the created work or opus) to return something to it. This particular psychological dynamic of the creative individual – "to be with and in the world" – indicates Rank's view about how to help people who break down due to difficulties with the inherent human task of finding a satisfying individual, socially-oriented, *and* organized way of life (for instance, neurotics and sociopaths).

Based on the assumption of this human relatedness, Rank takes psychotherapy theory beyond Freud's deterministic view of human nature and returns the focus on a person's most important attribute: namely, the capacity to make individual choices, especially in relation to the outside world:

"To live fully, even to survive, man must perform first of all an act of will, which includes even an act of surrendering, at first by a volitional affirmation of the obligatory; i.e., he must 'say yes' to life. This act of the individual will, saying yes to the obligatory, then becomes a crucial creative aspect of adjustment. Secondly, according to his own capacities and the specificity of each situation, man must effect change. He does this by bringing forth the new. This is the adaptive aspect of individual creation" (Menaker, 1972, p. 12).

Rank's philosophical and theoretical paradigm, similar to that of Perls et al. (1951), is guided by thinking about polarities and processes. Rank, however, groups all of these polarities entirely around the single creative life impulse which, in its conscious form, he calls the creative will. Gestalt therapy could greatly benefit from Rank's ideas on how individuals acquire the skill of ethical and aesthetic acts, which neither originates solely from outside nor from the superego.

I. Rank's Concept of Creative Will, Consciousness, the Creative Personality, and Will Therapy

Rank postulated the creative will as "a psychological factor of the first order" (Rank, 1929). He called his novel idea, in the years following his separation from Freud, the "neo-Copernican return to the conscious will" (ibid., p. 6): namely, the emphasis on the particular, free, and individual will as a fundamental biological disposition in each person, notwithstanding any specific stamp and childhood experience. For Rank, the individual creative will is the primary shaping or transforming force of the ego, of the individuality; it is also the decisive prerequisite for the individual's capacity to be responsible. According to Rank's dynamic and constructive volition psychology, the denial of the creative individual will forms the basis of all neuroses.

Although Rank still considers valid the notion that the human ego is shaped by earlier identifications, especially in respect to the mother, he also believes that it can be formed above all by its own will. By "will", Rank means the strength of this autonomous original force, which represents the individual (the ego). And this will becomes creative insofar as it shapes itself – through the ego, which perceives as well as becomes aware of itself consciously – into a self-affirmed superego, which then leads to the self-created formation of ideals, which in the last instance originally derives from the id and not from the outside (ibid., p. 7). In contrast to Freud's conception of the world, Rank sees human beings as more than determined; indeed, there is an original cause within the individual! He calls it "the dynamic causality of the individual will", which influences the development of an individual personality as well as the development of the immediate culture or civilization (ibid., p. 53).

In his cultural-theoretical work originally published in 1930 as *Seelenglaube und Psychologie* (*Psychology and the Soul*, 1998), Rank demonstrates, in a distinct way, how our entire cultural history should be explained as the history of the development and the repression of the creative will. And his response to one of the most central anthropological, theological, and psychological questions – "Where does 'the negative' in the world come from?" – is found in his thorough cultural history analysis of the soul: it is nothing else but the human counter- and self-will, which deny mortality.

Rank's thesis that the id no longer reigns primary is of special interest to Gestalt therapy. Indeed, as mentioned above, Rank's new psychological construct focuses on the equally independent and at times even tyrannical self-conscious and self-willed ego. In addition, the creative type and its more or less inhibited cousin, the neurotic, demonstrate that the ego is not simply a battlefield of polymorphously perverse drives (Rank, 1968), but should rather be viewed as a regulating and forming, dynamic original force. Rank understands "will" neither in the way of experimental volition psychology, as an intra-psychological, subjective entity, nor as a momentary, directing force; for him it is rather a progressive, differentiated, and dynamic process, formed by inner and outer intentions and counterforces (cf. the expositions on the ego function by Perls et al., 1951). For Rank, the psyche belongs above all to the present. The predominantly and individually co-determined acts of the will, in the context of the specific situation of their determination of meanings and goals, are continuously created anew (Rank, 1998).

It is only in the affirmation of the individual will that there exists a unique human phenomenon: direct creative and healing spontaneity. This flexible psychological functioning of the actual individual volition is thereby a decisively human quality, which defines humans as creators of their own selves and their relationship to the outside world. Strengthening this self-definition, above all in those suffering from psychopathologies, is the aim of Rank's will therapy.

In *Truth and Reality* (1936b) and in his three volumes entitled *Technik der Psychoanalyse I – III* (1926 – 31) (volumes two and three translated into English as *Will Therapy*, 1936a), Rank denotes "will" as: ego function, as an energy or forming psychological force, which allows the individual to select, reject, and make conscious decisions: that is, ultimately, to be creative.

In his posthumous collection of essays, *Beyond Psychology*, written and published in English, Rank arrives at his most comprehensive definition of will:

"[By will] I mean rather an autonomous organizing force in the individual which does not represent any particular biological impulse or social drive, but constitutes the creative expression of the total personality and distinguishes one individual from another. This individual will, as the united and balancing force between impulses and inhibition, is the decisive psychological factor in human behavior. Its duofold functioning, as an impulsive and likewise inhibiting force, accounts for the paradox that the will can manifest itself creatively or destructively, depending on the individual's attitude towards himself and life in general" (1941, p. 50).

In a very condensed and summarized form, Rank (1929) presented the development of the drive, will, consciousness and, what is so interesting in this context, formation of values (psychological categories), as follows:

At first, Rank perceived the self as dominated by instincts. Then the ego gradually emerges – initially, as an accompanying interpreter of that which is and what by virtue of its instincts must be. The first conflict arises when the previously and merely confirming "yes, I will what I must" becomes a "it should not be" or "it is not": in other words, the possibility of a denial of necessity determined by nature supervenes. The consequences of this is a change of the consciousness and of the will. The consciousness becomes an autonomous force, capable not only of supporting but also denying and inhibiting the instinctual will. And thus the will, up to now, with only an executing function, becomes creative for the first time: that is, initially creative *negatively* in the form of a denial, in the sense of "not to want something that is determined by nature". In short, Rank stresses the far-reaching consequences of the negative origins of the will.

Consciousness, on the other hand, is the midwife of the freely creative will. Rank begins with the general assumption that the consciousness was originally only a sense organ of awareness of outer qualities; then followed the capacity of awareness as well of inner sensitivities, out of which developed the psychological ability to differentiate between inner and outer, to delimit from one another, and also in part to control. Eventually, consciousness achieved the capacity of self-reflective realization and freed itself thereby not only from the control of surrounding forces of nature, but also from its own id. It influenced above all, increasingly positively, superego development as well as the concrete shaping of the outer world.

How, according to Rank, do ethical values and aesthetic standards – that is, the *what* of the concrete volition – develop, if actually (and thereby contrary to psychoanalytical conceptions) they are not thought to be exclusively shaped from the outside and through socialization (superego)? Consciousness itself – thus Rank further develops his theory based on polarities – in its development, is influenced in turn by the will. Therefore both of these phenomena (consciousness and will) can be understood only in their interplay and in their continuous changeability. With regard to the will, consciousness orients itself both inwardly and outwardly. Outwardly oriented, it acquires the quality of the conscious expression of the drive or of the intentional act. Inwardly oriented, it acquires the quality of the conscious perception of the drives, that is, the quality of feeling, which Rank describes as an index for the concrete *what* of the volition (1929).

This interplay takes place continually and impulsively. This is why every interpretation of this event, carried over from the outside, is a disturbing attempt to interrupt this spontaneous and reciprocal process of interpretation of the will and the consciousness. Furthermore, this type of external interpretation arises particularly from a reluctance to follow the flow of life and from a longing for a firm footing. No doubt, Gestalt therapy would agree with Rank on this critical point. It is not possible to arrive at insights – and even less possible to arrive at therapeutic effects – through external interpretation, but only as an immediate and conscious self-experience of this mutual process of will and consciousness. Rank correctly identifies his dynamic will therapy, in reference also to Einstein, as "the relativity theory of psychotherapy" (Rank, 1968).

With this, however, the focus of Rank's theoretical discourse in the present context has not yet been placed on the highly important development of the *what* and the *how*: that is, of the ethical and aesthetic aspects of the volition and action. Necessary for that development are the mental structures, autonomously created out of one's own ideals. Rank calls these structures psychological categories. Not only the will, but also consciousness, as an instance of realization, fundamentally goes in two directions; namely, turned inwardly, it searches for truth – or in Rank's words, "inner reality", as opposed to the outside truth of the senses, i.e., so-called reality.

Comparable to the twofold functioning of the consciousness on the volition (corresponding to the act of will and the awarenesss of feeling), the influence of the consciousness on the formation of ideals also has a double effect, namely:

- active, as creative expression in form of the ego ideal; and
- passive, in the creation of specific ethical and aesthetic norms for one's own action and creation: without the concrete acquiescence of the norms, as a rule, no deed is permitted.

It is therefore the inner-oriented force of consciousness which, through these self-made ethical and aesthetic norms, qualifies the content of the orginally purely instinctual according to a single possible form, in which the individual realizes the content of his or her respective drive tendencies. In short, the ego itself does the qualifying, through its own force of consciousness which, in the sphere of volition, raises drives to specific interests. Their accomplishment depends, however, once again, on the created mental forms out of the own formation of ideals (cf. Rank, 1929, p. 43). Through the influence of this norm-giving force of consciousness, the will succeeds – not only impulsively but also inhibitingly, which means, above all, that it has a regulating significance. It has a constructive effect not only in the mastering of reality, but also in the control of the life drive as such. In this way, the conscious will is an individual's decisively regulating and unifying force. Although many features of the concept of self from the viewpoint of Gestalt therapy remain unclear, especially the ego-aspect of the conscious contact-making, Rank's exposition provides some lucidity insofar as he describes extensively the interaction and the dynamic transformations from drive, will, and consciousness to the setting up of values and action in a concrete field. These ideas, through their philosophical and anthropological methods, approach those of Gestalt therapy. The fact that clinical psychotherapy concerns the loss of a capacity of a flexible and autonomous interplay among consciousness, will, and autonomous determination of values makes a detailed presentation about and understanding of this interplay very relevant for therapeutic success.

II. Creative Will and Guilt

In this brief section I will limit myself to the relevant question – as regards individual life and artistic creation – of guilt and the feeling of guilt as an example of the above-mentioned integrative theoretical and clinical relevance for Gestalt therapists.

Rank considers will and guilt complementary sides of the same phenomenon. This is because as soon as the above-described mechanism by the conscious ego to the ethical volition begins, feelings of guilt relentlessly follow. The psychological mechanism of the individually conscious volition produces, as it were, as frictional heat, exactly this feeling of guilt, which in part, however, veiledly manifests itself as a rationalization of the motive, as a distortion of the truth, and it is expressed in the form of doubts regarding the justification of the own volition.

For Rank, guilt, guilty consciousness, and guilt feeling are merely the consequences of the volition arising within the individual him- or herself. The function of guilt feeling and guilty consciousness is therefore to establish a balance between a giving and taking, the individual and the collective. It functions like a regulating thermostat with individual possibilities of adjustment. Rank emphasizes that it is not only possible that one owes something to others or to the collective, but also to oneself, as a result of not having done justice to oneself. To describe the experienced guilt directed vis-à-vis the collective, Rank uses the term "guilty consciousness" (*Schuldbewusstsein*), whereas to describe the experienced guilt directed vis-à-vis oneself he uses the term "guilt feeling" (*Schuldgefühl*).

As to the origin of how the guilty consciousness arises, Rank claims that it derives from the dynamic relationship between the will and the consciousness: "In the conscious awareness of volitional phenomena, the aspect of insight is emphasized, whereas in the present content of volition, it is the aspect of experience that is emphasized" (1929, p. 37). In other words, I become aware, first, *that* I want something, and then I become aware of *what* I want.

Yet, Rank continues,

"Only when a moral value in the form of 'bad', which the individual receives from outside, from the particular content of the volition, entirely transfers onto the will as such, does an inner ethical conflict in the individual arise out of an outer conflict of will which, ultimately, instead of leading to a simple rejection to the particular act of the volition and content, leads to a denial of one's own will altogether and, as a symptomatic lasting consequence, to guilt feelings" (ibid.).

This sweeping denial becomes determined from outside as well as from the direction of the individual's internal volition, because the will, in countering the predominance of the consciousness – which internally draws up for the individual ethical norms of right and wrong (not of good and evil) – reacts at times also by strongly and continuously condemning the consciousness when the norms are felt to inhibit its volitious actions.

These facts constitute what Rank describes as the decisive dynamics in the formation of the guilty consciousness. The consciousness, which inhibits the will through its ethical norms, is felt by the will to be bad – to the same extent that the individual self-will is felt to be bad by the consciousness. This mutual inhibition of will and consciousness is what, according to Rank, can manifest itself as guilty consciousness. And this dynamic still finds comprehensive expression in our present cultural history. For Rank, it is essential to permit the individual not only volition, but also to lead him or her to *autonomous* volition in order for the unavoidable guilt feeling, which accompanies one's volition, to at least be justified constructively: namely, through the creative accomplishment itself, which often follows the willed and self-affirmed action and which, after all, often has a social dimension. In Rank's will therapy, as well as in his expositions on artistic creation, special emphasis is placed on an acceptance of the guilty consciousness that inevitably goes hand in hand with the conscious volition.

III. Creative Will and Neurosis

It is but a small step from these elaborations on the connection among consciousness, will, and guilt to a description of the features of a neurotic person, whom Rank sees as someone in whom an equally strong will is manifested, such as an artist or a creative person in action. However, in neurotic
persons, this will in its original negative character is expressed as counter-
will and fatally inward-oriented; at the same time, it is particularly felt,
through conscious self-realization, as guilty consciousness: the "suffering
person is not capable of acting creatively because his or her self-conscious-
ness inhibits the will, which manifests itself in him or her as a guilt feeling
vis-à-vis the action as such" (Rank, 2000, p. 40).

What Rank is presenting here is the neurotic experience and behavior,
not as a form of psychopathology, but as a developmental phase of the individuality, in which the conscious, artistic self-will is still being denied (ibid.,
p. 66). Gestalt therapy later proposes the same idea.

A neurotic's cure is individually and socially possible only in one and the
same way: namely, by permitting the wanting of something and being the
one who wants to be him- or herself and is so. This person should not in any
way feel guilty or inferior, but rather be helped to become a creative and
transformed person of action.

The person suffering from so-called psychopathologies represents in
Rank's diagnostic conception, in simple terms, only the fundamental variations of today's type of person who, depending on which excessive predominance, is distinguished among one of four psychophysical basic elements:
the drive, the will, the consciousness, and the angst (anxiety), whereby the
dynamic relationship among these factors determines the respective psychological fundamental philosophy in a particular situation.

For Rank, a neurotic is very similar to an artist. Indeed, he calls the neurotic *artiste manqué*, a somewhat failed, inhibited personality, who does not
take full responsibility for his or her individuality. Neurotics basically suffer
because they cannot accept themselves, their own individualities, and their
personalities. On the one hand, they are too critical of themselves and, on
the other hand, they idealize themselves too much. They make claims of
perfection, the failure of which leads to increased self-criticism. According to
Rank, neurotics have such a bad and fixated attitude toward the past because they want, later, to re-create it rather than accept it.

Artists are thus in a certain sense analogous counterparts to neurotics. It
is not that artists fail to criticize themselves. But, in the acceptance of their
personalities, they demonstrate a certain ability, which neurotics strive for in
vain, and they also extend their already arrived-at limitations. In other
words, the prerequisite of the creative personality is not the self's acceptance
alone, but almost its glorification as such.

The emancipative and therapeutic task consists in accepting one's own
self with all the individual aspects of the ego and of the autonomy of will and
feeling. The goal of constructive volition therapy, for Rank – and later for
Gestalt therapy – is consistent: not in overcoming resistance, which he ob-

served as the phenomenon of will as well in its negative form, but in transforming the negative expression of will (counter-will, as an inhibition of drives and tendencies that are inwardly oriented) to one of self-regulated creative expression of personality.

IV. The Artist's Creative Urge

Artists and artistic creation cannot, according to Rank, be explained psychologically on an exclusively individual level (2000, p. 19): "The ideology of immortality is not only a result but also one of the most important basic prerequisites for artistic creation" (ibid., p. xxvi).

Through his anthropological investigations, Rank concluded that in all civilizations, the safeguarding of eternal life, as a rule, has been a much more important concern than that of happiness and prosperity in real life. This is shown, for example, today in our civilization through the enormous, if not cultish, importance given to life insurance, beauty, and extreme health care.

The ordinary citizen, according to Rank, behaves rather contentedly to safeguarding immortality by conforming to what is given and by identifying with collective forms, such as religion, belief in the government, family, and the next generation. The self-confident, strongly-willed and ably dissociative artist-personality strives nevertheless to find an individual solution to this fundamental problematic. An essential source of the individual creative urge lies in the impulse toward a personally individual – in any case not a collective – self-perpetuation (Rank, 1968).

Religion is formed through the collectively oriented belief in immortality. Art comes from the individual self-awareness of one's own personality, from which follows a striving toward the individual path of safeguarding immortality (ibid., p. 16). Naturally, both paths are not fundamentally divided. The collective needs an artist within it to make the abstract soul concrete and real through poetry, painting, and music. And the individual artist, who uses the collective – for example, cultural speech – for his individuality (for instance, to express himself in a poem), needs the cultural tradition and the confirmation of his fellow citizen or next generation in order to become immortal through their praise.

Creating art, like the human creative urge, according to Rank, is explained only by the constructive surmounting of the fundamental dualism between the collective and the individual (ibid., p. 2). The meaning and origin of all individuals and collective ideologies are also traced back to a common spiritual root, which Rank discovered in the belief in immortality:

"The essence of the artistic type lies therefore in this, that he can pass through his individual struggle, the conflict between individual and genus, between personal and collective immortality, in an *ideological* form, and that the peculiar quality of this conflict compels him, or enables him, to use an artistic ideology for the purpose" (1968, p. 369).

It is this capacity of symbolization, of forging an artistic ideology, that the neurotic person is not yet in a position to achieve the way the artist is.

Essential yet different particularities of the artist personality include, according to Rank, their capacity of (symbolic) representation of total experiences, their courage and ability to call themselves "artists", and especially the attitude to art itself.

The specialness of the artist is being able both to differentiate the intuitive playing child from the creative expert in the art of living and, along with aptitude, individual experience, and the id's spontaneous intuition, to use the culture and the artistic style of his or her period to create, in contrast, something individually new: "The artist, as it were, takes not only his canvas, his colours, or his model in order to paint, but also the art that is given him formally, technically, and ideologically, within his own culture" (ibid., p. 7). Artists use what is collectively inherited to dissociate themselves individually, and they need the collective to allow them, if nececessary, to confirm their new individual creations:

> "The artist, as a definite creative individual, uses the art-form that he finds at hand in order to express something personal; this personal must therefore be somehow connected with the prevailing artistic and cultural ideologies, since otherwise he could not make use of them; but it must also differ, since otherwise he would not need to use them in order to produce something of his own" (Rank, 2000, pp. 6–7).

The special feature about Rank's expositions on the creative personality is that this creation starts *with* the individual as well as *in* the individual, him- or herself: in other words, with the self-creation of the personality to the creative person or artist, whom Rank describes with the self-designation of artist. Thus, the first creation of the productive individual is the self-designation as an artistic personality, transcending the way one used to understand oneself. This basically remains the artist's most important creation, because all the others that follow represent in part an objectivized expression to the outside world of this original creation of the own self and, in part, a justification of the glorifying self-designation (ibid., p. 70).

The self-shaping and self-formation into the artist, however, is also closely connected with the life experience of the artist. Living and creating are reciprocal, because the human creative urge results in life experience and in producing art: Rank wrote that the artist had the tendency to flee from experience, that is, from the real, immediate life, which is also existentially threatened by death, therefore life is controlled by being shaped. In creation, the artist attempts to preserve or immortalize his or her transitory life. For this reason, creation and the process of life experience (everyday life) become opposites, and not only in the life of artists.

The artistic urge of the artist to create, which emerges out of a tendency to immortalize him- or herself, may become so powerful that the artist defends him- or herself against the transitory experience. The artist, with all his or her experience, flees from real life, which is predominantly transitory, whereas the experience, shaped by the artist, calms the consciousness of life's transitoriness and impresses as creation. As Rank thus dialectically summarizes:

> "In creation the artist tries to immortalize his mortal life. He desires to transform death into life, as it were, though actually he transforms life into death. For not only does the

created work not go on living; it is, in a sense, dead; both as regards the material, which renders it almost inorganic, and also spiritually and psychologically, in that it no longer has any significance for the creator, once he has produced it (...) [and] therefore again takes refuge in life, and again forms experience" (1968, p. 39).

V. Conclusion

Rank's investigations concerning the creative act and artistic personality, as well as his conclusions about the emergence and healing of psychological suffering, connect many fields of knowledge and are much too complex to outline in one brief chapter. I recommend the reader pick up Rank's writings directly and, as a way of introduction, not to forego reading Lieberman's (1985) dense and engagingly written Rank biography.

Rank's overflowing plea for creative, free, willful, and distinctive aspects of human beings has, I hope, become clear. In conclusion, therefore, let me add a few limited thoughts of Rank's on the creative acts of human beings.

Rank exposed the disseminated urge – and not only among Gestalt therapists – toward the excessive creative act and well-meaning help as a reaction formation of an unresolved Oedipus complex, which Rank naturally did not interpret sexually, but as ego-achievement in the sense of a reaction to the parents' restrictions against the child's own volition. Rank calls this the "Prometheus complex" in reference to the well-known Greek mythical figure, who on his own authority, i.e., against the Gods' will, wanted to help people and make them happy (Rank, 1928). The basic position of therapists, Rank indicates, is neither a passive mirror to the development of the repressed, nor active in the sense of a creative realization of the personality of therapists, but rather in the "middle mode" of the participating readiness (cf. Perls et al., 1951) and as "midwives", who help by grasping or also separating, there where mother and child would like and need. For instance, in his important work co-authored with Sandor Ferenczi (*Entwicklungsziele der Psychoanalyse* [*The Development of Psychoanalysis*], 1925), Rank warns not only against a mechanistic application of techniques, but also in particular against a self-image of the therapist that would be akin to a creative artist. Therapists do not heal through means and techniques: nor through simple or mere expressions of their creativity. They heal through their personality, which is professionally restrained and at the same time capable of spontaneous response. Above all, therapists in Rank's sense should allow themselves to be shaped by their patients and should let themselves be made into that which the patients want and need.

In the face of the abundance of knowledge, novelty and ever-new products, on the one hand, and the threateningly exhaustive exploitation of natural resources, on the other hand, which is caused by exaggerated productive human effects and transformations, Rank poses the question whether we have not already, some time ago, reached the limits of our individual and artistic productivity. As the artist Joseph Beuys formulated it, fifty years after Rank: "The mistake begins as soon as one buys a paintbrush and a canvas"

(Beuys, in Oman, 1998). To create less and instead change internally through the self-creative transformation of the own personality is possibly the most important work of art of future human beings for our survival. Or, as Rank, at the end of *Kunst und Künstler* [*Art and Artist*], wrote: "A man with creative power who can give up artistic expression in favour of the formation of personality – since he can no longer use art as an expression of an already developed personality – will remould the self-creative type and will be able to put his creativity directly in the service of his own personality" (1968, p. 430). This programmatic proposition by a post-metaphysical, post-religious, and still wildly behaving cultural epoch, is not easy to digest. Yet Rank also promises some comfort, as he continues:

"To reach this state of personal development will be for most a difficult task, because this would mean to overcome the fear of life. The fear of life and the wish to prevent danger and individual death has at the bottom of our psychic life led to the substation of artistic production for life. (...) For the artistic individual has lived in art-creation instead of actual life. (...) [T]he creative type who can renounce this protection by art and can devote his whole creative force to life and the formation of life will be the first representative of the new human type, and in return for this renunciation will enjoy, in personality-creation and expression, a greater happiness" (ibid., p. 431).

Thus for therapists and artists much remains to be done: namely, to contribute in our society means and ways to reduce the fear of the full life experience – in Gestalt terms the full contact, when the self is diminishing (Perls et al., 1951, p. 404) – through the support of the creative volition, which permits one to mature in one's own self-created, fully responsive personality.

References

Amendt-Lyon N (1999) Kunst und Kreativität in der Gestalttherapie. In: Fuhr R, Srekovic M, Gremmler-Fuhr (eds) Handbuch der Gestalttherapie. Hogrefe, Göttingen, pp. 857–877
Lieberman EJ (1985) Acts of will. The life and work of Otto Rank. Free Press, New York
Menaker E (1972) Adjustment and creation. J of the Otto Rank Association, 7(7): 12–25
Müller B (1993) Isadore From's contribution of the theory and practice of Gestalt therapy. Studies in Gestalt Therapy 2: 7–22
Oman H (1998) Joseph Beuys. Heyme Verlag, München
Perls F, Hefferline R, Goodman P (1951) Gestalt therapy: Excitement and growth in the human personality. Dell Publishing, New York
Rank O (1928) Gestaltung und Ausdruck der Persönlichkeit. Deuticke, Wien
Rank O (1929) Wahrheit und Wirklichkeit. Deuticke, Wien, and (1936b) Truth and reality. Knopf, New York
Rank O (1936a) Will therapy. Knopf, New York
Rank O (1941) Beyond psychology. Dover Publication, New York
Rank O (1968) Art and artist. Agathon Press, New York and (2000) Kunst und Künstler. Psychosozial-Verlag, Gießen
Rank O (1998) Psychology and the soul. The Johns Hopkins Press, London
Rank O, Ferenczi S (1925) The development of psychoanalysis. NMDMS, No. 40

Beauty and Creativity in Human Relationships

Joseph C. Zinker

The *Creative Process in Gestalt Therapy* was described by me in the book by the same title in 1977 (Zinker, 1977). This process is a breaking through toward the novel, the transcendent, the extraordinary, the surprising in human relationships.

Since its publication, I have become increasingly interested in how content contextualizes process. For me, however, process is primary for forming images and aesthetic configurations. I believe this was one of Perls' major discoveries. Namely, that his inquiries about a person's movements, gestures, and voice intonations led to the patient's discovery of meaning. It was not the story that contextualized the gestures, but the gestures that underlined new dimensions of the story. Almost always there is contrapuntal shuttling between content and process phenomena. For example, the patient says he is frightened while he is smiling.

Another dimension that has informed my work during these years is the powerful influence of the various social systems in which the person and family function. The same conversation of a couple in Saudi Arabia has a very different meaning in France; and, it is not even perceived as the same conversation. You have to constantly modify your perception of reality and how it is embedded and revealed in a given environment. Sonia Nevis taught us that we must perceive basic phenomenological data in a given context, followed by our perception of a system's competence and what is not fully developed. Then, learning can be "stretched" through experiment without mobilizing resistance (personal communication).

In this little paper I simply share my process observations, the emerging phenomena of people around me, the raw phenomenological data, and its intrinsic aesthetic qualities and beauty. The emerging meaning-making and its enrichment develop later in the therapeutic process.

Creativity is a *relational* process. It is aroused in our yearnings, our energy, and our impulse to move, sing, dance, and touch each other. Creativity is fuelled by love, anger, the pain of tragedy and loss, and our desire to become whole and fulfilled with each other. To be human is to be creative. And to be human is so astonishing, because only we are aware of our mortality, our temporary stay here on earth, and our yearning for total union with each other and with God.

Creating takes place between persons or between a person and something else. Creativity lives in the interactional space between us. The moment we begin to interact, something is liable to emerge that has the above-named elements. We claim that we were created by God, but our descriptions of God tell the many rich stories of our own creative nature.

Beauty is an aesthetic quality of objects or events. Beauty is not static. Both objects and events are created through interaction of persons with various materials or between groups of persons in speech, movement, and gesture. Beauty is in the eyes of the beholder. The object or process itself has no meaning without its relation to the looker/listener. These events are embroidered by variation of language, culture, historical and geographical events, values, and the structure of a particular aesthetic orientation. What is beautiful between people to some persons is ugly to others; what was beautiful to first century Greeks may or may not have been attractive to 12th century Indians. That brings to mind the factor of social class and education. Perception of beauty changes with education and class structure. Our tastes of beauty are modified by our parents, teachers, and peers.

Art is a broader concept than beauty. Its scope is enormous. Art covers things both beautiful and ugly, enlightening and darkly gloomy, cruel and evil, palatable and disgusting: in the theatre, choreography, the written word, and painting/sculpture. What is art changes from one generation to another. Art may or may not fall in line with or be related to ethical, religious, or political values.

For example, a mayor of New York recently threatened to cut off funds to the Brooklyn Museum because a photographic exhibit had an explicit homosexual theme. During World War II, modern painting was dismissed as trash by Stalin and Hitler. What one reader considers beautiful writing, another sees as excessively sentimental and therefore not qualified to be printed in an anthology.

Art, beauty, and creative process are not always congruent with societal norms and fashions of a given era. The artist or creative person is often a counter-cultural character. He often pushes the envelope of what is proper, beautiful, tasteful or "appropriate" in his culture. The artist or film producer may be a revolutionary, who pushes for significant changes in her society.

The psychotherapist as a creative person in the culture is often burdened by social pressures and norms of what is healthy, sick, or appropriate to hospital directors, the medical establishment, or ethics professors. The gifted psychotherapist has one foot in the professional establishment and the other in the creative process.

I. Yearning for the Transcendent

I am thinking here of my teacher, Abraham Maslow. He made some distinctions between physiological needs at one end of a continuum and self-actualizing needs at the other. Human beings struggle between simply surviving, sustaining themselves on one hand, and yearning for a beauteous, transcendent, and "conversion" experience on the other. Maslow theorized that deprivation and serious illness block creative activity and interaction and that we have to be able to satisfy needs for security, belonging, and love to enter the sphere of self-actualization and a creative life.

There is something in the essence of our creative spirit which, under the worst circumstances, pulls us forward toward the experience of feeling beauty, experiencing genuine love, and feeling union with each other. We yearn for transcendence. In my doctoral studies at Highland View Hospital, I met a poor black patient who was dying of cancer. I sat with her daily for six months, just talking. Together we found that in spite of her physical and psychological decline, she began to share with me a kind of transcendence and spiritual growth that she didn't have before. On the other hand, another patient with similar terminal disease steadily declined and consistently lost interest in people and life. This is a mystery. As much a mystery as people falling in love or becoming great actors, writers, or composers. But in almost all cases, people melt into an experience of connecting with nature, with an audience, with loved ones, or simply with an extended experience of tackling mathematical or philosophical problems.

Almost always these events have qualities of process, co-creation, immersion with others, context, and what feels to be "good form". We yearn to experience a sense of wholeness, completed form, and integration. Great mathematicians and physicists have been known to say that their discovered equations were truly "beautiful". Beauty is not sectarian. We find it in the most unexpected places. But we must have eyes and ears and sensations to seek and savor it.

II. Love

Love is "an intense feeling of deep affection or fondness for a person or thing" (Oxford dictionary). The loving experience is almost always an encounter. Beauty and creative process are born at the boundary between persons or, phenomenologically, in the fertile, thickened space between people. Physiologically, pheromones that are released in the process of mutual attraction, and endorphins, which are neurotransmitters, suppress pain and increase the pleasure of being with the other. We experience each other as "beautiful". The fragrance of the other's body is delicious and mouth-watering.

In the objective world, this sense of enhanced beauty is present, independent of what people actually look like. For me, this is God's gift to all mammals and human beings, a gift of experiencing beauty no matter how "beautiful" we actually are. We are filled in a kaleidoscope of liveliness; the world starts all over again with purity and brilliance. We feel transformed, immortal. We suffer when the other is absent or, at times, during forced separation or death.

Allowing ourselves to be loved is accompanied by heightened sensation and energy, and curiosity and surrender to each other. We find ourselves spontaneously singing, dancing around, and, of course, writing poems. Here again we encounter spontaneous creation, "good" or "bad":

Life in the sunshine
without you is cloudy ...
Dinners leave me hungry.
Laughter without you is a circus ...
Watching lovers kiss looks vulgar.
Racy novels are dull ...

Where are you, my love? (Zinker, 2001, p. 88)

The lover reads love poetry and, at times, enters into a kind of partnership with the poet in expressing his or her love – and sense of celebration. Here is an example:

My love came to my bed and slept –
I could hear her moist sensuous breath
Quiet, still, as if contemplating the
beginning of the universe.
My love slept and I sat at her side
reading Neruda
who instructed me about my hunger for
Silence in the infinite embrace of life.
Suddenly Neruda jumped out of his book
and stood above me smiling.
He put his hand gently on my shoulder,
saying softly (as not to wake her up) ...
He said softly,
"when a gift like this comes to you,
guard her with your life,
feed at her breast,
and most importantly, dance!
Dance your whole life with her,
And only her!"
Then Neruda vanished, leaving me alone,
To birth myself.

(Zinker, 2001, p. 180)

The loving experience wakes you up to a greater sense of connectedness with your partner, to your own inner life, and to meanings of life. It is a kind of rebirth of wonderment. This escalation of psychic energy pushes you to look with invested compassion at everything that the imagination can grasp: the remarkable cruelty in relationships, in families, between countries as well as the remarkable speed of new technologies and the evolution of theories, the nature of chaos, of politics, diplomacy, and economic behavior of nations.

Love invests itself in beauty, but it may also stimulate the darker side of humanity. The most cruel tortures and betrayals are carried out between intimates, not strangers. Yes, between strangers, also. But think of the ethnic/religious "cleansing" and atrocities in Poland, Ireland, Palestine, Yugoslavia, the Middle East, and Africa.

Love is not always beautiful. It is a paradoxical impulse that torments and moves us in many directions. Love may stimulate small, secure nest-building in the young, but it also tests older persons to take more responsibility for the future of our civilization.

III. Humor

Humor is one of the lubricants of social life. Humor is the first cousin of joy, surprise, and bemusement. Humor may hold important political and philosophical lessons, but not jokes. Jokes are canned episodes and can be told by humorless, joyless persons, and quite mechanically. Jokes have no soul, but they often have political and social relevance. Jokes are often funny (depending on culture and location), but humor is more complex and varied. Humor allows us to get together and turn the world upside down, to tolerate our mortality, bear the unbearable (as in the song "Springtime for Hitler" in the Broadway musical *The Producers*), see beauty in an ugly world, and appreciate the paradoxes of life. Humor releases joy and allows relief for those in illness or pain; humor is a creative process between people. It is an ego syntonic instrument that allows us to accept how foolish we can be, how we can deny the dying process. It helps us both accept and deny the inevitable disappointments in life. Humor is a beautiful human invention.

Many years ago, my 80-year-old father was hospitalized to undergo bypass surgery. It was one of the early attempts by a famous surgeon to perform the bypass heart technique with an octogenarian. The night before the operation, I sat alone with my father. He was immobilized by fear of the dangerous operation.

I tried to find some way of giving him relief. Then it occurred to me that my father was a teller of stories and jokes; I tried to find a solution to save the evening for him. I proposed a game to him, in which I would give him a "trigger" word and he would use it to tell a joke or story. My father accepted the proposal, and so it went:

> Joseph: St. Peter at the gates of heaven ...
> Father: A very rich man who was pious died and ...
> Joseph: A young man went to a prostitute ...
> Father: Oh! Yes, I have a good one ...

There were many jokes about wives, mothers-in-law, drunks, rabbis and priests, politicians, and professors.

The evening was filled with laughter and, at times, with tears. He told some of his favorite war stories and seemed to forget his operation. I really loved my father that evening. It was a beautiful, intimate contact between us.

This little story is not about joke-telling. It is about the healing power of humor and the sharing of common memories between an old man and his "baby" son. Now, as an old man myself, I still carry that memorable evening in my heart. This is also an example of a spontaneous creative image which developed into an experiment which carried poignancy and power.

IV. Improvisation

The daily process between people in ordinary life allows for little departure from established habits and rules of communication. One reason for this is efficiency and order. It has taken us thousands of years to just make ordinary talk with each other and get things done. Imagine that while negotiating the purchase of a house, the buyer begins to sing. Well, everything will stall, someone in the party will get upset, and the transaction will stop. At the same time, improvisations can be delightful in comedy, in the theatre or in difficult situations that may require the skill of making up stories on the spot.

Improvisation is the capacity to depart from a given theme that goes beyond a concrete definition of its conventional meaning. Many people are secure in knowing the world of meanings literally. This kind of "knowing", albeit secure, restricts their experience of the world to standard, "frozen" gestalten. Often anxiety, suffering, and neurosis are accompanied by the comfort of the standard meaning. A mother is a woman with children or a punitive witch.

Improvisation gives the person the flexibility to add images or musical themes that startle the other person. In a pseudo-autobiographical film by an American actor and producer, his mother appears as a great picture in the skies of New York City. She speaks to him: "I've been trying to find you, Melvin ... I keep calling you and you don't answer me." Crowds begin to gather in the streets and dialogue with her. One woman says back to her: "Yes, yes, I have a son like this ... Here, look at his photograph ... He is so handsome!" The mother answers from the sky: "Only *one* photograph?! What kind of mother are you?" Other people gather and exchange pictures.

Improvisation is the ability to consciously depart from given meanings, sounds, melodies, and literary forms into a kind of weaving and texture that only slightly touches what is *obvious*, but moves into complex *elaboration* that seems to enter other spheres, other connections that eventually return to the original theme, image or melody. These are conscious, deliberate departures of meaning – not unconscious ravings of psychotics or intoxicated persons. The distinction is that in mental illness, the so-called "improvisations" are generally static, often paranoid or grandiose *repetitive* themes lacking variety and complexity of meaning.

In psychotherapy, on the other hand, the creative practitioner *deliberately* introduces an improvisation that startles or surprises a client into thinking or feeling something original and often beneficial about the client's current worry or preoccupation. This gives relief to those who suffer constant obsessive and compulsive symptoms that plague them day and night. People can even laugh at themselves and recover their humor about events that previously "froze" their thinking and imagination.

V. Multi-Contextuality

When Freud introduced the notion of the various forces and polarities within the unconscious, he made possible a new sort of literature that was not logically positivistic, but multi-contextual. We can see many examples of this in modern literature: you can read T.S. Elliot's *Wasteland* and allow yourself the pleasure of seeing a variety of opposing images, "films", voices, religious metaphors, and other free associations. It is not straight, logical, and linear talk. The Russian poet Pushkin is straight talk. Rubens is more or less straight talk. They are beautifully literal. But Picasso is multi-contextual.

By multi-contextual I mean that any given human phenomenon or interaction is seen by the creative person as a collection of images and events that take place (and are seen) simultaneously – each image contributes to the whole perception of the person in a unique way. Together, they are a multi-dimensional "collage", a kind of "sculpture" that moves toward and "strives" to reveal itself in a completed, self-actualization form. The observer is constantly scanning the person(s) for movement toward "good form" and, having seen different dimensions, negotiates with the person or couple to produce an event or, as we call it, "experiment", in which the complete form can reveal itself in its new, satisfying "beauty".

In my writings over the past 35 years, I have given examples of these transformations taking place in groups, families, couples, and individuals. One must be able to focus sharply on the various "contexts", while observing a given phenomenon, and to fantasize its transformative potential. Metaphor is often used to describe an experience. A depressed young man is asked how he feels in his body at the moment. He says: "I feel like I am an old beggar." Would he consider acting: 1) like an old man or 2) like a beggar pleading for something from people in a group? 3) Would he consider shuffling with his shoes as he moves around? 4) Would he experiment, allowing his face to become mask-like (as in a case of advanced Parkinsonism)? and so on. His interest is peaked and, with the support of his wife, partner, or therapy group, he begins to reveal the multi-contextual aspects of his pain. He begins to "understand" his pain, and others are inspired to think about how they contribute to his discomfort, and even how they may act to lift the burden from his shoulders.

The *whole* field of human interaction is in motion and moves toward a potential outcome that teaches the client system to see itself in a *novel* way. This is a kind of transformative multi-contextual event that moves toward "good form", a resolution, a form that gives *relief* and satisfaction to those who suffer all their lives and are locked into static immobility and hopelessness.

Creative people like Picasso manage to communicate multi-contextually and yet stay understandable, colorful, possibly funny, possibly tragic, poignant, perceptually challenging, and even hilarious. T.S. Elliot's *The Wasteland* or James Joyce's *Ulysses* can move us deeply and teach us about life.

VI. Children

Children make spontaneous improvisations effortlessly.

Beatriz (age 6) and Rodrigo (age 10) were wandering around in a shopping center in Sao Paulo. They found themselves in a large furniture shop and, while their mother was discussing prices with a salesperson, they discovered a Japanese furniture section with low-standing, delicate tables and lamps. Without hesitation, they got down on their knees – as if in a tea ceremony – put their palms together, finger to finger, and began to sway and chant using "Chinese" intonations. They narrowed their eyes and swayed their little bodies. There was no malice or shaming in their behavior; no prejudicial shaming – just fun. It was beautiful, spontaneous improvisation. Their mother and the salesperson laughed with pleasure. It was a spontaneous experiment of some complexity, involving:

1. Changing the context of a store to a place of prayer
2. Changing the cultural context
3. Changing the habitual sounds of their voices
4. Using the props of the furniture to create a dialogue that had primitive synchrony of voices and gestures (these are Brazilian white, Catholic kids, whose parents are Brazilian and whose grandparents are Portuguese).

This is spontaneous improvisation. It requires a prerequisite sense of entitlement, freedom to make-believe, a non-punitive environment, and an experience of inner goodness and beauty. For the children, this was no big deal. They promptly moved on with their mother to another store without protest or theatrics.

VII. Adults

Recently, while on a trip to Sicily, I was walking with my little disposable camera down a narrow, ancient street. Approaching two stone masons out on a break, I wanted to connect with them; but my lack of Italian frustrated me. I stopped at a discreet distance and observed as both men started talking on their cellular phones. Don't ask "why", but my fantasy was that they called their mothers. Then I approached them more closely, turned my camera sideways, imitating a cell phone, and started chanting: "Mamma, oh! Mamma, where are you now?" It was a magical moment of connection between us. Both men turned toward me first with surprise, then bemusement, their faces melting first into smiles, then laughter: three strangers bursting into laughter. Later, they took me around an ancient building, showing me their restoration work, speaking Italian while I spoke with my hands and face. My wife, Sandra, who witnessed the whole event, did help a bit with the Italian. We wished them a happy celebration of the coming Santa Lucia procession and went on our way.

This is another example of spontaneous improvisation of an ordinary visitor with a camera passing two dusty stone masons in a ancient Mediterranean town. The "interventions" and motives for spontaneous improvisations are not necessarily therapeutic. They are the most primitive contact-making creations between people. At times like this, we know what it means that all of us are in the same family.

VIII. Movement and Gesture

Movement is most often relational and improvisational. People move in response and in relation to each other in a kind of huge cosmic dance. In the streets of Paris, people use their bodies differently than, say, in New York City or in Tel Aviv. In New York I feel seen in the sense that a certain personal space is created for my body by others (not always true in elevators and subways!). Although we may be very busy, the movement is created by a spatial choreography determined by how well people focus on each other and what motivates their urgency to "get there".

In Paris streets people appear to see each other as obstacles around which to negotiate one's body – unless, of course, they meet a friend in the street: then, all obstacle and personal space rules are suspended, and strangers take on the additional challenges of moving around more cramped spaces.

London is difficult during typically rainy, dark, rush hours. On just such an evening, I walked with my wife on a street adjoining the British Museum. Suddenly, I heard a baritone voice behind me and saw a tall black man practically stepping over me. As he pushed himself forward, he shouted sideways: "Can't you move yourself a bit faster!? You are blocking the flow ..." He was moving rapidly from one point to another, aggressively graceful, as if ready to toss a basketball into a basket. What speed! What grace! And no collision. His long, straight stride and his authoritarian baritone made me feel like a little prune of a "bag lady", fat and ungainly. His voice and body defined me.

Without much awareness, we create a choreography together, composed of measured gestures and rhythms that create an aesthetic, a modern ballet. The ballet both defines our body image and experience, and our relationship to each other.

IX. Culture

In some cultures, we can get so close to others, we smell their musty, rich, heavy odor as if they carry a dead animal or overripened exotic cheese under their shirts. People who live in these cultures may say to themselves in passing, "she has the whiff of a ripe bunch of figs mingled with crushed pomegranates". Odors, rhythms, and movements of bodies mingle like arranged instruments in a musical performance. Just look and listen!

However we move, we can't help feeling "aesthetically defined" as "a klutz" or as dancers floating dreamily with arms out like a Chagall painting, or as vertical marching puppets favoring one side of the body over the other. As we watch the street scene, we notice people tilting toward their cellular phones, talking enthusiastically. It is all part of a kind of communal ritual: each character's move is both a question and answer.

It is impossible not to see the beauty of the street dance, guided by one's alert eyes. However it works, there are no serious disturbances in the field; people manage their choreography beautifully. They are fascinating with their varied costumes, both drab and elegant, both relationally intimate or strategic. The scene "works" both functionally and aesthetically.

X. Contextual Qualities of Beauty and Creativity in Human Relationships

Beauty reveals itself in almost any process between people or in projects that call for an emotional investment of energy between ourselves and musical forms, reenactments of events, story-telling, dance, and playing with children. Each person's expression or gesture adds contextual richness to our experience. Beauty is sublime; it is deeply moving; it drives us to tears; it fulfills that which we yearned to complete inside of us and *between us*. Beauty surprises us and elevates us to a sense of joy when we lift each other beyond where individual expression falls flat and fails.

Martin Buber (1962) spoke of how when one person's voice strives toward heaven and fails to rise, only the joining of another person elevates us toward beauty. We need each other to awake joyful, deeply-moving experiences of beauty. The creative process is stimulated when we enter into meaningful contact. In this space, this thickened connectedness between us, beauty is born like the emergence of a baby from its mother's womb. We pray to God and we "make" beauty with chants for atonement and pleading for forgiveness. Beauty reveals itself when we admit our fragility, regret, and humility. Beauty favors our deepest articulated doubts and not our heroic superficiality. Together we make a process that coaxes the birth of beauty.

There are many more phenomenological dimensions of our humanness that can be described in the context of the creative process and the making of beauty. Here is a list of conditions and common qualities that may be helpful in examining these events:

1. Maintaining optimal energy for mutual stimulation (in a variety of forms).
2. Balance between strategic, "self-covering" and intimate connectedness. Once we enter the sphere of strategy, transparency of intimacy is clouded.
3. Balance between experiencing each other's darkness, hardness on one hand, and lyrical sweetness/radiance on the other.
4. To know each other's destructive power versus intent to do good.
5. Articulating and questioning each other's intentions and motives.
6. Balance between conflict and confluence: supporting adequate middle ground.
7. Acceptance of the drab, ordinary aspects of our lives – letting go.

8. Balance between our desire for growth and, on the other hand, recognition of deterioration/entropy.
9. Balance between denial of the tragic experiences of life and having the capacity to feel the profound, the heartache, compassion, and regret.
10. Capacity and persistence to begin, develop, and complete experiences together.
11. Balance between protecting each other from harm and at the same time allowing for autonomy and the freedom to falter.

So, what are creativity and beauty in our relationships all about? Can they really be defined in the shadow of a world in which people slaughter each other with great efficiency every day? A small part of the answer is that we develop tilting toward beauty or ugliness or, more likely, we desire to integrate, to balance these forces within us.

As we grow older, some of us harden our hearts, no doubt due to the hardness of our lives. Others, as if by a miracle of nature, remain open to the full range of human experiences. Some of us have found lovers, friends, and teachers who encouraged our pursuit of seeing, hearing, and creating beauty together.

It is a mystery of our development that some children, no matter how well-pampered, adored, and offered every opportunity to stay open to life, grow up as ordinary "beta" types who help us maintain the stability of our culture. (Ah! But watch them express tenderness with their children!) There are also persons who, after having been deprived, abused, and humiliated, move toward becoming beautiful human beings, or great artists, playwrights, or singers. A price is always paid. They may also be heartless persons incapable of intimacy and closeness. Trauma and deprivation may work differently with others. They are tenderized by pain. They suffer well – and somehow stay open to compassion and joy. We don't know much about these phenomena. We simply observe them in each other.

My own experience is that wholeness and grace in aesthetic development are hard to come by, and that for every blessing of beauty and creativity we receive, we are also robbed and cheated in other ways and remain incomplete forever.

References

Buber M (1962) Ten rungs: Hasidic sayings. Schocken Books, New York
Zinker J (1977) Creative process in Gestalt therapy. Vintage Books, New York
Zinker J (2001) Sketches. An anthology of essays, art, and poetry. GestaltPress/Analytic Press, Hillsdale New Jersey

The Aesthetics of Commitment:
What Gestalt Therapists Can Learn from
Cézanne and Miles Davis[1]

Michael Vincent Miller

I. Staying With ...

This essay is a meditation on a common Gestalt idiom – the expression "staying with" in the sense of staying with the truth of one's present experience, whether it feels positive or negative. This is such a common intervention from Gestalt therapists that it is almost a cliché. If you are a Gestalt therapist, it is hard to imagine a day of private practice going by without your suggesting to this or that client, "Stay with this angry feeling" or "with this fantasy of killing your mother" or "with this sensation in your chest" or "with the way you are perched on the edge of your chair". Like every idiomatic intervention in every school of psychotherapy, telling your client to stay with what is going on can harden into an empty and stereotyped technique when you can't think of anything else to do. But it has its roots in an important, original principle of Gestalt therapy – the replacement of the therapist's control of the client's experience, through such methods as interpretation or conditioning programs, with a basic respect for the client's subjectivity as a touchstone of psychotherapy.

In the early days of Gestalt therapy, the complementary notion for maintaining this sort of respect was the idea that the therapist must "stay with" the client, rather than go off on his or her own therapeutic agenda for what the client should experience. Nowadays, Gestalt therapy theory has begun to emphasize its ground in a conception of the emerging field, rather than starting out with two already well-defined figures or roles, called therapist and client, as though both already know what they are going to do. So, we might speak of "staying with" the unfolding process, as it surfaces, differentiates, melts, gives rise to differences again, and so on. We try to begin now more innocently and indefinitely, letting events assume their own proportions, even as we contribute to giving them form.

---

[1] This is a reprint of an article published in the International Gestalt Journal (2002) 25(1): 109–122.

Such an outlook is more related to wave theory in modern physics than to the older particle theory. Gestalt therapy has always assumed the therapeutic primacy of collaborative attention between therapist and client at the contact boundary, rather than within the psyche of either the client or the therapist. However, the newer perspective goes beyond the classical formulation of two well-differentiated beings meeting at the contact boundary; for there is a more complex shape-shifting and shape-giving going on than that. But discussing this further would take me too far afield.

Notice that this emphasis on staying with something that is unfolding brings in the dimension of time and therefore of change and development. "Staying with" begins in the present moment, but it is not about the moment. It is about the passing moment, which instantly turns into something else the minute you enter it. After all, we live in time, not in some timeless present moment, which doesn't exist anyway. To stay with a moment would be a neurotic fixation. Erving Polster introduces the temporal dimension of Gestalt therapy in the most direct manner by emphasizing how sequences, whether behavioral or narrative, are composed from the simple principle that "one thing leads to another" (Polster, personal communication).

When you stay with and ride such sequences, which sometimes can be like riding a bucking bronco, and sometimes like driving a sports car on an open highway, you will find that all roads lead to Rome. In other words, you can begin any place in therapy, and if you follow the process, you get to the heart of the matter. But the question remains: what is "Rome"? I would argue that Rome is neither the core of the personality nor the authentic self, nor even the important past traumas, though such issues might arise and become important on the way to Rome. What I would say is that Rome doesn't yet exist; it has to be made. The process of staying with the experience plays a central part in what one makes.

My intention here is to enlarge this question of "staying with" beyond a technical principle for psychotherapy. For me it has become both an aesthetic principle of transformation and an ethical position. I am going to call this a Gestalt therapy view of commitment. We talk a lot about commitment these days, but in a way that is deadening, as in "You should be more committed to this relationship" or "to this career". A common contemporary formula for the failure of relationships is that "men can't commit themselves to love". Would anyone want to commit himself or herself to love or a career dictated externally in this way? It turns commitment into a prison sentence, all too close to the word's meaning when psychiatrists "commit" someone to the locked ward of the asylum.

But there is a more organic and immediate sense of commitment, which goes something like this: if it feels good, important, or useful today, you will probably stay tomorrow. I believe it was the 19th-century American writer Ralph Waldo Emerson who said that a good life is an accumulation of good days. "Good" here does not mean necessarily happy or pleasurable but worthwhile, namely worthwhile to you. Neither Emerson's view nor mine is about what is often called the pursuit of happiness. You can't really pursue happiness or a good life, which can only be a projection – because it is an ideal of something complete – so either you can never catch up with it, or it has already passed you by. But if you stay with the vital actuality of this moment and the next one, you might look back one day and realize that you have had a good life – or at least a full one. As a matter of fact, nothing that is complete inspires commitment. It is done, so you want to leave it behind before you get bored to death. When you have a great conversation with a friend, one way you know it, is that when you say goodbye, you still feel you have a lot more to say. All the topics are still open and running. Healthy commitment is like this; you stay because what you are committed to still feels interestingly incomplete and thus alive.

In the case of these two artists I am going to discuss – Cézanne and Miles Davis – their art was always incomplete, so they kept searching. What I hope to show is that such a view leads to an aesthetics of commitment, and not a tyranny of commitment. It may even give rise to a vision of commitment as a kind of cure for ills, such as anxiety and depression, in place of Prozac and Zoloft and their relatives.

Whatever else commitment is, it involves a kind of discipline. The founders of Gestalt therapy were by no means indifferent to either commitment or discipline. For instance, Frederick "Fritz" Perls wasn't much given to social or cultural criticism, as Paul Goodman was, though both were anarchists. Perls was interested mainly in the quality of individual life. But now and then he would launch an attack on some aspect of American society that he felt was playing an important part in killing off people's lives. His most telling critique was aimed at the American pursuit of happiness, which Perls called hedonism. "We have made a 180-degree turn from puritanism and moralism to hedonism", he wrote in the opening pages of Gestalt Therapy Verbatim. "Suddenly everything has to be fun, pleasure, and any sincere involvement, any really being here, is discouraged" (1988, pp. 1–2).

Perls was not attacking hedonism in the usual sense, which suggests a life dedicated to voluptuous sensual pleasure. That might have been okay with Perls. But he regarded American hedonism as a shallow, plastic conception of a good time, which mostly amounted to avoiding pain. The only way to accomplish this was to desensitize oneself. As a result, there was a profound loss of awareness, because one gave up the capacity to feel anything, including love, joy, or pleasure. The pursuit of happiness led to the loss of the capacity to experience life fully. You can imagine what Perls would have thought of instant cures like giving medication to everyone who goes through a period of anxiety or depression. He went on to say in Verbatim: "There is only one way to regain our soul, or in American terms, to revive the American corpse and bring him back to life. The paradox is that in order to get this spontaneity we need, like in Zen, an utmost discipline" (ibid., p. 51).

Whereas for Fritz Perls, commitment and discipline meant staying with the moment-to-moment awareness of whatever was going on in one's actual situation, for Laura Perls, commitment and discipline meant staying with and accepting the limitations of one's actual circumstances and making the most creative use of what was available. In her beautiful little talk[2] on a Japanese movie, "The Woman in the Dunes", she says:

"As long as our man in the story cannot accept the limitations of the situation, he feels trapped. When he accepts his confinement, possibilities within its boundaries become re- alities: the desert becomes fertile, the woman a mother. This opens the trap, the bound- aries widen. By committing himself anew to the somewhat changed but still limited and difficult situation, the man takes responsibility for the *consequences* of his own creative activities (...) By accepting and coping with 'what is', he transforms and transcends the situation and achieves true freedom" (1986, p. 13).

Laura Perls' statement seems to me particularly important. Like Hegel, she is saying that there is no freedom without necessity. In other words, true freedom comes after commitment and discipline – in both the arts and in love. Most people seem to think it goes the other way around.

Which brings me to my two central characters or "case histories" in this narrative. Why Cézanne and Miles Davis? Largely because they are two of my great favorites. But there is a theme that I think they both exemplify (and it will be obvious I could have chosen any number of other artists). Both were frequently troubled and at times just plain miserable in their personal lives: Cézanne full of anxiety and self-doubt; Miles Davis full of dark rage and melancholy. What is important is that no matter how difficult things be- came, neither of them ever wandered far from their commitment to the con- tinual practice of their art and to the deepest search for personal truth within the framework of artistic expression.

II. Paul Cézanne

Cézanne's quest to give form to the subjective immediate truth of his per- ceptions never wavered once he left law school. He had gone to law school out of obedience to the wishes of his bourgeois father, who was a hat-maker and later became a banker. Leaving law school to paint was an act of rebel- lion against his family's way of life. It was not easy for him to do. It left him anxious, self-doubting, and angry for much of his life. He also remained ter- rified of his father. When he fell in love with a woman and moved in with her, he didn't have the nerve to tell his father, even after they had a child.

He was a difficult man. This is how John Rewald, his chief biographer and editor of his letters, describes him:

"Light-hearted and carefree in his youth, he later becomes suspicious and withdrawn. His expressions vary between tenderness, even humility, and arrogance; his self-reliance sometimes changes to bitterness and disappointment; his forgiveness and politeness can rapidly turn into rudeness" (in Cézanne, 1976, p. 6).

He was never satisfied. But he never stopped painting with the greatest intensity of focus. His suffering – his anxiety and anger – surely increased

---

[2] This talk was given on May 17, 1985, as an opening address to the 8th annual conference on the theory and practice of Gestalt therapy, published in The Gestalt Journal (1986), and re- printed in *Living at the Boundary* (Perls L, 1992, pp. 221–226) under the title "Commitment".

when the critics denounced his early paintings as trash and claimed that he had no talent. He suffered from this, but it never stopped him.

In 1874, when Cézanne exhibited his paintings at the first Impressionist exhibition, he was derided by the critics, as were most of the other Impressionists. But Cézanne got the worst of it. One critic described him as "a sort of madman who paints in delirium tremens" (Wechsler, 1975, p. 3). After three more years of this kind of reception, Cézanne withdrew from the public eye until 1889. In a state of relative isolation he kept on painting. If anything, he became more intensely committed to rendering the originality of his own vision, the truth of his perceptions.

By 1895, his reputation had changed: Cézanne had become known as a painter's painter – Pissarro, Renoir, Degas, and Monet were among those deeply impressed with his work – and by 1904, it was said that his influence was to be seen everywhere in the world of art (ibid., p. 5). By now, there has hardly been a modern intellectual movement that hasn't taken Cézanne to its bosom as a key figure and offered its own interpretation of his work. One art historian gives the following list: Naturalist, Symbolist, Neoclassical, perceptual, formalist, didactic, Marxist, psychoanalytic (both Freudian and Jungian), phenomenological and existentialist (ibid., p. 2). The English novelist D. H. Lawrence, the German poet Rilke, and the French philosopher Maurice Merleau-Ponty all wrote major commentaries on Cézanne.

Cézanne painted out of a loyalty to his subjectivity so pure that his paintings themselves became a way of seeing, rather than a way of adding feelings or symbols or meanings to what he saw. He single-handedly evolved a new language for painting, which influenced every painter in Western civilization who came after him. His withdrawal from society and public view may have been inspired partly by anxiety or depression or whatever, but he transformed his aloneness into a kind of epistemological research into the perceiving subject through the medium of painting. This was a profound act of commitment. A recent critic, Kurt Badt, has written:

"The mere fact that he took his own person and destiny as subject-matter for his art marked Cézanne out as a modern painter; his modernity was further demonstrated by the fact (not unconnected) that loneliness played a great and significant role in his art. By dedicating himself wholly to his art, he now accepted [around 1870] the fate of loneliness as an essential prerequisite of his work, surrendered to it, and thereby gained that new view of the world, which was expressed in all his work from now on" (in Wechsler, 1975, p. 142).

Badt regards this as something approaching a conversion of a religious nature. He contrasts it with the Impressionists who saw nature as lovely and consoling:

"Whereas other artists worked in an atmosphere of self-enjoyment, in a subjective and intimate relationship with the subjects which they were painting (...) Cézanne on the other hand painted in a state of self-oblivion, dedicating himself wholly to the objects in whose essential nature he sought to penetrate" (ibid., p. 143).

Meyer Schapiro, one of the great art historians and critics of our time, said of Cézanne, that "his work is a living proof that a painter can achieve a profound expression by giving form to his perceptions of the world around him without recourse to a guiding religion or myth or any explicit social aims" (1988, p. 29). D. H. Lawrence wrote that "the most interesting figure in modern art, and the only really interesting figure, is Cézanne: and that, not so much because of his achievement as because of his struggle" (1980, p. 571). Cézanne's aloneness, his struggle, and his devotion to his own perceptions are all facets of his commitment.

III. Miles Davis

Miles Davis was also an angry and distressed man. He was raised in a well-to-do African-American family in St. Louis (his father was a dentist), a background that made him all the more sensitive to and enraged by the racism he encountered everywhere outside the family. His life was often a hell, first because of addiction to heroin and alcohol, both of which he kicked, later because of renewed drug use and serious illness. But nothing swayed him from playing the trumpet from the time he was ten, and during his extraordinary jazz career, he never stopped searching for new ways to give musical expression to his vision of life.

He was not exactly an easy man to get along with, especially where race was concerned. He was known for turning his back on his audience in jazz clubs and playing his horn to the other members of his band. When his mind was scrambled by drugs or alcohol, he was given to staging outrageous scenes in public. Here is a not untypical anecdote from the poet Quincy Troupe's biography of Davis:

"There was the time when Miles abandoned his Ferrari in the middle of West End Avenue after spotting a policeman he thought was following him. He was so paranoid and high on cocaine that he ran into an apartment building and jumped into an elevator. A startled white woman was already inside the elevator; when he saw her, he slapped her face and asked her what she doing in his car. She ran screaming out of the elevator, and Miles took it up to the top floor, where he stayed, hiding in the garbage disposal room until late in the evening" (2000, p. 22).

But then, contrast this with Troupe's description of Mile's playing:

"Miles Davis was a great poet on his instrument. His horn could blow warm, round notes that spoke to the deepest human emotions. (...) Miles' sound always made us sit up and take notice. It was burnished, brooding, unforgettable. (...) When you heard Miles on the radio, you knew right away that it was him. You knew it by the sound because no one else ever sounded like that. Like Louis Armstrong's, Duke Ellington's, Thelonious Monk's, John Coltrane's, his voice was unmistakably unique" (ibid., p. 1).

How does one get from the mess of Miles Davis' life to the poetry of his jazz? The answer is the unshakeable disciplined commitment to the mastery of his art. The need to play his horn enabled him to overcome his addictions because they interfered too much. He took a lesson in the need for discipline from his lifelong love of boxing. As he explains in his autobiography (1989, p. 174), his model was the great prizefighter, Sugar Ray Robinson:

"Anyway, I really kicked my habit because of the example of Sugar Ray Robinson; I figured if he could, as disciplined as he was, then I could do it, too. (...) When he was in the ring, he was serious, all business. I decided that that was the way I was going to be, serious about taking care of my business and disciplined."

Davis was by no means unusual among jazz musicians in his involvement with drugs, his moodiness, even his frequent bizarre behavior in public or on the stage, although few performers have produced displays as dramatic as his. The habits or behavior of jazz musicians, combined with the fact that their performances are based on spontaneous improvisation, may lead one to imagine that they are undisciplined about their art. But this is a thoroughly mistaken idea. In his book surveying the impact of Miles Davis on American culture, Gerald Early (2001, p. 13) quotes the novelist Ralph Ellison, who knew jazz very well on this topic. Ellison makes it clear that he learned a good deal from jazz musicians about the commitment a writer needs:

"Now, I had learned from jazz musicians I had known as a boy in Oklahoma City something of the discipline and devotion to his art required of the artist. (...) These jazzmen, many of them now world-famous, lived for and with their music intensely. Their driving motivation was neither money nor fame, but the will to achieve the most eloquent expression of idea-emotions through the technical mastery of their instruments. (...) I had learned too that the end of all this discipline and technical mastery was the desire to express an affirmative way of life. (...) Life could be harsh, loud and wrong if it wished, but they lived it fully, and when they expressed their attitude toward the world it was with a fluid style that reduced the chaos of living to form."

IV. Expression of Subjectivity

Perhaps neither Cézanne nor Miles Davis led lives that we are likely to envy. Some of us may think there is nothing we would rather be than a great painter or jazz musician. But it wasn't easy to be Paul Cézanne or Miles Davis. Both their lives were filled with trouble. Out of their turmoil, both withdrew from public view for many years. In the practice of their art, however, they were both committed to an extraordinary degree to their search for the fullest expression of their unique subjectivity. Miles Davis listened to the world and listened to himself. He listened to the voices of black people expressing anguish, lamentation, and joy. He listened to the whole history of the music they made, and to every other kind of music, and he listened to the branches swept by wind, the ocean's monologue, and the sounds of the city. And he strove to shape all of it into music that gave expression to what he heard as it made its way through his own existence. Cézanne looked at his world with an absolute absorption and then worked and worked at painting the experience of what he saw without resorting to ideology, convention, symbolism, or any external props. Neither of them ever rested on their accomplishments, because they never felt that the task was complete.

By virtue of their disciplined, undivided attention to and absorption in the subjective truth of their experience, each of these artists created new forms that changed the course of everything that followed. Neither painting nor jazz was ever again the same after them. Cézanne, leaving impressionism behind, almost single-handedly created modern art. Miles Davis, who came of age during the be-bop era, invented almost single-handedly "cool jazz" and then went on to create most of the new possibilities that have shaped jazz to this day.

How would one apply this ideal of disciplined commitment to an intimate relationship, for example? As far as I'm concerned, no one gives us a better sense of this than D. H. Lawrence, whom I still regard as a wise authority on love. In a fine essay called "We Need One Another", Lawrence writes the following about the relationship between commitment and sexual desire:

"And what is sex, after all, but the symbol of the relation of man to woman, woman to man? And the relation of man to woman is wide as all life. It consists in infinite different flows between the two beings, different, even apparently contrary. Chastity is part of the flow between man and woman, as to physical passion. And beyond these, an infinite range of subtle communication, which we know nothing about. I should say that the relation between any two decently married people changes profoundly every few years, often without their knowing anything about it; though every change causes pain, even if it brings a certain joy. The long course of marriage is a long event of perpetual change, in which a man and a woman mutually build up their souls and make themselves whole. It is like rivers flowing on through new country, always unknown.

But we are so foolish, and fixed by our limited ideas. A man says: "I don't love my wife any more, I no longer want to sleep with her." But why should he always want to sleep with her? How does he know what other subtle and vital interchange is going on between him and her, making them both whole, in this period when he doesn't want to sleep with her? And she, instead of jibbing and saying that all is over and she must find another man and get a divorce – why doesn't she pause, and listen for a new rhythm in her soul, and look for the new movement in the man? With every change, a new being emerges, a new rhythm establishes itself; we renew our life as we grow older, and there is real peace. Why, oh, why do we want one another to be always the same, fixed, like a menu card that is never changed?

If only we had more sense. But we are held by a few fixed ideas, like sex, money, what a person 'ought' to be, and so forth, and we miss the whole of life. Sex is a changing thing, now alive, now quiescent, now fiery, now apparently quite gone, quite gone. But the ordinary man and woman haven't the gumption to take it in all its changes. They demand crass, crude sex-desire, they demand it always, and when it isn't forthcoming, then – smash-bash! smash up the whole show. Divorce! Divorce!" (1933, pp. 36–38).

I have been reflecting on these themes for a long time – beginning with an old article called "Notes On Art and Symptoms" (Miller, 1980). There I spoke about the aesthetic transformation of mental suffering in psychotherapy, taking the model from what artists do. This has led me to an idea not only of transformation as the outcome but commitment as the process that does not deny one's pain or difficulty in life, but achieves a kind of "cure" by making productive use of it. To my thinking, this sort of commitment is love in the broadest sense, whether in an intimate relationship or in pursuit of one's calling. It's a way of staying connected to life in a difficult and imperfect world, rather than withdrawing into depression, which often is just the other side of a demand that one's life be paradise and a refusal to settle for anything less ("Paradise or nothing", goes the depressive's cry). As I have already pointed out in agreement with Perls and Lawrence, such commitments oppose the shallow "pursuit of happiness", in which one throws out a relationship and seeks another as soon as there are problems, or takes a pill in the hope of abolishing anxiety and depression without any effort at self-exploration or any taking of responsibility.

I'm not one who likes to mix psychotherapy and spiritual questions. But I have to confess that an aesthetic understanding of commitment, rooted in the quest to give form to the truth of one's experience, sometimes makes me wonder if their relationship can be ignored. The aesthetics of commitment is as close as I can come to an ideal of faith or spiritual devotion that might direct one toward a higher freedom. For me, artists like Cézanne and Davis exemplify the idea expressed in Kierkegaard's title: *Purity of Heart is to Will One Thing* (1956). This doesn't mean being a monomaniac or an obsessive; it means giving your full attention to what you are doing at the moment and bestowing the fullest true form on the moment that you can give it. Kierkegaard here contrasts this with what he calls "doublemindedness", by which he means denial, self-deception, evasion or anesthetization of anxiety and depression. To give your wholehearted attention and creativity to the truth, even to the truth of suffering, leads to transcendence and transformation of it, as Laura Perls points out. Kierkegaard calls this willing the Good. True enough, artists have often led questionable or terrible lives; but in their work, they seem to discover how to will the Good. As models of how to live from day to day, their lives tend to be of little use; but, their ways of working can teach us a great deal about the paths to a better life.

References

Cézanne P (1976) Letters. Hacker Art Books, New York

Davis M, Troupe Q (1989) Miles: The autobiography. Simon and Schuster, New York

Early G (ed) (2001) Miles Davis and American culture. Missouri Historical Society Press, Saint Louis

Kierkegaard S (1956) Purity of heart is to will one thing. (Translation by DV Steere) Harper Torchbooks, New York

Lawrence DH (1980) Phoenix: The posthumous papers, 1936. (Translation by E McDonald) Penguin Books, New York

Lawrence DH (1933) We need one another. Equinox, New York

Miller MV (1980) Notes on art and symptoms. In: Rosenblatt D (ed) A Festschrift for Laura Perls. Special Issue. The Gestalt J 3(1): 86–98

Perls FS (1988) Gestalt therapy verbatim: With a new introduction by Michael V Miller. Gestalt J Press, Highland, New York

Perls L (1986) Commitment: Opening Address, 8th Annual Conference on the Theory and Practice of Gestalt Therapy, May 17, 1985. In: The Gestalt J 9(1): 12–15

Perls L (1992) Living at the boundary. Gestalt J Press, Highland, New York

Schapiro M (1988) Cézanne. Harry N Abrams, Inc., New York

Troupe Q (2000) Miles and me. Univ of California Press, Berkeley

Wechsler J (ed) (1975) Cézanne in perspective. Prentice-Hall, Englewood Cliffs, New Jersey

Contact and Creativity:
The Gestalt Cycle in Context

Gordon Wheeler

Creativity may be usefully defined as the capacity to generate novel solutions to problems, which includes of course the ability to see the world in problem-solving terms in the first place. Clearly, this creative capacity is the defining characteristic of our species, an extremely young branch of the primate order, which has managed to arise and then spread over the entire planet in the course of only 3000 or so generations, a mere blink of evolutionary time. This capacity, in turn, rests in some way on our biological history: specifically, the remarkably rapid expansion of brain tissue in our ancestral line, in which the neocortex together with its infoldings has multiplied some fourfold in surface area in the brief evolutionary window of only a couple of million years (Calvin, 2002). Plainly, a pace this rapid points to a strong positive feedback loop between adaptation and evolutionary pressure, one in which each new degree of development opens up new environmental territory, which then exerts strong selective pressure for expansion of that new capacity, in the recursive way of evolution. It is this expansion, together with accompanying reorganization, that has both permitted and been driven by the growth and elaboration of imaginal power and the nesting of active and long-term memory, which are key to our ability to *experiment* – i.e., to create and try out these novel solutions flexibly, both "in our heads" and in the "real world".

To achieve all this, we are evolutionarily "hard-wired" (to use the current cybernetic metaphor) to live by and through a more or less continuous problem-solving process, generating novelty by engaging in an ongoing recursive sequence of near-constant scanning of our world (both "inner" and "outer"), registering contrasts and differences, elaborating an organized picture or map as we go (the "best available gestalt"), relating that map to an emotional valence, running "scenarios" in our head on the basis of those scans and that valence, estimating outcome probabilities, and using the integrated whole of this process as a ground for experiment and action, and all the rest of that flexible, recombinant organization of perception that we know as *experience* (see Wheeler, 2000). This is our ongoing human-process strategy for surviving, meeting challenges, and seeking to grow, given our biological nature as low-instinct, high-learning animals, who aren't good at much of anything except this creative problem-solving ability itself. With it, we have managed to outperform and outlast rival hominid and other species across the entire variable range of planetary (and now some extra-planetary) environments.

At the same time, this recursive sequence also amounts to a description of our inborn *gestalt-process nature*, the basic data and subject matter of our Gestalt model of understanding and intervention for change. Thus creativity, seen in this way, is no more than our *gestalt nature in action* – what in the Gestalt model is meant by the rich term *contact*, the construction of meaningful (i.e., useful, experimental/predictive) whole pictures of understanding in the integrated field of experience and living (Lewin, 1936; Perls et al., 1951).

How this process of contact works – the unfolding of a creative sequence – has been explored and elaborated in a number of ways in Gestalt teaching and literature. Prominent among them is the heuristic/diagnostic model known as the Contact Cycle, or Cycle of Experience, which outlines the life history of an impulse or desire, tracing a path from sensation and awareness (the formation of a sense of need), through the heightening of energy and mobilization (gathering attentional focus and muscular tonus preparatory to moving), action toward the goal, "contact" in the sense of transaction or resolution, withdrawal/closure, and then on to the next sensation and need (see Fig. 1). Whether the contact/solution achieved is then novel/creative or familiar and routine is not addressed by the model: if anything, examples in the literature tend to be simple biological urges that are relatively unproblematic in the field (see Wheeler, 1991). Either way, the implication here is that this sequence is natural and "organismic", basically biological in nature; thus, left to itself, it should simply run out to a series of satisfying outcomes (barring internal interruptions or "resistances"), and presumably also coordinate those goals and paths with the sometimes nested, sometimes contradictory unfolding of other goals (and the goals of others!) – all somewhere outside the borders of the schematic, by a homeostatic process of "organismic self-regulation" (Perls et al., 1951).

And yet, biological underpinnings and organismic self-regulation, however important, can only be part of the story of creativity. For by the same terms of our high-flexibility, high-learning, and low-instinct animal nature, we are also the most intensely and richly *social* of animals, the animal most characterized by extreme neotony (immature birth) and consequent long period of childhood dependency and concentrated social learning. Thus, too, we are *relational* by our very nature, "pre-wired" again for interpersonal orientation and *intersubjectivity*, that capacity for looking at others as well as ourselves in terms of our shared motivational process (which is another way of saying our integrated gestalt/constructivist nature, or flexible organization of the experiential field in terms of our felt needs [Wheeler, 2000]). That is, we don't just look at others: we look at others *looking at us*. Of course, to be used at all well, this capacity for knowing and using the social field intersubjectively must be learned in development; but our prepotent ability to learn it is itself inborn and basic to our beings, in that infinite recursion of nature and nurture that characterizes all of life, but is the very hallmark of

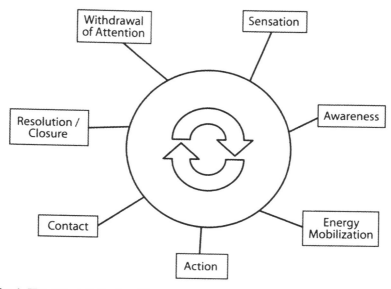

Fig. 1. The "Gestalt Cycle of Experience: Flow of an Uninterrupted Sequence" (from Nevis, 1987, used by permission)

our species. For humans, as the biologist Paul Ehrlich [2000] observes, nature *is* nurture.

Unfortunately, little or nothing of this social, relational ground of our being is evident in our familiar Gestalt Cycle models. As customarily drawn (Fig. 1), the Cycle gives us a schematic of the life history of an impulse in isolation, as if existing separately from its "inner" context of competing or overlapping desires and background of beliefs, expectations, and values – and separately as well from the "outer" context (which is also a living part of our "inner" life) of *other people*, who make up our relevant landscape and our contextual world. Now, certainly, every abstracted model plays on a necessary tradeoff between lifelike complexity, on the one hand, and clarity and simplicity of use on the other: a map, as we know, is not the territory being mapped – nor would it be useful if it were. Rather, a model is no more (and no less) than a lens, which serves to bring certain features into sharper focus while inevitably obscuring others; and as long as this model is held and used as it should be, as a diagnostic and heuristic tool (and not in any sense a full, normative picture of the real flow of human process and experience), then we may hope to avoid the more reductionistic implications of the diagram. Alas, examples of such normative, reductionistic teaching and applications of the Cycle model abound, amounting at times to a trivialization of the Gestalt perspective itself, and of its unique power for clarifying our interventions and our understanding of human affairs.[1]

---

[1] Exceptions to this oversimplification include the work of E. Nevis, Zinker, Melnick, and S. Nevis, all of whom make important steps in the direction of an interpersonal or relational version of the model.

In particular, the Cycle models, as usually drawn, may often seem to imply that the only significant place to look for the dynamics driving human behavior is basically "inside" the person. Such a sharply individualistic bias distorts and constricts our understanding of human process in social field in general, and creative process in particular. Viewed in terms of this diagram, creativity would then have to be seen as an essentially mystical business, arising somehow solely from within – more or less the "genius" or inspiration model of the Romantic tradition (deriving in turn from the hypertrophied individualism of the Greeks. In the Greek version, remember, creativity was ascribed to the Muses, those female deities whose job it was to give inspiration or breath to creative genius – which was itself of course *male*, in the misogynistic reading so often found in hyper-individualistic cultures). Recontextualizing and redrawing the model in its living context can then serve to shed light on some quite different, often neglected features of our human landscape, with a corresponding expansion of its power to clarify the dynamics of creative experience and behavior.

I. The Cycle in Context

And yet, the various Cycle models have proved highly durable and useful in a variety of applications (perhaps most of all in interpersonal and systemic analyses, where it is much harder to confound this schematic map with any ideal of personal experience and process [see Nevis, 1987; Zinker, 1977]). How then can we embed the model more clearly in its natural ground of the living social field, making it more "experience-near", and then using it to shed light on the dynamics of creative process? First of all, focusing on the social context in this way points to a *hidden discontinuity* in the model as traditionally drawn, at the stage where the cycle moves from mobilization to action (see Fig. 2). What is obscured here is a *state or phase transition*, from the "inner" world of more or less private thoughts, feelings, impulses, and desires, to the "outer" world of public action, with a sharply discontinuous rise in perils, stakes, and possibilities for satisfaction or otherwise. Let us then redraw the diagram with this in mind, "uncurling" the circle into a wavy line (somewhat as Nevis [1987] does) and placing it in its *experiential field context*, with that field organized around this rough "me/not-me" boundary (to use Sullivan's language [1953]) – which is the pre-organization Stern (1985), Fogel (1993) and others point to as a prepotent categorizing principle of our development from birth on.[2] At the same time, in place of a one-dimensional line, we will indicate a gathering stream or channel of attentional focus, with felt boundaries between what lies inside and outside that particular organizing concern.

---

[2] But note that this is still a highly Western, individualized way of putting this field differential, as if my community, relationships, and other commitments were clearly "not me". A less culturally biased labeling might be "body-self"/"field self" – or perhaps personal/transpersonal, as in many religious and other spiritual perspectives.

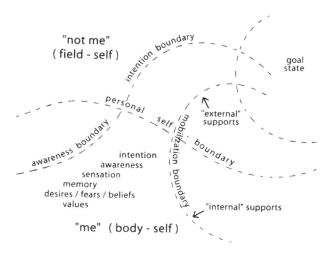

Fig. 2. The Cycle in Context: Organizing/Managing the Experiential Field
(from Wheeler, in press, used by permission[3])

Here (Fig. 2) the phase transition we spoke of above, from private to public, becomes the chief organizing principle of the diagram as it is in development and in so much of our lived and felt experience. Below the dotted line, we have all the "inner" realm of desires, fears, intentions, past experience both encouraging and discouraging, and integrated learning, which form the "inner ground" of belief and action. Above it, on the diagram, lies the "outside world", the world of resources and risks, supports and obstacles, most significantly in the form of *other people*. All of us know the sharp intake of breath or deep sigh that can precede that moment of boundary-crossing or "plunging into" this outer world, a moment signaled at times by phrases like "Here goes nothing", or even "Cover my back", spoken to oneself or aloud to an onlooker/supporter. Drawing the picture in this way helps clarify a number of experiential issues and processes that were passed over in the circle diagram: for example, *attentional dynamics and process* (by showing more clearly how attentional boundaries must be energized and supported: see Kent-Ferraro and Wheeler, 2003); *play* (see Mortola P, Wheeler G, *Play*. The Analytic Press/Gestalt Press, Hillsdale, New Jersey, in press), and above all the crucial issue of *support* (Wheeler, 2000). In each case, insight and intervention power are gained by relocating these processes in the social field, which is their dynamic contextual home.

For our purposes here, let us then "zero in" on that moment or space of transition itself, the place where my field-organizing process takes the fate-

---

[3] Wheeler G (in press) Experiment and play: The cycle reconsidered. In: Mortola P, Wheeler G (eds) Play. The Analytic Press/GestaltPress, Hillsdale, New Jersey.

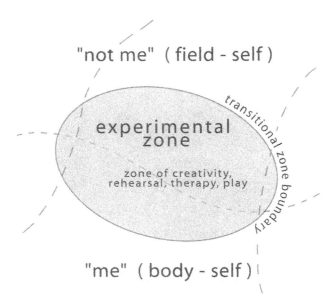

Fig. 3. The "Experimental Zone" Phase-transitional Space

ful step out of the world of feelings, fantasy, and the physical body, and into the wider, more perilous world of nurturance, rich resources, rich satisfactions and potential disasters (Fig. 3).

Here we focus specifically on the "space-between" the inner and outer worlds of experience (at this point we will drop the quotation marks around these quite problematic terms, *inner* and *outer*, which are often used in a sharply individualistic sense, as if the two realms were rigidly separate rather than highly interpenetrable and mutually informing, as they actually are in lived experience). The interpenetration of the two experiential worlds is indicated here by the heavy dotted line across the diagram in Fig. 3, which both distinguishes *and joins* the individual with the social surround. The infant is born, to be sure, "preprogrammed" to begin integrating self-experience in terms of this basic field-organizational difference, "me/not-me" (or better, again, "body-self/field-self"), but still that boundary is always flexible, situational, highly mobile, and varyingly flexed or relaxed depending on the degree of perceived danger, safety, and support.

The first thing we can note about this zone, as we have drawn it here, is how that crossover space *partakes of both worlds*, both the inner and the outer. At the same time, by drawing a boundary around it, we mark a *third space*, a transitional zone which draws freely on *both* the feelings and fantasies of the private zone *and* the physical reality of the public zone, while still being relatively protected from the high stakes and life-threatening risks that can characterize that outer realm, the "real world". Even physical objects in this third space have the character of Winnicott's (1965) "transitional

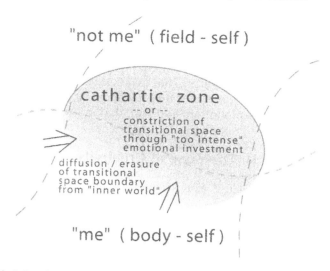

Fig. 4. Aristotle's Cathartic Theory of Drama: Full Dissolution of Boundary between "Inner Space" and the "Play World"

objects", items which have tangible reality while still embodying issues and meanings from the inner, imaginal world. Children's toys, such as teddy bears, dolls, and comfort objects such as blankets often have this dual character, but so too do many of the tools, toys, and commitments or activities of adulthood – what Kohut (1977) termed "self-objects", a term which points (from a different perspective) to their dual nature, as well as their role in serving the maintenance of a coherent sense of self.

This zone is then the particular arena of *rehearsal, experiment, and play.* Games, which are *formally bounded play*, belong by definition to this transitional zone – with the boundary of the space coinciding with the boundary of the game. That is, a game, like all play, is simultaneously *both real and not real.* If it is not felt as real enough – if the play does not partake of "inner space" – then I have no investment in it, I don't care enough to be "really playing" (the kind of reproach children may sometimes make if one is only "going through the motions", when what they wanted was a "real playmate"). On the other hand, if I lose all sense of boundary between the game space and the "real world", then I become a problematic game partner, one who is "overinvolved", in a competitive sport for example, forgetting that the activity was "only a game" (for further discussion of play from a Gestalt perspective, see Mortola and Wheeler, in press).

This is also the space of *story-telling, drama and, by extension, all of art.* Aristotle's cathartic theory of drama, the communal emotional purging of the audience, depends on a momentary forgetting of the fact that what we are watching is "not real", i.e., the temporary loss of that distinction, which is represented on the diagram by the lower arc of the oval (see Fig. 4). When we cry, or experience terror, or feel ennobled in a movie, play, or novel, we are enacting Aristotle's view of dramatic art, "losing ourselves" for a time in the experience.[4] By the same reasoning, Brecht (1967) objected to this kind of drama, as serving to lull the audience into complacency by containing and draining away their empathy and political outrage in the artificial space of theater: this is the rationale of his political "theater of alienation", in which he reminds the audience constantly that this is only a play, that happy endings are not real for real people, and that it is the real political world outside the theater, of poverty, exploitation, and war, that matters.

II. The Zone of Creativity

Thus, this transitional space is also the zone of *imagination*, which is to say the *zone of creativity*. What we do in this transitional space is by definition experimental: we try out novel combinations of elements, features, problems, and solutions – all that imaginal activity which we have said it is our special human nature to be able to do. Indeed, generally speaking we *cannot not* do this, much or most of the time, barring serious trauma. And here, trauma itself may be defined as those events which resist integration and thus are not available to the creative zone: i.e., they become "frozen gestalts", patterns and sequences that then are not susceptible to this kind of deconstruction, creative recombination, and play. Such events may be said to have been *undergone* without being fully *experienced* – i.e., integrated into an *organized, flexible, and usable narrative whole of meaning*. The hallmark of such fully integrated experience is then precisely that it may be *played with* – which is to say, manipulated creatively.

   In order to be capable of this, our brain/minds are necessarily organized *narratively* – i.e., as mutually embedded *gestalts with a time dimension* (see Wheeler, 2000). In Gestalt terms, narrative is the structure of ground, the organization of experience into story-telling units suitable for recombination, manipulation, and recall. That is, we run scenarios in our heads – trial narratives or "what if's" – that play out different scenes and sequences, various combinations of imagined outcomes, wishes, fears, and other considerations, all in imaginary or experimental space. We are able to do this specifically because of the felt difference represented by the upper boundary line in the diagram, which distinguishes the trial narrative zone – i.e., *creative space* – from the zone of "real-life" stakes. Thus we begin to see how protecting this space is an essential field condition for creative process.

   As long as the experiment remains purely imaginary, we are still in the lower region of the oval on the diagram, the zone of daydreams (and night dreams) and fantasies, memories and hopes, regrets and fears – but also of mental rehearsal, reflection (including theory – the novel combination of concepts and ideas), and philosophy. Ultimately, all of our behavior that is choiceful, and not merely routine, grows out of this space: selection of one scenario

---

[4] Note here that this loss of separate-self sense is temporary, with the time boundary serving to replace the blurred distinction between felt emotion and the fantasy world. If the blurring is permanent, then we speak not of imagination, but delusion.

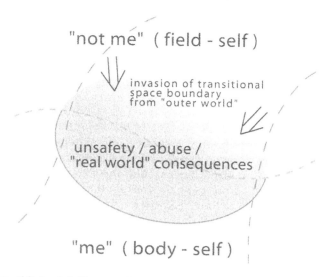

"not me" (field - self)

invasion of transitional
space boundary
from "outer world"

unsafety / abuse /
"real world" consequences

"me" (body - self)

Fig. 5. Space of Potential Abuse in Therapy: Upper Boundary Effaced (by Therapist):
Invaded Creative Space Becomes "Real Space"

over another indicates readiness to cross the dotted line – first to the upper part of the oval, *enacted experiment*, and then on to fully public space.

Or we may take that next step, crossing the dotted line to experiment with tangible materials in some way – in dialogue, in the lab, in artistic media, or in rehearsals and other kinds of trial and practice sessions. Therapy takes place in this zone, which Goodman (2003) aptly characterized as a space of "safe emergency", capturing exactly the dual nature of all creative/experimental process. Here again, therapy, like all serious play, all activity in this space, is at the same time *both real and not real* – this is what makes it a creative space, a zone for experimentation, under any model (and this is true whether or not the particular school or theory focuses, as Gestalt does, on this experimental process itself). As with game space, if the therapy is "too unreal", too *unfelt* (as, for example, through denial of the present relational validity of the encounter, in the way of the classical psychoanalytic model), then much of the activity of the client's inner world – specifically, everything having to do with present relational perceptions and feelings, the organization of the present inner/outer field – is discounted or denied, with a resulting impoverishment of the space's potential for fostering creative experiment. On the other hand, if the therapy becomes "too real", and is taken (by the therapist) as wholly taking place in the outer relational zone, then the useful distinction between the real therapeutic relationship and other kinds of "real-world" relationships is sacrificed – with the door then opened for abuse (Fig. 5). Either way, the creative potential of the process is lost, as a space specifically devoted to experiencing new relational meanings and trying out new relational sequences, under safe-enough conditions of relatively low stakes – the prerequisite for all creative process and experiment.

III. Field Conditions of Creativity

This brings us to the question of the provision and support of *field conditions for creative process* itself – always remembering that in the Gestalt model, when we speak of field, we are referring to the *whole experiential world*, both the inner *and* outer zones of perception and experience. What drawing the diagram in this way supports us to see is how *creativity depends on and is supported by the assertion/protection of the boundary around this "third space,"* the space of experimental process itself. Whenever the consequences of any trial activity or novel combination of elements and ideas threaten to become "real world" consequences, then the experimental zone is compromised to that extent, if not cancelled altogether. The higher the stakes, the more I am constrained to limit risk, sticking to familiar response patterns, even when those patterns are deeply unsatisfying. This is, after all, what we come to therapy for: because our familiar habit patterns are unsatisfying. And locked in as we are by the apparently high stakes of stepping outside them, we can find neither the perspective to see them for the learned patterns they are, nor the corrective experience to suggest there might be other ways, together with a safe-enough space for making these experiments. Therapy, we may find when we get there, is especially designed to offer this safe-enough creative space, one in which the therapist her- or himself can become a "transitional object" in this sense, for intersubjective exploration by partaking enough – but not too much – of both worlds (or better, a "transitional *subject*", a partner for a time in the transitional space of experiment and creativity). And thus, too, the therapist's special responsibility to protect the upper boundary of the oval zone on the diagram for the client, the boundary that represents the difference between this particular "real relationship" and other "real-world" relationships, thereby maintaining the *experimental, low-stakes nature* of the encounter.

These field conditions for therapeutic growth are then the same, dynamically speaking, as the field conditions for all creativity. In all these different kinds of cases – the generation of novel combinations and new trial solutions in art, science, "free play", games, theory, psychotherapy, and other relationships alike – the creative process itself depends on *field conditions of protection and support for this transitional space*, which is the essential space for experiment and novelty, and which can then partake of both experiential realms, the outer/public and the inner/private, without being overwhelmed by either. For the developing child, this support necessarily comes from adult caretakers, who affirm the child's experimental process and products, and receive and respond to trial interpretations of the world, and of relational experience – even as they may teach and steer the child toward progressively more complex, ambitious solutions. Without this support, the child has no experiential base for exploring and learning to value experimental space itself.

For the adult, support for creative space and meaningful experiment depends crucially on both 1) knowledge/validation of our inner worlds (feelings, desires, fears, and the like), so that we have new material, new imaginative combinations to work with, and 2) the identification of a *significant social group of reference*, where our own experimental combinations and trial meanings can be received and in some sense understood (as at least intelligible, if not necessarily successful or desirable). Each of these will be taken up in more detail below, as we consider how creative space is inhibited or blocked, when either or both of these essential supports are not available and felt.

IV. Shame and the Constriction of Creative Space

Any field condition that is the opposite of this support then works in the opposite way, limiting or canceling out the space where experiment and creativity arise and are played out. By "the opposite of support", in a field-self model (as distinguished from an individualist model), it is important to be clear that we do not mean just active opposition, but far more insidiously, all that complex social/emotional field dynamic we know as *shame*. Resistance, after all, is a form of engagement: when we are met with active resistance in the outside world, we may often be able to react with a redoubling of energy and an increase of creativity, including the creative organization of more support in some part of our social field. Where we cannot respond to opposition in this way, oftentimes the problem may be that support is itself tinged with feelings of shameful dependency – feelings that are themselves then material for therapy.

Engaged resistance, which may be energizing and even inspiring, becomes debilitating shame when our social world moves from opposition to our *actions*, to withdrawal and shunning of our *inner states of being, our desires, fears, feelings, and dreams*. When this is chronically or severely the case in our early years then, eventually, the developing child ceases to energize whole parts of the "inner world" at all – thereby ceasing to know, explore, try out, and develop those whole dimensions of the self. The result is that the experimental zone itself is not fully supported and energized from "below" (on the diagram): with prolonged or severe shaming, we literally don't *dare to dream*. The inevitable consequence is to shrink and weaken that zone, which is the essential space of creative process.

These problems are compounded in a hyper-individualistic culture such as ours in "the West" today, and perhaps most of all in U.S. culture, where the individualist tradition is most entrenched. In an individualistic self-model and ideology, where a rigid autonomy is often held up as the developmental ideal, support itself is necessarily pictured as weak and regressive, with sensitivity to the lack of basic social affirmation, or shame-sensitivity, typed as particularly shameful (see Wheeler, 1996, 2000). At the same time, since maximum individual self-expression is supposedly also an ideal of the system, a kind of double bind dynamic is set up, where high pressure for creative self-expression and "originality" competes with inhibited access to the inner world of free impulse and feeling, and the outer world of social belonging and support. With the experimental or creative zone weakened to that extent, and pressure to "produce" creatively still high, the result is likely to be a kind of creativity that is jerky and impulsive, asocial or anti-social, unrooted in a community of shared belongingness and meaning. Creativity in the arts may then be expected to be divorced, oftentimes, from politics, ethics, and authentic feeling. While creativity in economics and technology may easily burst forth without concern for social, political, and ecological consequences, creativity in politics and social forms themselves may seem to dry up altogether. An ancient and inherent linkage between personal ambition and the collective welfare is severed, with "self versus other" coming to be regarded as the natural order of social relations, evolution, and nature itself. Meanwhile, since the drive to integrate and resolve the whole experiential field remains the basic imperative of our human nature and process, dominance and submission may easily become the basic ordering principles of our society and the basic energetic fuel of our creative process itself. That all of this is a fair (if not universal) description of the world we actually do live in today, is an indication of the persistence of creativity in the face of adverse conditions – and of the inseparability of creative expression and form from those social field conditions themselves.

V. Expanding/Constricting the Zone of Creativity

How then do we then support and expand the creative zone, enhancing both the range and vibrancy of the arena of novel combination, low-cost trials, and new solutions and growth? Such support and enhancement must always attend to issues and sources of shame, in both the inner and outer worlds. First of all, support is always needed for the inner world of experience – all that realm we have been referring to, loosely, as private (though, of course, that privacy is relative; we often "betray" our own fears and desires, revealing things we meant to keep safely to ourselves). This support is provided automatically in healthy development through the normal process of intersubjective interaction: that is, interaction where our integrative experiential process is seen, met, and validated – even in cases when our desires or actions themselves are opposed. Again, it is not just resistance in the world of action *per se* that inhibits creativity; rather, my essential energetic zone for creative experiment shrinks when I live with the sense that my own experience, my sense of self and the world, and my attempts to integrate that sense into meaning, can find no witness, no accompaniment, no resonance in the crucial outer field of *other selves*. I find no vital belonging in my natural social environment; the world I am given is *not my world*.

And here we see how that sense of inner/outer, which serves at times to organize my self-experience so usefully for action, and which is perhaps most strongly clear in states of opposition, is only a flexion of a boundary that remains always interpenetrable, always just one possible organizing dynamic of a vital, living whole. In adulthood, the remedy for a lack of that affirming resonance, that support for novel organization of at least the inner world of experience, always involves identifying and identifying with a *dif-*

ferent social group of reference. Underneath the romantic Western cultural image of the solitary hero on *his* intrepid quest (the image is heavily gender-typed) lies a reality of rich social support, whether from a present affirming group of fellow-dissenters, and/or from a more distant reference group of meaning, through identification and inspiration. Thus Mandela finds creative inspiration through identification with M. L. King and others, King with Gandhi, Gandhi with Thoreau, Thoreau with early American Puritan dissidents, who themselves identified with Jesus, and so on. Indeed, we may think of maturity and mature "autonomy" not, as Perls famously remarked, as the transition from "other-supports to self-supports," but rather much more complexly and intersubjectively, as the transition from *dependence on and identification with immediately present others* (as the child on/with its care-takers), to the richer autonomy of an adult capacity to *select those social supports and contexts* that best integrate with our wider adult goals and deeper adult values. We do not "outgrow" our need for socially resonant others in favor of an isolated "autonomous self" to support our own creative learning and growth: rather, we become more able to carry this essential, referential social support with us, and use it to protect and support the "creative zone," which is where that experimentation and growth take place.

VI. Creativity and "Internalized Shame"

But what if the absence of that essential context for contact and intersubjective resonance was so severe and prolonged in development as to amount to an ongoing trauma or post-trauma condition (remembering that trauma, in a Gestalt view, may be understood as that which chronically resists integration, substituting pattern repetition or "frozen gestalts" for our normal, creative capacity for novel integration of the experiential field)? This is then the self/field-condition known as "internalized shame", (Kaufman, 1980), "shame-binds" (ibid.), or a "shame attack" (Lee, 1994). Here the presence of an active "shaming other" is no longer required to trigger a significant reaction of shame, constricting the creative zone or even paralyzing our ability to respond at all, in other than completely repetitive ways. Rather, the original source of shaming has been internalized, most often into a well-integrated schema of sensation, emotion, behavior, and belief (Fodor, 1996), and then oftentimes forgotten. (Here I am thinking of one group member in particular, who referred ruefully to this automatic, self-paralyzing response to expression and free desire as his "inner Rottweiler".)

This is what we discussed above as a constriction or collapse of the zone of creativity "from below" (again diagrammatically), i.e., a condition where sensations, desires, and perceptions from the inner world, which are the necessary dynamic elements of new creative syntheses, cannot be energized or flow freely into the experimental arena. Novel combinations of thoughts, feelings, and desires cannot even be perceived and held long and energetically enough to fuel the creative zone, bringing experiment and novel trial combinations to life under relatively safe conditions.

Here, too, the loosening of this constriction and restoration of creativity and growth will depend critically on the *reintroduction of an affirming social world for contact*, the location or relocation of a *reference group of support* of the kind discussed above. This support, which generally needs to be immediately and tangibly present, at least for a time, in the person of a caring, intersubjectively resonant other, is often first found in the therapist. But, eventually, almost always, it also must be found in a *reference group of identification*, a group of other people who have experienced the same kind of shaming for some similar kinds of inner experiences and/or group memberships. Think, for example, of a "heterosexual-identified" therapist working with a homosexual-identified client, one who has been traumatically shamed in development for "wrong" erotic responses and orientation. Eventually, the client will almost always need to form some connections with others who share that experience, until the identification is robust enough to be portable – i.e., to serve, again much like Kohut's "self-objects" (1977), to mirror/resonate with the person's experiential world, so that his or her creative processes can then go on, even in the absence of those affirming others. Again, our need for resonant affirmation by others for our experiential creativity and for the validity of our self-process itself is not something to be gotten over or outgrown in mature adulthood. What develops, in the healthy, creative case, is not a progression toward indifference toward the social field, but rather our capacity to invoke and evoke that necessary reference group of identification and "carry it with us", making use of it to support our creative process, when such support is missing in our immediate social surround.

VII. Conclusions

To analyze the *field conditions for creative process*, as we have been doing here, is still not to reduce that process and mystery to those conditions or to their component parts. When we have finished our analysis (at least provisionally), that mystery remains, the alchemy of creativity itself, through which existing elements, under certain conditions, become *reordered* into something new in the universe, a pattern which did not exist before and which, by existing now, necessarily affects in some way every other pattern in the field, both now and in the future. Goodman (Perls et al., 1951) knew that alchemy as *middle mode*, a mystical union, fundamentally erotic in nature, in which the distinction between self and other becomes suspended, or, as we might say, is relaxed into its natural creative whole, which is the germ of life itself. The alternate flexing and relaxing of that boundary of distinction in the field is itself the fundamental erotic act, which gives birth to the experiential universe, and is life and creativity itself.

That creativity comes to life, experientially, in a *transitional zone*, which partakes of both the inner and outer domains that make up our experiential field. This "space between" is the special arena of *experiment, rehearsal, art, games, and other play – and therapy*. To support creative process, we must support this zone itself, the zone of safe emergency, both by freeing up the flow of energy and material from the larger domains of which it is a part, and by protecting this third space from too much invasion or collapse into the larger surrounding domains. Protecting this space and enriching this flow are the special concerns of psychotherapy, under any model, with a resultant increase (in successful therapy) in the client's ability to find new creative solutions in work, art, relationships, and life.

Strong shame inhibits and potentially vitiates this essential transitional zone, which becomes impoverished from "below" (through constriction of imagination and desire) and invaded from "above" (by too many "real world" consequences for experimental trials and rehearsals). As a dynamic field condition, which is the functional opposite of support, shame shrinks the creative zone, in effect shrinking the self. Restoration of creative self-process necessarily involves the reconstruction of that missing support – including the identification of a significant social group of reference, with whom and in whom the client can find and feel resonance and validation for her or his integrative, creative self-process itself, which are chronically missing in cases of traumatic shame. The restoration of a freely energized self-process is then the restoration and enhancement of creativity, eros in action, the inspiration and respiration of our very lives and selves.

References

Brecht B (1967) Die Dialektik auf dem Theater. In: Schriften zum Theater, Suhrkamp Verlag, Frankfurt a.Main, pp 867–941

Calvin W (2002) A brain for all seasons. Univ of Chicago Press, Chicago

Ehrlich P (2000) Human natures: Genes, cultures, and the human prospect. Island Press, Washington DC

Fodor I (1996) A woman and her body: The cycles of pride and shame. In: Lee R, Wheeler G (eds) The voice of shame: Silence and connection in psychotherapy. Jossey-Bass, San Francisco, pp 229–268

Fogel A (1993) Developing through relationship. Univ of Chicago Press, Chicago

Goodman P (2003) Novelty, excitement and growth (volume 2 of Gestalt therapy). In: Wheeler G (ed) Reading Paul Goodman: Gestalt for our times. The Analytic Press/GestaltPress, Hillsdale, New Jersey, pp 201–423

Kaufman G (1980) Shame: The power of caring. Shenckman, Rochester Vermont

Kent-Ferraro J, Wheeler G (2003) ADD: A Gestalt perspective. In: Wheeler G, McConville M (eds) The heart of development: Gestalt approaches to working with children, adolescents & their worlds, vol I: Childhood. The Analytic Press/GestaltPress, Hillsdale New Jersey, pp 199–238

Kohut H (1977) The restoration of self. International Universities Press, New York

Lee R (1994) Couples' shame: The unaddressed issue. In: Wheeler G, Backman S (eds) On intimate ground: A Gestalt approach to working with couples. Jossey-Bass, San Francisco, pp 262–290

Lewin K (1936) Principles of topological psychology. McGraw-Hill, New York

Melnick J, Nevis S (1994) Intimacy and power in long-term relationships: A Gestalt therapy-systems perspective. In: Wheeler G, Backman S (eds) On intimate ground: A Gestalt approach to working with couples. Jossey-Bass, San Francisco, pp 291–308

Nevis E (1987) Organizational consulting: A Gestalt approach. Gardner Press, New York

Perls F, Hefferline R, Goodman P (1951) Gestalt therapy: Excitement and growth in the
    human personality. Julian Press, New York
Stern D (1985) The interpersonal world of the infant. Basic Books, New York
Sullivan HS (1953) Interpersonal theory of psychiatry. Norton, New York
Wheeler G (1991) Gestalt reconsidered: A new approach to contact and resistance. Gard-
    ner Press, New York
Wheeler G (1996) Self and shame: A new paradigm for psychotherapy. In: Lee R, Wheeler
    G (eds) The voice of shame: Silence and connection in psychotherapy. Jossey-Bass,
    San Francisco, pp 23–60
Wheeler G (2000) Beyond individualism: Toward a new understanding of self, relation-
    ship, & experience. The Analytic Press/GestaltPress, Hillsdale, New Jersey
Winnicott D (1965) The child, the family, & the outside world. Penguin, Harmondsworth,
    United Kingdom
Zinker J (1977) Creative process in Gestalt therapy. Brunner/Mazel, New York

Part III
Connecting Theory and Practice: Case Examples

Embodying Creativity, Developing Experience: The Therapy Process and Its Developmental Foundation

Ruella Frank

I. Introduction

It is the intention of each human organism to seek relationship within its environment. Through this dynamic interaction, the organism changes and grows, "assimilating from the environment what it needs for its very growth" (Perls F et al., 1990, p. viii). *How* the organism incorporates what is vital to its developing is through the creativity of adjusting or the spontaneous interacting of one with another to create something different and new. Any adjusting is creative insofar as it leads to integration: the unification of two unlike essences that are now made into a more inclusive whole. This is the experience of contacting – the quality of connecting with oneself and within the environment.

To understand the nature of a human organism's relationships, the work of psychology, we must always locate organism as part of environment. *How* relationships function becomes most apparent through experiences of adjusting. It is here that organism and environment meet and form the experience that is self.

The self is fluid and relational. For the baby, the mother affords a secure environment from which he can garner nourishment and support. Simultaneously, the baby offers the mother an environment in which she can express her love. One adjusts *along with* an other and creates a whole of experience. The self is not a "thing" that exists as independent of the other, nor does it exist a priori to relationship. The self is process, coming into being through contactful experiences of creating and adjusting.

In a process-oriented therapy, such as Gestalt, we therapists investigate the processes of adjusting and analyze how our clients experience themselves within the relational field. Diagnosing phenomenologically, we attend to what our clients (and ourselves) sense, perceive, and therefore, know. And, *how* one knows, first and foremost, is through movement. The movement explorations of one's own body within a particular environment creates dynamic input in the form of prioprioceptive feedback. Proprioception, the sensing of one's movements, allows us to know *that*, *where*, and *how* we experience ourselves within or as part of that specific environment.

When our environment changes, we sense the difference in our bodies. Similarly, when we experience some difference in our bodies, however subtle, we feel a shift in our relationship within the environment. It is not possible to know ourselves apart from our surroundings. Experiencing movement, we sense the other existing within our own aware response.

Input from proprioceptive awareness supports our ability to explore freely, which allows the differentiation of one part of our body from the other *and* from the surrounding environment (Frank, 2001). The more clearly parts of the field can be differentiated, the greater the clarity of our interest and the greater the precision to select what is of concern to us. What is found and selected is then assimilated through spontaneous adjusting. Assimilating, making what was *unlike*, *like*, allows one to grow and change as more relevant aspects of field are embodied.

Our ability to sharply perceive differences within the field – to create bright figures as they emerge from the background – is reliant upon fluid, creative adjusting. As our body – "*that part of the environment which also proprioceives*" (Kitzler, personal communication, 2001) – moves unrestrained and uninhibited within the field, it readily contributes to the processes of contacting or the fluid forming of self. In the process of spontaneous and creative adjusting, we sense what was *external* as, now, *inside* ourselves – a harmonious part of experience.

This chapter explores the fundamental role of proprioception in all creative adjustments, first in the infant and then the adult therapy client. It further identifies and examines several necessary contexts, or attributes of field, that are always part of adjusting processes for the infant throughout the time span of traditional development and for the adult in the here and now of therapy. Later in the chapter, two clinical case vignettes illustrate and illuminate the usefulness of these contexts within psychotherapy.

II. The Creativity of Infancy

Nowhere are the processes of creative adjusting seen more clearly than in the developing explorations of infants. Throughout, we see continuous experimenting for seeking, finding, and incorporating the other as part of experience. Movement towards the object of interest, in general, is definite in its intention and clear in its meaning. In their lively responses to an other, infants create a progressive differentiation of me from not me, and organize the ability to *separate from while including the other* in experience, which is the essence of contacting. The self evolves through a series of these ongoing coordinated interactions within the field.

The following is an analysis of the movement patterns of an infant captured on video tape. The reader will observe how the infant, experimenting with a variety of alternatives, continuously discovers the best choice possible to solve her problem. Each meeting of infant/environment offers her precise and necessary proprioceptive information regarding her relationships within the field. In this playful process, the infant's manipulation of her toy reveals and even clarifies her intention toward it. In the here and now of exploration, experiences in creative adjusting change this infant into something more than she was before. Moreover, it will become obvious how the preceding sequence of creative adjustments forms the ground for the next sequence to unfold. The reader will see a series of creative sequential adjustments as the infant grows in her ability to forge more and more flexible relations, developing ever greater fluidity of self.

A. The Infant and the Interlocking Chains

Propping up on her elbows and forearms, a four-and-a-half-month-old infant rests on the floor as she plays with a chain of four interlocking colored links – red, yellow, blue, and green. 1) With her left hand, she grasps the red link, at one end of the chain. With her right hand, she grasps the green link, at the other end of the chain. 2) The infant draws her forearms and hands together, making the links into a pile. 3) She lifts her left hand, holding the red link, and brings it to her mouth. All the while, she is gazing at the yellow link resting on the floor, just near her other hand. 4) Now she pulls both hands apart and the red link drops out of her mouth. 5) Her head drops forward, and she gazes at this same link. 6) Once more, she draws her forearms and hands together and constructs a pile of links. She reaches her head toward the red link in her hand and grasps onto it with her mouth. 7) After sucking for a few moments, she again pulls her hands apart, stretching the links before her. 8) She now gazes at the yellow link. 9) For several tries, she brings her hands together and apart, while dunking her head up and down, attempting to grasp the yellow link with her mouth. 10) Finally, she accomplishes her task. The yellow link is captured, and she begins to suck. But, because she is not able to stabilize the yellow link with her hand as well as her mouth (her hands still remain fisted around the red and green links at the ends of the interlocking chain), the yellow link falls out. 11) The infant then lets loose of the red link, which frees her left hand. 12) She extends her left hand to the side and practices pinching movements with her thumb and index finger. 13) The infant now draws her forearms together in an effort to again gather the links. Quickly, she applies her newly acquired pinching skill to pick up the yellow link with her thumb and forefinger. She then draws it toward her mouth and sucks on it. 14) Happily sucking her yellow link, she looks up and toward her mother, who has been quietly sitting next to her, and smiles. She knows she has achieved something marvelous. (I distilled these steps from close observation of Beverly Stokes' "Amazing Babies", video tape, 1995.)

The above description illustrates lucidly the precision with which the infant purposely explores her toy and, in the process, invents a novel experience of self. With each experiment, the baby creates proprioceptive feedback that is crucial to positioning her body in clear relation to the object of her keen attention. In sequence #1, the links have grabbed hold of the infant's attention and excite her. She responds through a rising level of energy. Tension of her organic, nervous, and muscular tones shift to create a change in her attitude. The baby senses this difference in experience as a readiness to respond. The ongoing changes in her musculature, her newly forming attitude, shapes her movements toward the object as well as her orientation in space. The stimulating object has beckoned her to action.

In sequence #2, she draws the links together, revealing new and different properties of the object, building the relationship further. Grasping onto the red link and drawing it into her mouth (sequence #3), she explores its qualities – its taste, texture, and contours. At the same time, her eyes focus on the yellow link, which feeds her further information. In sequence #4, she pulls the links apart, scattering them, thereby deconstructing what she has just made. The movements of drawing her forearms together and apart, and the proprioceptive feedback that she receives from the condensing and dispersing motions, are crucial to the processes of differentiation. The movements are, in fact, the precursors to the more subtle pincher movements, also variations of condensing and dispersing experiences that she will make with her thumb and index finger later in the experiment. With some practice (sequence #12), these more sharply articulated pincher movements prepare the way for the final experience in this series, as she grasps onto the yellow link with her thumb and index finger (#13) and brings it into her mouth to suck.

In this fluid dance, many figures of interest are organized and reorganized, created and destroyed, moving toward integration and assimilation. Here, it is clearly seen how the earlier figure formations become ground for later organizing figures to emerge. The series of emerging adjustments progresses spiral-like as the actions that bring the infant in sharp relation to the object (yellow link) appear to collapse in on themselves, providing the perceptual foundation for the next emerging act (Mead, 1938). The condensing and dispersing that are involved in the first phase of experimenting suddenly consolidate in experience and form the background from which more precise movements – such as the pincher movements – can emerge. In addition, all the varied means by which the infant explored the rings through touching/moving, which enhanced the possibilities of tasting, seeing and, though less obvious, smelling and hearing, were key to the processes of creating new experiences.

Finally, a further consolidating of experience occurred as the accomplished infant looked toward her mother for confirmation and support. The experiments were, after all, conducted within a larger social field. It is the mother who gave the infant the links to begin with, thereby affording the baby the opportunity to practice her skills. The varied possibilities that the links held emerged only in relation to the infant's developing potentialities. In the above scenario, *how* the movement patterns took shape – what the infant's body could and could not do – was relative to the conditions presented by the object (the environment). What the environment could and could not offer the infant was created by and with the structure of the organism. In other words, both infant and object were constructed in experience. It could easily be seen that with her greater differentiated movements, the infant's proprioceptive awareness heightened, and the clarity of figure grew stronger.

III. Five Necessary Contexts for Assimilating the Novel in Infant Development[1]

The following contexts are part of the organic explorations within the infant/ environment field, enabling and simplifying the process of dynamic and creative adjustments. Each of these contexts interacts with the others to provide the infant flexibility and stability within the continually changing field. The property of flexibility allows fluidity of adjustment – the infant's ability to easily move in a variety of ways in relation to the other. At the same time, the property of stability – the capacity to find and experience equilibrium – allows the infant to assimilate what has just occurred.

These same contexts are significant in understanding and guiding the adult psychotherapy process. They are of particular value in organizing experiments within the therapy session and toward greater integration and, therefore, growth within the client/therapist field.

A. The Caregiving Presence

First and foremost is the social context, that is, the caregiving presence. The primary caregiver is generally experienced as a consistent, available, and predictable enough *presence* from which the infant can take support. The caregiver's presence is active and in the foreground, so that the infant is not left to deal with a frustration that is beyond her developmental scope. The caregiver's presence also provides a near-background stability, which permits the infant to exercise her faculties independently in order to accomplish the task at hand. Often times, the caregiver joins the infant, spontaneously supporting her emerging capabilities as well as making the new task a social event. In each case, and unless thwarted or perverted, the caregiving presence serves to provide a *safe enough* environment so that the infant can take risks and gradually move beyond what she already knows. The relational field is mutual, but not necessarily equal (Kitzler, personal communication, 2002).

When the presence of the caregiver is such that the infant feels sufficiently secure in her explorations, the input from proprioceptive feedback is

---

[1] These contexts have been inspired by Feldenkrais practitioner and teacher, Mark Reese, Ph.D., whose article, "Notes on lines of convergence between the Feldenkrais Method and Dynamic Systems Principles" discusses the techniques Moshe Feldenkrais used in order to heighten his students' learning potential. They include: novel tasks, novel environments, novel spatial orientation, and effort substitutions.

experienced as clear and becomes a useful guide to further adventures within the field. When the caregiving presence is chronically inconsistent, unavailable, and unpredictable, the infant is reticent to fully explore, proprioceptive feedback is muted, and further investigations and information gathering within the field are limited.

B. The Supporting Surface

Though frequently not part of awareness, the very ground upon which infants sit, crawl, roll, or walk provides a solidity of surface and continuity of support. From here, all movements and affective interactions emerge. Stimulation from the underlying surface (the earth) presses into the tissues of the infant's body, and the infant senses that which *is* his periphery. He feels bounded by something other than himself – something that is separate from, yet included in his experience. The degree to which this underlying support is felt by each infant varies according to the shifting conditions of the field. If, for example, the caregiving presence is sufficiently distressed, angry, or anxious, the infant will react by either a heightening or diminishing of his overall muscle tone. The level of tension within the muscles at any given moment affects how infants rest upon the earth as well as move up and away from it. It affects, in other words, how they respond and relate within the field. Any shift, however momentary, in the caregiver's ability to provide a supportive environment, influences the infant's muscle tone and, thereby, his capacity to experience the support of the underlying surface. Where the support surface does not feel sufficiently stable, the infant's fluid explorations within the field are impeded. Where the caregiving environment affords ample psychological and emotional support, the infant experiences the surface support as constant, and he gracefully moves through the world. The experience of an adequate surface support, so necessary for easy explorations and fluid creative adjusting, therefore, is dependent upon the supportive caregiving presence, as well as the *capacity* of the infant to experience that support. This varies from one situation to the next and from one infant to another.

C. The Co-Created Task

The task appears as the stirring environment, *and* the infant's exciting *internal* needs dynamically interact. The emerging task must be stimulating enough to hold and maintain the infant's curiosity as she engages with and completes it. An environmental stimulus of weakened intensity will not captivate the infant, and the level of excitement necessary to respond and relate to the object will not develop. If the stimulus is too intense, the infant's arousal builds too quickly and is not tolerable. The infant cannot support this level of excitation and must avoid it by averting her gaze and finding something else to focus on. Averting her eyes and focusing elsewhere gives her time to recuperate, as the level of excitement diminishes and it is more easily contained and supported. The now freed energy and excitement is used to find and make something else – the next emerging task. At times, the stimulating environment is so intense that the infant can and must shut out what is intolerable. The infant's excitement now constricts and, anxiously, she contracts away from her surroundings. In these moments, it takes even longer for the infant to recover her curiosity. But if the intensity of stimulation is neither weak nor overwhelming, the infant becomes transfixed (Stern, 1990). Her level of arousal immediately and easily builds, as the object of attention draws her in. As a steady and fluid rhythm rises and diminishes, the stimulating other *and* the excited infant maintain their engaging. The task, in this case, a smooth coordinating of infant and environment, organizes easily and can be simply completed.

D. The State of the Nervous System

Just as the infant relies on an adequately stimulating environment to draw him in, so too must his nervous system be in a state of ready response. This means that the infant's level of arousal is able to effortlessly build and attend to the developing task. In fact, an infant's level of arousal will determine *how* his interest in the task develops. The degree to which the infant feels stimulated is the degree to which he is enlivened and energetically available to create and tackle the task at hand.

The state of the nervous system is reflected and expressed through the infant's overall muscular tone. If the general state of the nervous system is overly active, the infant will appear *high in tone*. This means that he will startle easily, quickly react to stimulating events, and use more effort to explore his environment than is necessary. His movements may seem excessive, and he may look agitated. The hyper-state of the nervous system and hyper-tone of the muscular system do not encourage an easy articulation of one part of the infant's body with another, and proprioception is inhibited. Important parts of the environment that facilitate spontaneous and creative adjusting, therefore, are not clearly differentiated and perceived.

If the general state of the infant's nervous system is overly passive, he will be *low in tone and* require more stimulation before he responds and more time in which to respond. Applying little effort to explore his surrounding environment, his movements will appear slowed and even lethargic. The impressions from the environment are not easily absorbed by the infant's body, nor readily used in the service of adjusting. Again, proprioception is dulled, and discriminating within the field is retarded.

When the state of the nervous system is appropriately active, however, and the infant is alerted to the adequately stimulating environment, he appears *balanced in tone*. In this condition, discrete muscular changes necessary for graceful movement explorations can be clearly sensed against a background of relatively relaxed effort. Here, spontaneous explorations of the field are supported.

While the state of the nervous system may appear *as if* it is purely organismic, and the intensity of the stimulation may appear *as if* it is purely environmental, this is far from true. In reality, they meet in the act of creative adjusting where each influences and co-creates the other. The sensitivity of the infant discovers the stimulating object while, at the very same time, the possibilities of the stimulating object bring forth those very sensitivities (Mead, 1938).

E. Flexibility in Orienting Capacity

For every new task to emerge, the infant must have the flexibility to spontaneously redirect herself in relation to the changing demands of environment. This happens through subtle head movements, initiated by the sense organs: mouth, eyes, nose, and ears, in reaching toward or moving away from the other. An almost simultaneous shuttling back and forth between sensory input and movement response exists such that *internal* organismic and *external* environmental processes are made one in experience. Flexibility in the infant's orienting capacity, demonstrated by the delicate shifting of the head on the neck, continually changes the spatial relationship of the infant to the object. In this way, perceptions are fluidly organized, disorganized, and re-organized, allowing the infant a variety of responses to either similar or different environmental stimuli. Such variation in response enables fluid and creative adjusting to novel conditions. And, the greater potential for *response-ability* allows a wider range of novel interactions. The possibilities of proprioceptive and exteroceptive (from the sensory organs) feedback are enhanced; there is much more to discover, select, and make one's own. Without the flexibility of the head on the neck, perceiving would clearly be limited in range and depth. These five interrelating contexts – caregiving presence, supporting surface, co-created task, state of the nervous system, and flexibility in orienting capacity – always exist as part of the organism/environment field and play a critical role, either as foreground or background, in the processes of creative adjusting. We will now examine the psychotherapy session from the perspective of these contexts.

IV. Experimenting in Creativity: The Adult Therapy Session

Gestalt therapy is best differentiated from other therapies by its understanding and use of the experimental process. In fact, the whole of the Gestalt session can be thought of as an experiment, where the process itself enhances awareness. There is no specific outcome of the therapy experiment, only a moment-to-moment heightening of what is real and what is true. The "actual living through" of a situation allows the client to experience him or herself in relation to the world and, therefore, to realize his or her own authenticity. As the experiment continues, clients are encouraged to become more and more themselves (Perls F et al., 1990). This is seen as an uninterrupted

completing of the act, the result of which leaves each client with a personally validated experience of self in the world. The experiential validation is
the experimental proof. With the fluid completion of an action – sensing,
moving, perceiving, feeling – and the meaning that is constructed from these
interrelated structures are assimilated as a whole of experience and can now
serve as background support. That is, the assimilated action (a smooth coordinating of organism and environment) is integrated in a way that provides
balance and equilibrium. From here, further experiments in creative and
spontaneous living emerge, both within and outside of the therapy relationship. The validating of any experience is proven in this unobstructed living
through or completing of the act (Kitzler, personal communication, 2002). It
is the process of creative adjusting or of contacting.

   Within the whole of the experiment that is therapy, many smaller experiments are created by both client and therapist. These *co-created tasks* are
offered to clients for the purpose of discovering their essential truths. The
tasks allow clients to move from their rigidified positions, to better see themselves and to bear responsibility for their behaviors (Perls L, 1993). The experimental task must be of sufficient interest to the client as to warrant attention: "The experiment allows the explorations of difference" (ibid., p. 3).
And it must be different enough from clients' habitual behaviors to maintain
their attention and allow awareness to develop incrementally. The task
brings what was formerly background and unaware into the foreground as
aware response.

   Observing the client, the therapist creates a task inspired from the most
obvious phenomena – tilting of the client's head, holding of his or her breath,
tensing of shoulders, or shifting of position. The therapist knows that in staying with what is obvious, the client's most relevant, existential concern – that
is, the unfelt predicament – will easily emerge. This is because any aware
exploration enables some release of the client's former muscular holding,
such that the habitual experience is already interrupted. During the experimental task, it becomes apparent (for both therapist and clients) how clients
return to their former habit of fixing, revealing the organizing of their behaviors in the here and the now. In addition, the experiment can also enhance
the clients' recent successes and further validate what already functions
well.

   The experiment has only two goals: to heighten aware response to whatever exists here and now and, while doing so, to free up the client's vitality
or healthy aggressive energy. The level of the client's healthy aggression can
be measured by the amount of effort needed to complete the task – no more
and no less. In general, the therapist invites her client to stay with the task,
"to inspect it, try it for fit, work it over, and to some extent work oneself over.
In this way, the already known and the new knowledge are *actually assimilated to each other*" (Perls F et al., 1990, p. 119). The experiment, then, is itself an exploration in creative adjustment.

   Every therapy experiment is tailored to the needs of each client. To do
this well, the therapist must take into consideration the client's organizing
capacity, that is, the *state of the nervous system*. This is reflected most

clearly by the client's overall muscular tension as expressed in the quality of his or her movements. Sometimes, the experiment encourages a reduction in the client's tension by releasing the fixations of the neuromuscular system, so that the client can experience *how* he fixes himself and, thereby, *how* he blocks, unaware, a fluid completing of the act. At other times, the experimental task encourages an increase in overall neuromuscular tension for similar purposes. In either case, the task will hold the client's attention only insofar as he or she is available and can attend to it.

Thus, in the broadest sense, the therapy task is created by the therapist and offered to the client to enhance proprioceptive awareness. The client then returns the experiment to the therapist in the form of feedback (Bloom, personal communication, 2002). The feedback may be expressed verbally or through the sometimes elusive, yet obvious, language of the body: shifts in muscular tension and in gestural, breathing, or postural patterns. The therapist, in turn, may feed back her response to the client by sharing the client's postural pattern as well as sharing changes in muscular tension and breathing rhythm – basic kinesthetic attuning. For example, if the client is excited and sitting at the edge of his seat, the therapist's vocal, breathing, muscular tension, and movement patterns will kinesthetically and empathetically adjust to the client's experience. The process is felt and shared.

The experimental task graduates so that both client and therapist keenly notice when an aware interrupting or healthy checking of experience moves out of awareness. This can be observed, again, through the client's breathing, postural, and gestural patterns. For example, the client may be freely moving with his excitement and, in the next moment, begin to hold his breath and tense his neck and throat. If the client does not notice this interruption of experience, the therapist will likely bring it forward for further exploration.

Both the task and the *therapist's presence* are modulated in relation to the reciprocal processes of feedback. Attuned to this primary level of experience, the therapist builds the experiment step-by-step, so that the client can maintain his position at the boundary – "a temporary lack of balance (...) at the growing edge where we have one foot on familiar and one foot on unfamiliar ground, the very boundary experience itself" (Perls L, 1993, p. 155). The therapist moves from an active and foreground position – one taken to structure and guide the experiment – to a sitting back and waiting to see what happens position. The novelty of experience generally elicits discomfort from the client, as the creativity and spontaneity of adjusting requires a de-structuring of previously held notions and their accompanying muscular fixations. As the experiment advances, with the client's emerging levels of anxious embarrassment and awkward excitement – which the therapist is sensitive to – the therapist offers her active support judiciously and only insofar as the client cannot tolerate his uncertainty. When the experiment moves along without interruption, the therapist takes a background position, allowing the client to fully exercise his growing faculties.

The experimental task invites and encourages the client to creatively adjust, which also develops the client's *flexibility in orienting capacity*. That is, the client, more alive to himself and his surroundings, now demonstrates a wider range of responses. No longer dulled to his senses, his ability to spontaneously orient himself to the demands of the environment expands, promising even more novel experiences. The therapist monitors her client's growing flexibility by observing the highly subtle changes in the client's relationship of eyes to head, head to neck, and neck to torso. Knowing that fixed patterns in these particular areas of the body indicate the petrifaction of orienting capability, any freedom of these habitual fixations immediately restores the client's creativity and vitality.

To maximize the potential for creative adjusting within the therapy session, the therapist must be a consistent, available, and predictable presence, so that the client feels supported enough to experiment with behaviors that are new and different, sometimes surprisingly so. As the client perceives the *therapist's presence*, the client's capacity to experience the underlying and *supporting surface* of the earth changes. This can be observed by the therapist and experienced by the client as a change in breathing (deeper and fuller breaths), a change in muscular tone (shoulders once held tight are now relaxed), and a change in gestural patterns (from jerky or twitching to smooth). The client's relation to the underlying surface upon which he or she rests is a primary diagnosis of the relations within the field and indicates how the therapy experiment is unfolding.

By the nature of the experiment, the client is encouraged to disengage from what has become customary and banal and to create something new. The novelty now challenges what was formerly believed impossible. This is elucidated in the following two clinical case vignettes. Every therapy experiment necessarily reflects and relies upon the contexts, as presented above, for assimilating the novel. By being aware of these contexts, the therapist is equipped to tailor experiments toward each client's unique needs.

For Michele, the earlier experiments diagnose her difficulty in proprioceptive awareness, while the later ones enhance her growing sense of self. The experiments for Lara are designed to hold her attention, thereby enabling her to bypass her deeply routine and neurotic behaviors. At the end of the session, she is able to validate her experience of self in the world with clarity, if only for a moment.

A. Michele

Michele bounces into the therapy room wearing a brightly colored, oversized, and long-sleeved T-shirt and baggy sweat pants. She "flops" onto the large, soft arm-chair, pulls her legs up onto the seat, and crosses her bared-feet, yoga-style. Michele is petite with a full face and round body. This morning her hair is swept back in a long, curly pony tail, which makes her look younger than her twenty-five years. Because of her generally good humor and infectious laugh, at times, Michele looks cherubic. Having worked together weekly for almost three years, Michele and I have developed a warm affection for one another.

A talented performer, Michele, has just come from an audition and is eager to fill me in on all the details. Her story, as usual, is funny and entertaining. As she tells me what happened, Michele begins moving restlessly from one position to another. She places her legs up and under her; next she tucks them to one side; then she plants her feet on the seat of the chair, while her knees are pressed onto her chest. Watching her fidget, I discover my breathing becoming slower and deeper and surmise it is my attempt to counteract her agitated and breathless pace.

Once her story is finished, I ask Michele what she notices about herself in the moment. "I feel pretty hyper", she says. "Yes", I add, "you seem to be very excited. Your speaking became faster and faster as your story continued." "Oh really", she says, "I never noticed that." I suggest an experiment and invite Michele to talk to me as fast as she can. This is an easy task for her, and when she does so, she says, "This isn't too different than my normal pace", and I agree. Her self-revelation interests her and she confesses that although her friends have brought this to her attention, she never really knows that she is "talking too fast".

I propose a different experiment for her. I ask her to pay close attention to how her body rests on the chair and to tell me of any sensations that she might feel. After a few seconds, Michele reports, "My stomach is so fat! When I notice myself, I notice my fat ... UGH!" I remind her that to make an evaluation is far different than to notice a sensation. At the same time, we both realize how difficult it is for Michele to notice her body without hating herself. I tell her that I have another plan in mind.

I ask Michele to press her spine into the back of the chair and to wiggle around until she is sure that her spine and the back cushion are connected. Then I ask her to lift and drop her arms and hands, one at a time, onto the chair's armrests. Once done, I ask Michele what she notices. "I feel my spine against the back cushion of the chair, but I don't feel my arms or hands", she says.

I give Michele two soft, round, and small balls and ask her to squeeze them in her hands. But when she tries this, she says that her hands and fingers are weak and that she can hardly squeeze the balls. Explaining my next experiment to her, and having received her permission, I now take a soft, bristle brush and slowly begin to stroke downward on both sides of her arms, from elbow to hand. She enjoys the feeling of the brush on her skin, and I notice that her breathing has deepened, as has mine. When I have finished, she says, "Now, I can feel my arms and hands." More aware of these areas of her body, I give Michele another ball and ask her to explore it with her hands and fingers in order to sense its texture, weight, and volume. From here, she experiments with a series of balls of different shapes, sizes, and textures – hard, heavy, soft, light, coarse, quilted, squishy, etc. With apparent interest and dedication, Michele explores them: poking some with her fingers, rolling or squashing others between the palms of her hands, and bouncing one on the floor and then tossing it up in the air and catching it. Watching her playful actions, I pick up a ball, one that changes its shape when it is squeezed, and I toss it to her. Soon we are engaged in a game of catch: first squeezing the ball, then tossing it back and forth. "I don't use my hands very much", Michele discloses, "I constantly worry about germs and I wash my hands a lot, so I don't touch many things. Except boys … does that count? I love touching boys." I tell her that if she limits and restricts what she touches, she will lose touch with herself. A moment later I add, "Yes! Touching boys absolutely counts."

When we are finished, Michele tells me that she can feel her arms and hands and that they now seem attached to her body. I ask her to notice the weight of her body resting on the chair as well as to notice her breathing. This time, she allows herself to remain still, and she appears able to focus on her body for a longer period of time – approximately one minute. "I feel really calm now", she says. After a few more moments of sitting quietly, she adds, "Now I'm worried that I'll be so different, I won't recognize myself." I ask Michele what sensations she notices, now that she's worried, and she reports a mild tension in her shoulders and belly. I respond, "Sometimes being different makes us anxious and we close somewhere in our body, and sometimes being different makes us curious, and we open." We continue in silence for a few more moments, and I watch Michele taking deeper and deeper breaths. We have ten minutes remaining in the session, and I realize, aloud, that Michele will probably want to wash her hands after touching the balls, so I ask if we can make her hand washing an experiment. She smiles and says, "Sure!"

In the bathroom, Michele rolls up her sleeves and shows me how rough the skin of her arms and hands has become as a result of frequent and compulsive hand washings, and I suddenly feel sad. At the edge of the wash basin in the bathroom sits a marble-colored, coarse bar of soap. Michele grabs it and begins to quickly lather up. I encourage her to slow her tempo enough so that she can notice both the touch of one hand caressing the other and the feel of the warm water. Slowing down considerably, she says that she likes the lavender odor of the soap; she also comments on its unusual color. I watch as Michele carefully washes every finger and under each nail, and I am impressed with her thoroughness.

We return to our chairs, and I give her a bottle of creamy lotion to rub into her hands, which she enjoys, and I do the same. It is the end of the session, and I suggest to Michele that when she is home she continue our experiment in "aware hand washing". I say, "When you feel your hands touch one another, you might also think to yourself, 'These are *my* hands. This is *my* body'."

B. Shaping the Experiment

Unaware of her habitually rapid-paced speech, Michele is out-of-touch with her experience. Her excitement and anxiety build quickly and do not easily dissipate, indicating that her nervous system is high in tone. Her overall muscular tone, however, is flaccid. This indicates an imbalance in muscle tissue, creating *holding patterns* in other areas of her body. The holding, I surmise, is most likely to be found in specific muscles that lie closest to her bones, in her connective tissues, and in her organ system. Michele, in fact, has suffered from irritable bowel syndrome, sudden and explosive diarrhea after eating, since she was a teenager and has learned from our therapy how she automatically holds down her unwanted feelings by tensing her abdomen.

A series of graded sensorimotor experiments allowed the heightening of Michele's proprioception, a necessity for becoming more in touch with herself, and therefore, her surroundings. As is true with infants throughout their development, over time, each preceding creative adjustment in the here and now of Michele's therapy formed the ground for later and more elaborate adjustments to spontaneously emerge.

In the first experiment, Michele was invited to speak as fast as she could. But she already had been speaking so quickly that she simply felt unable to talk any faster. From a background of such heightened nervous tension, it was not possible for Michele to experience the subtleties of her building excitements or anxieties. The experiment served as a diagnostic tool, and I soon realized that I needed to design experiments for Michele that would, at first, reduce her overall background tension as well as minimize the *over-efforting* she habitually used in all her interactions. I believed that a decrease in tension would enable her to sense the more subtle changes of experience necessary to fluidly adjust from one situation to another.

We began with Michele sensing herself as she rested in the chair. This basic experiment, I thought, would bring to awareness the surface below her and *how* she utilized it as an underlying support. The task led to Michele's negative self-evaluation – "Fat!!! Ugh!!!" – rather than an experience. I knew then that I needed to structure the experiment more tightly in order to disorganize her predictably negative responses to herself. I gave Michele two tasks: to wiggle in the chair and feel her spine touching the cushion, and to lift and drop her arms onto the arm-rests of the chair. I chose these areas of her body, spine and hands, as I believed that they were less likely to bring up uncomfortable feelings and the disapproving judgments necessary to avoid them. Further, I imagined that this more active task would capture her attention, such that her body would become more clarified in experience. And it did. Michele was able to notice the difference between what she did feel – her spine – and what she did not – her arms and hands. Now she was engaged in the subtle processes of differentiation – one part of her body from another and from the immediate environment of the chair. In the process, Michele experienced the chair backing her – the now aware and supporting surface – providing the beginnings of a reliable foundation from which her foreground activities, the proprioception of her arms and hands, emerged. Although she did not sense her arms and hands clearly, I knew that the experience of *no feeling* was the beginning of *some feeling* for Michele. As proprioceptive awareness was gained and heightened, more areas of her body could then be incorporated into further spontaneous and creative adjustments.

In the next experiment, Michele squeezed the balls that I had placed in each of her hands, and she noticed her weakness. This may have been the result of too much tension held in her shoulder area, such that she did not have the requisite strength to use her hands well for manipulating objects. I speculated that after years of anxiously pulling away from objects, including the intrusive touching from her "anxious and needy" mother, Michele's shoulders had tensed and locked, further inhibiting her free explorations/manipulations. I stroked her arms and hands with the soft brush and stimulated her sense of touch, bringing them sharply alive. Vitality in these formerly deadened areas, I believed, would immediately reduce some of the tension that she carried in her shoulders. As her localized muscle tension dissolved somewhat, her high in tone nervous system became subdued. Soothing her overly-stimulated nervous system would allow Michele's excitements to build incrementally. Excitement that lacks support moves easily into anxiety.

I was well aware that I had taken a risk by touching Michele, an intimate experience for both of us, and so I explained the experiment beforehand. And, although I was confident in her ability to tell me what she wanted or did not want to do in session, I carefully monitored her experience, and my own, knowing that any subtle pulling away or holding of breath on her part would need further inquiry into our experience, and that any discomfort I might feel would indicate a need to explore what was going on between us as well. I might have had Michele brush her own limbs, but I chose to use myself as a more active presence from which she could draw support. It was, after all, an earlier relational field which Michele spontaneously had pulled away from: the mother of her childhood. Moving toward reparation, therefore, I felt it was necessary to introduce the greater social field as a more active part of the experiment. Focused on the enjoyable stroking sensations, Michele rediscovered *herself and me* through a heightening of kinesthetic sensitivity.

Once her sensory system was brought to attention through the stroking, Michele's movement repertoire was able to expand. My invitation to explore the different shaped and textured balls allowed her to actively engage her senses, and a fuller range of experiences surfaced as *the balls enticed her to use them* in a variety of ways. Now her orientation shifted as she followed the trajectory of the balls upward, downward, and from one hand to another with the shifting of her head and eyes. Michele flowed easily in relation to her task, and used as much effort as was necessary to complete it. In the organic and fluid coordination of her movements, an inherent creative adjusting emerged. Playing upon the spontaneity of her interactions with the balls, I interjected myself into the experiment, once again, and we played catch.

Before the session's end, I invited Michele to experiment again and to notice herself doing a task that she does all too frequently. She and I had spent sessions discussing her fear of germs and her constant hand washing – a creative adjustment she had developed in her childhood as an attempt to soothe her anxiety. This time, I wanted to use her methodical and compulsive behavior in a new way, refining and tuning this adaptive pattern, such that it could become as spontaneous and creative as her prior exploration with the balls. The habitual task was explored within a new circumstance: I was in the room with her – an experience of support that is lacking in the isolated anxiety of compulsive behaviors. And, instead of focusing on getting rid of the germs, something Michele has dedicated large parts of her life to, she grew interested in sensing the water, smelling the soap, and feeling one hand upon the other. The final experiment, sharing my hand lotion with her at the end of the session, further enhanced our relationship through a mutual and caring task. The homework assignment (aware hand-washing) was a way to integrate the creativity and novelty of experiment into her everyday life. Adding the phrase, "These are *my* hands. This is *my* body", makes aware what had been formerly disowned: the fullness of embodied experience.

In the next case vignette, the goals for Lara were basically the same as for Michele – to heighten awareness and free healthy aggressive energy so that adjusting is creative and spontaneous – although the kinds of experiments that I devised were quite different. The reader will see how drawing upon the five contexts that accompany creative adjusting shape and refine the experiment.

C. Lara

Lara walks into the therapy room even more slowly than usual this morning and collapses onto the big, green chair. She is of medium height and average weight, with an overall structure that looks weakened, as if impotent. While her upper torso and arms are thin and delicate, her lower body and legs appear slightly swollen.

Lara's liquid eyes have a gentle quality, cool and luminous and, as in most of our sessions, they do not meet mine. Instead, her pelvis and lower legs face me directly, while her upper body twists to her right, allowing her to wilt over the chair's arm. Her head faces in the direction of her rotated torso, as do her eyes, which are focused downward. Lara stares at the pile of pillows in the corner of the room, and we are silent for some time.

In the two years that we have been together, Lara and I have spent a good deal of time working with her tendency to look away from me. I have commented that when she looks away and stares at "nothing in particular", she seems lonely. Once noticed and appreciated, Lara feels a "distant sadness". She has said, "It seems impossible" for her to look directly at me. When she has attempted to do this, she feels anxious; she then fills herself with an unrelenting shame. Lara stays with her anxious shame for only a moment, before she immediately transforms the feeling into fixed ideas and habitual expressions of self-loathing. Because Lara is unable to stay with her experience, she never really learns what is so anxiety-making or so shaming, for her, about our seeing one another. Instead, she occupies herself with denigrating remarks. She is "stupid", because she cannot look directly at me without feeling uncomfortable. "Anyone with half a brain", she says, "would be able to do this. It's so simple." Lara's self-hate turns immediately into depression. The entire process takes no more than thirty seconds.

Lara and I have spent time deciphering this process, and we are both taken with how quickly it occurs. To her dismay, however, she can not get rid of that shameful, anxious part of herself. And, because she is unable to be anything but herself – a self that is unacceptable to her – she falls into a depressed collapse. Lara's depression, always present somewhere in experience, is so deeply entrenched that it is difficult for anything novel to emerge in therapy or elsewhere.

In this session, I need to create a sufficiently interesting experiment for Lara, which will bypass her extremely well-organized set of systematic and defeating behaviors. So, I ask her to become aware of her posture. "I'm all twisted to one side", she says. "Yes, that's an interesting position you've gotten yourself into." I say this holding my breath, as I anticipate her potential self-hating remark. But Lara becomes intrigued by my remark. "What's so interesting?" she says. I tell Lara that if she wants, we can investigate her position and discover what might be of interest to her.

Lara is willing to explore herself, and when she does, she notices several things. For one, although the lower half of her body faces me directly, she says that the weight of it is placed only on the right half of her buttock bone. In addition, her upper body is "pushed over and leaning toward the right, and collapsing onto the arm of the chair" and that her spine and her rib cage seem to fall into her pelvis. She further notices that her head faces downward and toward the corner of the room and that her eyes do the same.

We are now both silent, and I wait with curiosity for what will happen next. Lara takes her time, as if digesting some heavy meal, and then says, "I'm in the shape of a question mark!" For a brief moment, I think that she just might enjoy her self-revelation; but instead, she begins her familiar attack. "That's typical", she says, "I'm always so confused. That's why I never make decisions. I hate that about me."

Ignoring her pathological self-diagnosis, I tell Lara that I am interested in her experience, and I devise a task for her. I ask if she will experiment with her position by pushing her left buttock bone onto the seat of the chair. To execute this new position, Lara notices that she must straighten out her pelvis and twisted torso so that she faces more directly toward me. I encourage her to do this as much as possible, while still leaving her head and eyes facing the corner of the room and down. Now, Lara says, "I feel a little anxious." "That's good", I tell her, "it's the beginning of something different. You will have to feel some anxiety on the way to becoming less depressed."

Hoping that my comment has not stimulated her mind too much, I immediately ask Lara to sense the chair under her pelvis. Once she becomes aware of this, I invite her to keep her eyes facing the corner, while she turns her head in my direction. This is a difficult, awkward task for her, but one that she is willing to try. I then ask Lara to glide her eyes, which are placed in the far right corner of their respective sockets, all the way to the left corners of their sockets, without moving her head, and then to shift them back again toward her favored right side. "I've never moved like this before", she says with a laugh, "I'm getting dizzy." I say, "I'm sure you are."

Without my instruction, Lara shifts her eyes side to side a few more times and says, "This feels strange, but good somehow." Then, I ask her if she will move her head (which still directly faces me) to the right one more time and bring her eyes in line with her head. Once her head and eyes face the same direction, I ask her to shift her head even further to the right and to let her eyes shift, again, to the left sides of their sockets. This last move is an even more difficult task, and Lara becomes slightly agitated. "What's the point? Why am I doing this?" she rightfully wants to know. I imagine that now Lara is beginning to feel the seeds of a potentially lively embarrassment. But because she almost always drowns her embarrassment, leaving an habitual self-hate in its wake, I say to her, "You are doing these crazy movements, because you have a crazy therapist", and ask, "Please humor me." We both laugh. Lara takes a deeper breath and continues her task as the seeds of spontaneous play emerge.

For some time, Lara shifts her eyes and head in a variety of combinations: her eyes reach upward, while her head presses downward; her head presses upward, while her eyes rotate down, and so on. Lara now invents experiments on her own. I watch as she moves her torso into the action, consciously twisting it in the opposite direction from both her head and eyes.

As her energy continues to build, I ask Lara to move her head, eyes, and torso toward me. Now, she looks directly at me, and for quite some time. A pensive Lara says that she feels it is somehow easier to see me, and that I look very clear to her. Suddenly she startles. Lara realizes that it has been difficult to look at me before, because she does not like to be seen. "What if you see something you don't like about me?" she says. "I don't want to see that in your eyes." We are both taken with the spontaneity of her brilliant revelation. "What do you see in my eyes right now?" I ask. "Kindness", Lara says, and begins to tear. "I see kindness."

D. Shaping the Experiment

Overall, Lara's superficial muscles appear to recede away from her skin and are soft, indicating their low tone. Her nervous system, characterized by Lara's collapsed posture as well as her prevalent slowness to react and respond, is low in tone as well. To have gained her attention, a precursor to developing proprioception, I needed to create experiments that were stimulating enough to intrigue her, thus building tolerable excitement, but not so stirring that she would become overwhelmed and have to shut down defensively. Only when Lara's nervous system became appropriately active could any prescribed task build with clarity and continue to hold her interest.

The first experiment, investigating her seated position, brought Lara's attention to her body, instead of, as usual, being focused on her thoughts. Although she was able to notice herself with some interest at first, she quickly doused the fires of curiosity and continued to assess rather than experience herself. Lara's ability to so quickly dismiss her experience and to admonish herself had come from years of practice under the tutelage of her brilliant, successful, and critical father, who continually instructed/demanded her to *"be somebody!"* Her strong desire to brutally criticize herself, and to consequently collapse, seemed the better alternative to the overwhelming pressures of being the person her father had thought she *should* be. Although her depression, the result of telling herself that she was *wrong* or *bad*, had integrity – it kept her world predictable and stable – it also contributed to her misery.

I considered two different experiments for Lara. In one, I asked her to exaggerate her folded posture and to discover what she felt in the process. But, I quickly decided that by her doing so, she would have collapsed even more, and that was already too familiar a position for her. Falling in on herself, even with awareness, would not have sufficiently stimulated her excitement. In this case, nothing new would have emerged. Instead, I invited her to experiment with shifting the weight of her body, which ultimately shifted the placement of her pelvis and torso. This movement now positioned us in a very different relational configuration (her pelvis and torso met me more directly) than is our norm. In doing something different, her appropriate and often dampened anxiety moved foreground.

Intending to support her risk-taking and help her remain at the boundary of experience, I told Lara that feeling her anxiety was a necessary step out of her depression. I knew that unless she were able to feel and tolerate the slow build-up of her anxiety, she would not be able to maintain the excitement held captive to it. I instantly had her notice the chair beneath her. This stable surface, when given attention, supported her feelings of discomfort and awkwardness. These often avoided experiences had to be accepted by Lara in order for her to transition from habitual to fluid behaviors.

When Lara moved her head all the way to the right side and her eyes all the way to the left, she became agitated and asked, "What's the point?" I offered my playful support, again wanting her to continue at the edge of excitement and novelty, "you have a crazy therapist", and asked for her indulgence. I hoped a lighter moment would again discourage an all too well-known collapse into self-hate and prevent this vestigial part from dominating the whole of her experience.

Once emerged, Lara's now supported anxiety moved quickly into excitement and was used to freely explore, as she spontaneously discovered and invented her own orienting experiments. Executing the non-routine tasks required much concerted effort from Lara. It was the kind of concentration that became fascination over time and seemed similar to a trance. In this state, stimulation, such as my presence, which often made her painfully self-conscious, as well as her debilitating thoughts, receded sufficiently into the background. As she was so deeply absorbed, any extraneous efforts that she might have applied to the task ordinarily were kept at a minimum. At the same time, the reduction in her overall muscular tone supported her growing fascination.

The highly differentiated movements of her head, eyes, and then torso in a variety of directions challenged Lara's basic and routine pattern of orientation and required her to remain present and alert. "In the now you use what is available, and you are bound to be creative" (Perls F, 1959, p. 54). The shift in her orienting capacity, a growing fluidity in the relationship between her eyes, head, neck, and torso, heightened proprioceptive awareness, enabling Lara's formerly methodical, perceptual patterns to expand and change. I asked Lara to look at me directly. Because the shift was executed so effortlessly, it took her by surprise. Now that she was not avoiding her feeling, the deeper meaning of her behavior emerged: *If I look at you, I will see that you don't like me.* In the present, Lara possessed the freedom to boldly discover more creative configurations of self – "I see kindness."

A solid understanding of the five contexts that accompany spontaneous creative adjusting and their relationship to proprioception enabled me to design effective experiments for Michele and Lara. Every experiment reinforced each client's ability to move with greater flexibility in relation to the changing environment. And the integration of such fluid adjustments became a part of the stable background from which subsequent adjustments could emerge.

Embodying their experience through experimenting, Michele and Lara felt a gradual sense of excitement build as they spontaneously adjusted themselves to the novelty of each task. In the end, both grew, in their capacities and their selves.

References

Frank R. (2001) Body of awareness: A somatic and developmental approach to psychotherapy. GestaltPress/Analytic Press, Hillsdale, New Jersey

Mead GH (1938) The philosophy of the act. Univ of Chicago Press, Chicago

Perls F (1959) Gestalt therapy verbatim. Real People Press, Utah

Perls F, Hefferline R, Goodman P (1990) Gestalt therapy: Excitement and growth in the human personality. Souvenir Press, London

Perls L (1993) Living at the boundary. Gestalt J Press, New York

Stern D (1990) Diary of a baby. Harper Collins/Basic Books, New York

One Therapy Session:
Dialogue and Co-Creation in Child Therapy

Sandra Cardoso-Zinker

Imagine a fragile little boy, sitting on the floor in a corner of a waiting room, looking at some magazines. He is alone. He is three years old. I am going to describe his story. First, I will share some basic theoretical ideas with you, and as I do so, the text will alternate between male and female gender, so as not to emphasize one gender or the other.

I. Gestalt Therapy and Human Growth

In 1951, Perls, Hefferline, and Goodman spoke of human growth in the following context:

"The field as a whole tends to complete itself, to reach the simplest equilibrium possible for that level of field. But since the conditions are always changing, the partial equilibrium achieved is always novel; it must be grown to. An organism preserves itself only by growing. Self-preserving and growing are polar, for it is only what continually assimilates novelty that can preserve itself and not degenerate. So the materials and energy of growth are: the conservative attempt of the organism to remain as it has been, the novel environment, the destruction of previous partial equilibrium, and the assimilation of something new" (Perls et al., 1994, p. 155).

A child is born to grow. This optimistic view of the human being had a fundamental impact on my work. To receive a client with the perspective that she would move toward a new place in life, no matter which way this would be, gave me the freedom to enter into contact with my client. There would not be a goal to achieve. My job would be to transform my client's experience into a lively dialogue between herself and everything else that is part of her relational world.

We are in the process of constant change. Perls, Hefferline, and Goodman say that:

"Contact, the work that results in assimilation and growth, is the forming of a figure of interest against a ground or context of the organism/environment field. The process of figure/background formation is a dynamic one in which the urgencies and resources of the field progressively lend their powers to the interest, brightness and force of the dominant figure" (ibid., p. 7).

We are in constant relation with the environment. Each child has his unique way of assimilating the experience, one that at the same time creates a unique way of responding to the outside world. As Gary Yontef describes: *"Creative Adjustment* is a relationship between person and environment in which the person [1] responsibly contacts, acknowledges and copes with his life space, and [2] takes responsibility for creating conditions conducive to his own well being"(1993, p. 195).

These basic ideas of Gestalt therapy are related to a dynamic flow of contact and contact-making. The basic way of being in contact is through living experience. In our work, we pay attention to how the energy of our client flows in relation to the interchange of experiences with others and the world. When the energy is potent and full of color, there is growth. But sometimes, this energy is influenced by experiences that are assimilated in a negative way, paralyzing or weakening the investment of energy into new experiences. In this moment, there is a lack of spontaneous creativity and narrowed awareness. The child becomes desensitized to her own sensations and feelings. The different possibilities that the field offers to fulfill a child's needs are not sensed or are prematurely abandoned.

Very often the experience of pain and struggle to mobilize the vitality that moves us forward is lost. The sense of being fully there is muted. A child needs help and support to recover the flow of the energy that keeps him in constant movement of growth. At this moment, the child needs the experience of a creative therapist, who is able to stimulate his client to experience the environment with liveliness and increased curiosity:

"The creative therapist sees the client in his completeness: his plasticity and rigidity, brilliance and dullness, fluidity and stasis, cognitive punctuality and passion. The creative therapist is a choreographer, historian, phenomenologist, a student of the body, a dramatist, a thinker, a theologian, a visionary" (Zinker, 1977, p. 17).

We are able to join our clients with open hearts and minds in the experience of the moment. We can make meaning of the child's existential dilemmas with our compassion and attentiveness. Our clients will get in touch with their own resources as competent human beings through the "filter" of our presence. A child is almost always in a state of "play" or spontaneous experimentation and improvisation. The child therapist is able to track the clients' awareness and activity without putting herself into the foreground.

Zinker reminds us:

"Gestalt therapy is really permission to be creative. Our basic methodological tool is the experiment, a behaviorist approach to moving into novel functioning. The experiment moves to the heart of resistance, transforming rigidity into an elastic support system for the person. It does not have to be heavy, serious, or even precisely fitting; it can be theatrical, hilarious, crazy, transcendent, metaphysical, humorous. The experiment gives us permission to be priest, whore, faggot, holy man, wise witch, magician – all the things, beings and notions hidden within us. Experiments don't have to grow out of concepts; they may move from simple playfulness into profound conceptual revelations" (ibid., p. 18).

The therapist supports the child's grounded experimentation to stay connected with his environment.

All these basic ideas and Gestalt methodology are in the background of my work with children. Here is one example of such work with one child.

II. Working with Children: An Exciting Challenge

"The young person is experiencing the world with unique perspective, in a process of developing the awareness of himself and the environment, in constant change and transformation, physically, cognitively and emotionally. He is developing his style of communication, learning how to assimilate his experiences, to express his internal world and to make himself present. It is a special experience to witness how the child develops his style of contact making and creative adjustments and how he responds to the novelty of the moment. One must be open to the child's adventure with the unknown with pure eyes to see what is there" (Cardoso-Zinker, unpublished manuscript[1]).

In the process of becoming adults, we are in danger of alienating the children around us, abandoning them in their struggle of growing up. When neglected, when not seen and heard, children are not able to move forward and stop their process of contacting the world: "The child needs the stimuli from the environment to develop his abilities and expand his experiential field. This is a relational dynamic: the child assimilates and integrates the stimuli through experience" (ibid.).

At a certain moment of great stress, children stop experimenting with the world and the freedom of creativity and expressiveness. The naturally authentic movement is overtaken by an overwhelming experience of containment. The act of experimenting is abandoned in favor of stereotyped behavior, usually supported by cultural and social demands of the environment. The Gestalt therapist's vision is to stimulate the rebirth of the child's continuous experimentation.

The child needs support and affirmation. The child needs to experience his ability and competence to explore the world around him (this principle will be concretized in the forthcoming session). The child needs somebody to validate his learning experience. An ordinary child is in constant process, driven by a seemingly endless flow of energy. In order to save himself, the child stops this flow, holds his breath, and freezes his movement. All these physical phenomena are masterful ways in which the child preserves himself from further punishment and/or painful interaction with the environment.

Every child is a master in both self-preservation and protection of the adults who take care of him. The child assimilates the unspoken culture of his family system and intuitively "plays by the rules" in order to both protect himself and his family from pain. For example, if the child senses that continuing to cry may result in great harm to himself or to his parental system, he will tend to suppress the gasping sounds of wailing, and if necessary, will "play dead" in order to survive. This is both a "symptom" and a victory of

---

[1] Taken from my article entitled "The Story of Daniel: Gestalt Therapy Principles and Values", forthcoming in Lee R (ed) The values of connection: A field perspective on ethics, as well as in Gestalt Review.

the child's creative adjustment. In this case, the energy that would have been used for gasping and crying is used instead in the service of making silence and peace in the field inside of himself, and between himself and those around him. The therapist is aware of that phenomenon and gradually helps this child to free the energy that returns him back to his expression.

We therapists facilitate the child to reconnect himself with a magical moment of his process of being alive and reaching forward toward mastering his connectedness with life.

III. The Story of Pedro

I met Pedro when he was three years old. He did not speak, play, or interact with other children or adults. Communication was made through his mother, who would give social meaning for subtle sounds or gestures that he would express and with unexplained crying. His bond with his mother was obviously strong. The father was distant and saw him as a handicapped child. This fragile little boy had an older sister (three years older), described by her mother as being jealous of her brother's attention.

Pedro was referred to me by his speech and physical therapists, who were not making progress with him in their therapy sessions; there was no emotional connection between them. When I met Pedro and his family, the atmosphere of failure and helplessness permeated their lives. I was very touched by their pain and struggle to overcome a very difficult moment.

Thinking about Pedro, I remembered the first time I met him in my office waiting room: he was in the corner of the big room, almost behind a couch, when I entered and greeted him and his mother. He turned his face, stared at me for two seconds without moving one muscle in his face, and then he turned his face away, toward the wall. In that moment, he expressed himself looking at me and moving away. He expressed the fibrillation between feeling safe and scared. The two seconds of looking at me and looking away is the result of his creative adjustment.

My understanding is not to look for something that is pathological in his attitude, but I consider that every expression of a child is a dynamic interchange between various aspects of his experience. Every time the child senses, sees, and feels, a creative adjustment takes place. A child is assimilating the environment in a circular and dynamic way. There is no definition for me of one behavior that is more creative than another; or, I don't look for an attitude that is well-adjusted or not adjusted in a specific context. I see the competence of a child who, at any moment in space and time, lets us know in a most original and unique way, the impact of the world on him; as he does this, he is also changing the world around him with his presence. Every child's presence is a creative adjustment in the world.

Back to the waiting room, I am looking at Pedro. His two seconds of attention, his way of protecting himself, gave me the sense that he had potential to re-create his experience; and, as any other child, he had the capacity of exploring the world. My belief in him would not create another expectation that he might fail once more, but would give me strength and support to work with him day after day. I could accept what he was capable of doing in that moment and help him to feel safe and confident as he moved into the future; his future contained all the possibilities of modifying his existence in the world.

The session I am going to describe took place three years after the beginning of our therapeutic work. Pedro was at a very important moment of his life: one of his biggest challenges was to go to a regular school and interact with other children and teachers. For the first time in his life he was to experience an environment that was different from his home and the offices of therapists.

This session will show how support, trust, and respect are important in our work as facilitators. The challenge is to learn how to follow the creative process that the child naturally brings to us and, as therapists, to pay attention to the child's world, joining him with our emotional freedom; we do not impose rules or pre-definitions of what is "creative". We do not make the child fit into our concept of what he should be. Every child has his unique way of expressing himself. Our job is to listen, respect, and help him become more of what he is as a human being, struggling in life.

The therapist has a powerful evocative presence, hopefully a fully developed one, which elicits the child's best efforts to enter the world and eventually to shine in it.

A. The Session Description: Phenomenological-Existential Approach in Therapy with Children

The moment the child is born, his world is in constant change. His abilities and possibilities are in the process of maturation. He is learning about himself and the world through a continuous process of experimentation.

Being a child therapist means to stay with him in an existential moment where the experience is lived fully in the moment. Nothing else is more important than what exists here between the therapist and the child. The energy of life reverberates between them.

We validate the child's experience again and again. We accept his language, his fantasies, his fears, and the way he chooses to express his frustrations and understandings. We accept his grimaces and body movements. The child carries the wisdom of how to survive in his specific environment. Very early, he starts his process of learning the rules of social behavior and its codes. We need to identify that, accepting the way he is assimilating all this information and how he uses it.

Our pleasure is to listen to his stories, to learn about his experience, and to accompany him in his journey of meaning-making. First and foremost we join the child in *his* world, using his language, metaphors, and images. Then we offer him our world that will bring the novelty and challenges of a creative dialogue between us. The session is a co-creative event.

The session with Pedro is presented in four separate sequences.

Sequence One

Pedro enters the therapy room, looks at the toys, and quickly suggests that we play the "spaghetti game", a game we had played before. I say okay and remind him about the rules. We play the game for a while and *he wins!*

Afterwards Pedro says: "Let's pretend that we are going to eat the spaghetti!"
Therapist: "Yes, good idea!"
We make the gestures as if we were eating the spaghetti with our hands. We move our mouths, eating with gusto.
A little while later Pedro says: "Let's play that I am your 'daddy' and you are my daughter!"
T: "Okay, you are my daddy, and I am your daughter; okay, let's do it ..."
[End of sequence one.]

Let's examine and summarize my behavior with Pedro. When Pedro enters the room, I wait for him to choose something to do. I don't have an agenda. We have a process together, but each session is a new session, giving him the chance to bring something that is important that day for him to experience while being with me. I trust that something will emerge from our meeting that will be meaningful for him. I put aside my expectations and feel myself free and open to his process. I mobilize my psychic energy to receive him.

I genuinely agree with his proposals; I don't ask him questions in advance to find the meaning of what he is asking for. I don't ask why he wants to play "daddy". I simply join him in this journey, and we don't know how it is going to end; but, we are together in this adventure. And I believe that he is going to a place from which he will eventually benefit.

I am fully here, validating his experience of being a *winner and the owner of his choices*. In that moment, he is experiencing his competence in my presence.

B. The Art of the Encounter between the Child and the Therapist

Usually there is a room where the action takes place: the play, the games, the story-telling, the actual sharing. The therapist owns the room. The child comes for frequent visits. In the beginning, everything looks strange and uncomfortable for both. But soon the uncomfortable feelings change to a sense of familiarity and easiness.

The therapist and child develop a dance. The dance of their encounter, creating their rhythm together, each one of them contributing their best to that moment. In this dance, the child takes risks, creating a different reality when he expresses his fantasies. The therapist takes the risk of opening the space for the child's imagery and actions, joining the client in an adventure of the unknown.

By now the child feels free to share confidences or to open her mind and heart during the session. *The therapist supports the child's view of reality. The therapist does not judge, interpret, or impose her or his personal beliefs onto the child.*

The child brings out her fantasies and joy. She creates her own world. The therapist takes the "playing" very seriously, knowing that this is not only a game for having fun, but the complex struggle of a child trying to make sense of her suffering.

Sequence Two

Pedro, as daddy, is yelling at me: "You stay there. Stay quiet!"
Therapist: "What?"
P: "Stay quiet. I told you!"
T: "But I did not say anything ..."
P: "I told you, stay quiet. You are always disobeying me!"
T: [I stay in silence, looking puzzled and frightened.]
Pedro looks at me intently. Then, he smiles.
T: [I remember that he cries a lot, so I start "crying".]
P: "Shut up, stop crying!"
T: "But I ..."
P: "Stop disobeying me. Why do you have to disobey me?"
T: "But I am getting angry ..."
P: "I told you to stay quiet. Okay, go to your room now ... You are going to be alone. Come here right now, but I don't want to hear you talking." [He takes me to the corner in the room, locks the "door", and takes the "key" with him.]

In this moment of the session, I am not a strange adult who intimidates Pedro. I am part of his world of fantasy. I am an instrument for his process. At that moment, I am focusing on Pedro's experience and expression of his feelings. I put myself in his place, imagining how he would feel in that situation, and I offer him my understanding of his emotions.

The room is transformed into a territory of possibilities for the imaginary, and I am immersed in that. It is not my imaginary world, but Pedro's. He is comfortable in using the space in the way he wants to, and I am comfortable surrendering to his needs. And then, we are taking risks, creating a different reality and dancing ... two people in the same rhythm. We are together in a dance in which the rhythm is defined by the rich and complex understanding that Pedro is forming about his experiences in the world, of his father, mother, and sister. I am his instrument in this moment. I am the embodiment of acceptable, yet risk-fluid boundaries.

C. The Richness of Improvisation

Sequence Three

Pedro: "I don't want to hear you saying anything else ..."
[He brings me a "bottle" and says that I have to drink the milk, which contains poison.]
P: "You will drink and die."
Therapist: "But Daddy, are you going to kill me?"
P: "Yes, and stay quiet. Drink now!"

I drink the milk and fall on the floor, as if I were dead. He laughs, and after a while, he asks me to stand up and go near the table where he and Mum are going to send me away from home, and I will become a poor little girl.

T: "But Mum also does not like me?"

P: "No, and stay quiet: don't say anything. You are going to leave home now and be very poor. Go away now!"

T: "Daddy, what did I do to make you so angry?"

He doesn't let me finish talking, tells me to shut up. Then he gives me the following instructions: go to where the armchair is, and while you are on your way, a hunter is going to kill you. I play out that image and he has a lot of fun with that.

T: "Daddy, did you kill me?"

P: "Yes, shut up!"

T: "Did you want me to come into the world?"

P: "No, it was your mother who wanted you to be born. Nobody else wanted you!"

T: "And what is going to happen now that I am dead?"

P: "Now I am going to be with your mom!"

I am lying down on the floor, and he puts a big teddy bear over my body, saying that I am afraid of teddy bears and I will be scared.

T: "Oh! What is this monster over my body? Daddy, did you put this here?"

P: "Yes, shut up." [He pretends to slap me in the face and gags me.]

My heart is beating fast. I am restrained. I have the feeling that this event will be memorable for Pedro.

Experimentation is part of the children's world. They are in constant movement when playing. To play is part of their routine; but when playing is happening in a therapy session, it is transformed into an enactment of the child's struggle. The benefit of the use of playing as an experiment is the opportunity for the child to make sense of her reality.

In the experiment, the child has the possibility of behaving in a different way from the way he is used to in a safe environment. Pedro is experimenting to be in a position of controlling the situation. He changes from being helpless to being powerful. His intention is not to "kill me", but he is expressing and exaggerating the experience of being in his family. He can bring out his fantasies of being oppressed while keeping his integrity. We are co-creating this whole experiment based on improvisations. Pedro creates something in the moment, following the energy that is created by the two of us.

Even after three years of therapy sessions, I still surprise Pedro with my questions, my reactions, and with how my voice and body change after he speaks. The surprise has the effect of reorganizing the way he thinks about himself. For example, Pedro thinking to himself: "I have no voice to express my anger." Therapist: "Did you kill me?" Pedro answers: "Yes, shut up!" Suddenly he hears his own angry voice. He is a different boy. In the balance between evocative and provocative interventions, I keep the flow of tension and movement between us.

The use of experiment with children is the use of our bodies, energy, gestures, and voices. Our whole being is involved. Pedro and I are using the whole space around us. We walk around; we are on the floor. We integrate our voices and gestures to bring to life an image; we are in contact with feelings, sensations, and movements. We use metaphors.

The experiment is a way of transforming the world of concrete images into a lively and meaningful experience. Pedro is integrating his body, sensations, emotions, and understandings. Working with different aspects when the child is playing, we are giving him the possibility of experiencing competence. That is the ultimate function of the experiment in child therapy. Pedro does not leave the session being falsely victorious. He leaves taking ownership of his competence.

D. Discoveries and Affirmation: The Process of Meaning-Making

While therapist and child are developing the experiment, a high level of energy is generated. Their emphasis is on the action and contact, once the theme is developed during the session. Generally, this is also happening when a child is playing in his daily life.

However, in therapy, it is necessary for the child to reach a different level of comprehension about his experience. An important aspect of this work is *timing*. We need to pay attention to what will be the appropriate moment to stop the action and bring the awareness to the moment. The interruptions are meaning-making events.

The therapist assists the child in giving a significant meaning to what he is experiencing, integrating what is known with the novelty. It is not an interpretation of what had happened in the session, but a new clarity for what was experienced, without losing the impact of the present moment. The emerging clarity of thinking and understanding helps the child deal with his suffering. We accept his pain and provide a new context, a new frame for his experiences. Pain is transformed into meaning.

Sequence Four

Pedro throws more animals around me to make me scared. He is having fun. A couple of minutes later, I tell him I am no longer his daughter, and that I would like to talk to him as the father. He agrees with the proposal for such a dialogue:

T: "You get very angry with your daughter ..."
P: "Yes, I did not want to have a daughter like that. She disobeys me all the time. She is worthless."
T: "You are seeing all the bad things, but could she have good things, also?"
P: (Pedro looks down for a minute, then looks at me again, and now begins, as Pedro, to talk. He expresses insight about his own father.) "Yes, he could raise the son, couldn't he?"
T: "Yes, raising the son will be really good. It would be really good having your father closer to you ..."
There is a long silence, and the session ends.

The moment I interrupt Pedro's flow of action I am aware that if we stay too long with his excitement his energy will begin to dissipate, and he will lose an important insight. The moment I slow him down and talk to him on a different level, I am giving him the chance to examine and become aware of what had happened. He is able to bring cognitive closure to the whole event. I support his evolving wisdom.

Even if some interventions are challenging for Pedro, they also evoke new feelings in him. They help him to make contact with himself and to express his inner truth. I did not take him to a place that I thought would be better for him. I followed him without interfering in his process of expressing what he wanted and could do. The evocative intervention strengthens and empowers the child's self.

Integrating what is there, in the experience, with new discoveries is an exciting trajectory toward becoming a person, a mature person.

E. Support and the Beauty of Respecting a Child's Existence

In the moment of silence right after the last dialogue I had with Pedro, when he could express his feelings toward his father, I looked at him. His eyes were open, bright, and shining. He was not crying.

His face was relaxed; there was no tension in his mouth. His cheeks, usually pale, had a light pink color. He was sitting on a chair next to me. His slim arms were resting over his long legs. He was breathing deeply.

I looked back into his eyes, and they were alive, looking into my eyes. We were sitting together and he was alive, right in front of me.

For a couple of seconds, I thought about all the things we had passed through together in the last thirty minutes of our lives. So many things to be analyzed or synthesized. So many different nuances of the work that could be discussed.

But I came back to his eyes, and they were alive!

Meeting Pedro's eyes, a boy, six years old, who for a period of his life had chosen not to exist, not to be present, not to be in contact, and not to give his energy to the world, made my eyes alive, my heart beat; my eyes were warm and open.

And I was deeply moved by those eyes. I felt a profound respect and love for Pedro. In the moment of shared silence, his eyes were alive!

References

Perls F, Hefferline R, Goodman P (1994) Gestalt therapy: Excitement and growth in the human personality. The Gestalt J Press, Highland, New York
Yontef G (1993) Awareness, dialogue & process. The Gestalt J Press, Highland, New York
Zinker J (1977) Creative process in Gestalt therapy. Vintage Books, New York

Memorable Moments
in the Therapeutic Relationship

Nancy Amendt-Lyon

Recently I have felt the desire to document some of the memorable moments that I have been able to experience as a Gestalt therapist, both in individual and group therapy.[1] These memorable moments are among the peak experiences that I remember as having been particularly daring, productive, and fulfilling to both the patients and myself. Recounting these vignettes now, after some time has expired, runs the risk of sounding trite or trivial to the noninvolved reader. Nonetheless, I will take this risk and describe several moments of encounter when I was especially challenged by the therapeutic situation and mustered all my intuition and theoretical knowledge to create an appropriate and unique intervention. The custom-made interventions that I will attempt to describe in their respective contexts were intended to fit the demands of each relational field; they were also aimed at producing something novel and valuable to those involved (see Amendt-Lyon, 1999, 2001a, b). The writing experience brought home to me how difficult it is to best capture the essence of creative interaction in the therapeutic setting and to define creativity.

I. Connecting the Theoretical and Practical Aspects
of the Method

For the identity of Gestalt therapists, or of colleagues from other schools of psychotherapy, mutual stimulation of the theoretical and practical aspects of the method is crucial. Actively accessing our theory nearly always triggers us to reorganize our practice. Applying theory provides us with signs and reminders which allow fresh approaches to emerge, whereas by practicing psychotherapy, we accumulate the resources of experience through which we adjust existing theory and stimulate new directions.

---

[1] Daniel Stern, in his chapter in this volume, refers to "moments of meeting" and addresses an analogous phenomenon.

By connecting various aspects of theory to daily professional practice, we allow our historical identity to resurface and be accessible. Insights from experienced, contemporary practitioners should also be assimilated into the new directions of our theory. My assumption is that this active, conscious connection can both help prevent younger generations of Gestalt therapists from drifting away from or negating the historical roots of their theory and impede the process by which "professionalization" runs the risk of deteriorating into the perfection of techniques and rehashed exercises with new, unsuspecting patients.

Actively and consciously connecting theory and practice would also refresh older generations' approaches, especially those who were trainees when certain streams of Gestalt therapy experienced a phase of negating the relevance of theory and when little was written in the field of Gestalt therapy. For those of us in private practice, this approach would prevent us from calcifying in the common solipsistic mode of practicing Gestalt therapy as lone wolves, isolated in the solitude of our offices. A further aspect I address deals with the implications of our therapeutic work for the future of our patients. Particularly when an expressive medium is used, it is important for both therapist and patient to understand the implications and intentionality inherent in what has been expressed. Beyond such well-tried interventions as "How does that make you feel?" and "Where are you now?", we must probe into fantasies and thoughts pertaining to the near and remote future. For example, "What does this new insight imply to you?", "What do you imagine will happen next?", "Where does this take us?", or "Where do we go from here?"

The following vignettes attempt to illustrate the interaction between theoretical background, intuition, and use of artistic media that stimulate my practice of Gestalt therapy. All names and important identifying features have been changed to protect the persons involved.

II. Katarina's Ten Commandments

One particularly memorable moment I had was experienced with Katarina, a young singer who had withdrawn from professional life for a few years after having her first child. Soon after giving birth, she separated from her husband, who suffered from alcohol dependency, and then divorced him. When we began our work, she ruminated over her own erratic alcohol excesses, especially when she was alone, and obsessed over her fears of being able to perform as a singer again. Her parents taught her to take pride in her working class background, which she left when she pursued a successful career and entered middle class. Now she was afraid she'd never be able to take up her profession, and she doubted if she would be able to support herself. After maternity leave, she continued to live on social welfare subsidies. Katarina was overly strict and merciless with herself; if something went wrong, she was to blame. In her unsparing and disciplined family of origin, according to Katarina, she played the role of the clown and mediator, whereas her older sister played the role of the academically inclined beauty. Based on Katarina's descriptions, her mother was chronically depressed, and her father was the unquestioned, proud patriarch of the family. Katarina compensated many of her narcissistic deficits professionally, but when she temporarily left singing to become a mother, her self-esteem and confidence nose-dived.

During one particular session, she was beside herself and fell into a frenzy. I agonized over how to interrupt her familiar vicious circle of self-effacing behavior and allow her to tap into the rich resources of her own effective experiences, family background, and social network. I knew from our past work that she enjoyed my theatrical vein, so I stood up from my chair and, assuming a different position in the room, asked her to tell me what rules for life she was given by her family. Katarina looked up at me somewhat perplexed. Then I asked her to stand up as well and to define the "ten commandments" that she learned from her family of origin. I fantasized that this would help her to connect with her supporting background and available resources, and that they could accompany and guide her through this uncertain phase of her life. My assumption was also that the hidden agenda of her ruminations, that is, the introjects, would come to the fore. The "ten commandments" she came up with were as follows: 1) Katarina doesn't have to starve 2) Katarina will always have a roof over her head 3) Katarina has a healthy child 4) Katarina hides her "hinterlands" 5) Katarina should be wary of those who have lots of money 6) Katarina should never forget the ten commandments of her family 7) Katarina should not reach for more happiness than she is entitled to 8) Katarina should never play unfairly with her advantages 9) Katarina should never be happier and more successful than her relatives, and 10) Katarina must never aggravate critical situations – she should rather assuage them!

When she finished this experiment, Katarina was beaming and had taken on a self-confident stance. It was as if she had regained her backbone! She laughingly wrote down what she had verbally just formulated. These ten statements were the basis for her self-understanding and her mode of relating to the world. Articulating them with me as her witness enabled Katarina to connect with those aspects of herself that function well. Moreover, it became evident that by adhering to all the commandments, she impeded herself in various ways from functioning well and living healthily.

Suddenly, I realized that I was in her hinterlands with her, and a spell was broken that had previously kept me from understanding where she was coming from, figuratively and literally. This brief experiential moment of creative writing also showed me how the dynamics of the therapist-patient relationship can be deduced from our reaching out to the arts. Creative expression within relationship points to a new meaning or function of art. It is that which developed and emerged between us and reflected something novel and valuable to both Katharina and myself in this specific context. We delighted in playing with the ten personalized commandments, and we often referred to them in future work. This memorable moment transformed our therapeutic relationship and produced a new level of understanding.

III. "Make a Wish for Your Birthday!"

Hildegard was referred to me after having been discharged from in-patient psychiatric treatment, diagnosed as borderline, depressive, and suffering from post-traumatic stress disorder. She had a history of childhood abuse and neglect, and for years she had practiced self-mutilation: cutting herself with a razor and burning herself with a cigarette lighter. She obviously showed strong suicidal tendencies, indulged in alcohol excesses and excessive spending, had virtually no impulse control, had few friends, and clutched on to her immediate family members – yet was highly ambivalent toward her mother, who was addicted to alcohol and various medications. Hildegard had numerous, indiscriminate sexual contacts, and she suffered from flashbacks of being gang raped, which had occurred several years before. When we began to work together, she voiced the desire to be heard and taken seriously. Although close to thirty at the time, she exhibited the behavior of a teenager or sometimes that of a small child, and I soon realized that I had to meet her on this emotional-developmental level for our therapeutic alliance to function. We drew pictures together, e.g. Winnicott's squiggle drawings. She drew comic-like pictures of her arguments with her mother, and she loved it when we had dialogues using hand puppets or stuffed animals. Her favorite choice of a stuffed animal was a cuddly, disheveled dog. Her suicide threats and attempts continued throughout our four years of therapy. We agreed that she could call me on my private phone if she felt endangered. My main tasks were to help her to process what was happening in her life in simple, concrete terms, to facilitate her learning to accept her feelings of ambivalence, and to explore alternatives to her self-destructive behavior. I found myself soothing and comforting her a lot, too.

One night, she called and told me that she was standing at her open window (she lived on the fourth floor) and that she didn't feel safe. I spoke calmly to her for about 45 minutes and convinced her to check herself into the hospital for psychiatric treatment. She reluctantly agreed, on the condition that I bring her there myself, which I did. And I stayed with her, consulting with the medical doctor on duty, until she finally fell asleep. The comforting effect that this had on her was very important, most likely a corrective emotional experience for a woman who was often neglected as a child. During her six-week stay in the hospital, we phoned regularly, and I visited her once.

When she resumed therapy, it was spring, and she entered my office one day when there were more flower arrangements in the room than usual. She immediately asked if it was my birthday today. I generally prefer not to reveal personal data to any of my patients, but I intuitively felt that it was important at this moment not to ask her such questions as "What gives you that impression?" or "What would it mean to you if it were?" but, rather, to disclose this fact about myself in a straightforward manner. I felt compelled to take a risk of self-revelation in order to maintain her trust, a main issue for those who suffer from borderline disorders. "Yes, it is", I replied simply. She smiled slowly, withdrew into her thoughts for a while, and then exclaimed:

"Make a wish for your birthday!" Again, in light of her history of double-binds and abuse, I realized that a direct and honest answer was called for, an answer that would at the same time allow me to be selectively authentic. In addition, I wanted my answer to be relevant to the here-and-now of our working alliance: working through and finding a healthy solution to her self-destructive and suicidal tendencies. I said: "My wish is that my children out-live me!" She looked into my face, and I held my breath for a moment, be-fore adding: "And that goes for you, too, Hildegard, since you are twenty-five years younger than I am, and I want you to outlive me, too!" Unexpect-edly, I felt a surge of emotion swell up in my chest, and I fought back tears as I looked into her eyes. She, too – who had never shed a tear while working on her heart-rending experiences in all her years in therapy – had tears in her eyes. She looked at me with a mixture of satisfaction and disbelief, fell silent for a few minutes, and then picked up the thread of our dialogue and began to deal with her self-destructive behavior. Hildegard realized that she mattered to me and that it made a difference to me if she lived or not. I also learned, in the course of later sessions, not to panic if she showed me her most recent cuts and burns. Slowly we began to comprehend that Hilde-gard's injuring herself physically meant that she was avoiding the more dev-astating psychological pain involved in dealing with explosive issues. Our dialogue had gained significant depth along these lines.

IV. Painting the Indescribable and Unimaginable in Yellow and Green

Crisis intervention was why Karin, who worked in public relations, entered therapy. Her mother had committed suicide, not quite unexpectedly, but nonetheless a tremendous shock for Karin and her siblings. Karin's relation-ship to her self-absorbed, distanced mother was highly ambivalent. Being confronted with her suicide brought many unresolved issues to the surface, and Karin was shaken by a mixture of emotions from her sudden loss, in-cluding anger toward her mother for leaving her children this legacy and shame for being angry at someone who could not see any alternative to sui-cide. This crisis brought out hysterical processes in Karin, who tried to cope by changing jobs, participating in numerous esoteric workshops, having an extensive horoscope done, and engaging in a series of short-lived affairs. It was difficult to arrange a therapeutic commitment with her. Either she ideal-ized me and wanted to stay for intensive continuous treatment, or she would doubt whether therapy could help her at all. Similar to the circumstances with her mother, Karin's relationship to me was colored by feelings of envy and rivalry. Appearances were very important to her, and I realized that we were entering a new phase in our relationship when we could work on the negative, unattractive aspects of appearances, which, naturally, we both have. Toward the end of one session, Karin withdrew into silence. My query as to what was happening drew a pensive response from her. The indescrib-able and unimaginable aspects of her mother's suicide were consuming her.

She was plagued by the image she had when she discovered her mother's lifeless body. The image that represented this horrific experience was of yellow-green bile. Instead of coming to our next session, Karin called to cancel and told me it was overwhelming for her come to therapy today, since it was the anniversary of her mother's death. The next few sessions were noticeably slow-paced and cautious. Karin was engaged in "talking about" events in her life, and my efforts to understand their significance and in which direction they were taking her proved fruitless. Queries as to which medium she could employ to communicate her experiences rolled off her like water off a duck's back. I decided to state the obvious and conveyed to Karin my impression that a certain stagnation had set in. We were at an impasse. Karin agreed, chiding me that "nothing" was happening and that she considered terminating therapy. I fought with feelings of being inept at connecting to her adequately.

When she entered my office the next week she immediately zeroed in on the painting materials in the corner. Karin expressed the urge to paint the yellow-green bile she had previously imagined with finger-paints. Her main theme was the bile within her, representing the experience of her mother's suicide. The narcissistic wounds, unexpressed anger, and reproaches were well-expressed on a big sheet of paper. Karin not only dared to create something that she considered to be sloppy, ugly, and disgusting, but she also shared it with me. In our reflection of her finger-painting process, we began to fathom what she experienced as being "indescribable" and "unimaginable", which injuries she suffered, and which movements she felt were taking place. A certain peace and composure came over her face, and I sighed with relief. Karin could adequately express her inner experiences within our relationship, and together we risked exploring ugliness and shame-laden issues. The patterns in her finger painting began to connect to her inner experience, and they made sense. Her anger toward me for not being a magician and helping her out of her crisis immediately could be worked through, and our relationship was no longer tainted by destructive aspects of rivalry and envy.

V. "Coming Down to Earth"

The therapeutic relationship with George, a medical student from Germany who had been studying in Vienna for several years, presented me with a considerable challenge. He had been diagnosed as suffering from extreme manic-depressive episodes before he was referred to me. He requested that I recommend a psychiatrist so that he could take medication in addition to being in therapy. I kept in contact with the psychiatrist throughout George's therapy, and this cooperation was productive for our process. With me, George presented the manic aspects of his personality; the depressive aspects were negligible. Actually, the main figures in our relational field were his obsessive-compulsive thoughts and behaviors. During the first few months of therapy, George spoke "at" me like a machine gun, and he kept changing the subject if our dialogue entered realms he wished to avoid. He was always equipped with sensational stories that filled our sessions and enabled him to avoid what was bothering him most. He had difficulty keeping eye contact and broke off in the middle of sentences. I mentioned this pattern of speediness and avoidance to him and tried to connect it to his reasons for entering therapy. In a charming and witty manner, he comforted me and asked me to be patient with him. My curiosity about the other end of the manic-depressive polarity grew, and I began to doubt the validity of the original diagnosis. At the same time, we explored the concrete situations in which he began to obsess and gain speed.

Humor and pantomime were my means of interrupting the well-tried monologues he tended to hold during our sessions, allowing us to enjoy brief moments of dialogue. Then I began to respond to his speediness by literally changing our working level. I sat down on the carpet and handed him modeling dough to knead. Or I told him to look around the office and see what interested him. He immediately grabbed a Nepalese drum and began to play simple, moving rhythms. I intended to explore the opposite pole of his escalating spiral of predominantly rational-verbal processes by supporting such sensory-motor and nonverbal activities as sculpting and playing percussion instruments. My interventions took him by surprise, yet he accepted these small risks. In fact, he appeared to be relieved. When kneading modeling dough or playing the drum, his breathing slowed down, his eyes were concentrated, and George fell silent. After he had enough of sculpting or drumming, we remained sitting on the carpet and talking about what he had just experienced and what had changed for him. I was fascinated by the qualitative difference in our dialogue. He could look me in the eye, speak more slowly and in complete sentences, and briefly be uninterested in impressing me with a flood of hair-raising stories.

About two years into our therapeutic work, George began working during his vacation at an old-age home, where he was very popular among the elderly and the staff. He had been relatively composed at this time, and I could meet his occasional initial speediness, usually coupled with endless monologues and fantasies about himself in superlative terms, with a humorous comment or the direct question: "Is this your idea of a dialogue?" He would laugh at this as if he expected it, and he began to talk with, not at me. One particular day he shared a daydream that caused us both to giggle. He told me that he imagined himself as the medical director of this old-age home and thought about how he would treat the residents and subordinates. I decided to take the transferential cue he gave me in his fantasy, connecting it to the here-and-now of our relationship and to the superlative self-image he often presented to me. By doing this, I stepped into his daydream, joining him in the no man's land of common fantasies with images of my own. I acknowledged: "Yes, I can just see you in your white coat with a stethoscope around your neck and all the young doctors following you on your rounds. By that time, I'll be a resident of the home, old and frail. And I'll drive all the doctors crazy, because I will demand that only *my boy* George be allowed to treat me!" He scrutinized my face to see if I were serious, then we both broke out in loud laughter. Whereupon George spoke to me in a confidential manner: "I sure have delusions of grandeur, don't I?" I replied that I certainly have witnessed him taking off on fantasies, that these tend to get speedier as he goes along, and that there are preconditions for all this happening. This made sense to him. I dared to tread on unknown territory by taking up his fantasy and continuing with my own images, emphasizing his fantasies of greatness and desire for power, as well as issues of dependency in his relationship with me. George and I agreed how vital it was for him to "come down to earth" more often and for longer periods of time. We developed various signals for situations requiring this, such as merely sitting down on the carpet, indicating a downward spiral with an index finger, and raising a hand to indicate that I want to speak, as if I were in a classroom. Our experiments and signals have helped George appreciate the comedy within the tragedy: that is, not to be so dead serious and to participate in dialogue. Engaging in a process-oriented method of diagnosis helped us to correct the stigma of the initial diagnosis, which George feared was a permanent burden. Manic behavior and obsessive-compulsive patterns were our focus, but the depressive aspects of the supposed bipolar disorder were not manifest.

VI. "Neither Victims nor Perpetrators"

The following vignette is taken from an advanced Gestalt therapy training group. My co-therapist and I were leading one of our three-day weekends and collecting possible themes from the participants for our day's work. The day before we had worked on issues dealing with sexual abuse, speechlessness, and taboos in the family and society at large, especially with regard to National Socialism. These topics had also accompanied us in various forms during weekends past. Lydia recounted a dream she had had the night before. The dream was very moving and upsetting to us all. We were fascinated by the fact that in dealing with National Socialism on both the collective and individual levels of society, the question of responsibility was posed. Lydia's dream was entitled "Neither victims nor perpetrators".

To begin with, Lydia narrated the dream in detail, as if it were unfolding again before her eyes. She described the atmosphere, the scenes, the action, and the persons and objects involved, which was quite a chore, because the dream was complicated and consisted of three seemingly unconnected scenes. Since Lydia described predominantly scenes and atmospheres, hardly remembering any dialogues, I suggested that the entire group enact the dream as if it were a play, thus emphasizing the moods and emotional tones involved. Everyone agreed, and Lydia first slipped into roles of different persons and objects, then assigned the roles as well as designated places and actions in the dream to the group members. She described the emotional atmospheres and suggested appropriate sentences and nonverbal communication to fit the plot that she had created in her dream. The group members were to initially take these affective cues and eventually extemporize according to the flow of the group process.

The first scene of Lydia's dream began in a narrow, uncomfortable garden with catlike animals. These creatures were part tiger, lively, and yet somehow timid. Their attributed sentence was: "We are fearful, but we will fight!" The catlike creatures prowled around cautiously and were friendly to Lydia. The second scene took place in a loud, confusing airport in South Africa. There were airplanes, a table with various items, and three boxes with a wreath in each of them. Lydia wanted to buy the wreaths, but she didn't have the proper currency. She sent the person accompanying her to get the right money, although she knew that he wouldn't succeed. Nonetheless, she said to the escort: "Bring me the money!" This was possibly to keep up a certain appearance with the merchants. The merchant who was selling the wreaths was described by Lydia as nonrelating and unfamiliar to her. Yet, surprisingly, he said to her: "Take them! I'll gladly give them to you, and you don't need to get money for them." In the third scene, Lydia concentrated on the three wreaths, shyly choosing those group members to enact them whose family histories were most relevant to the historical issue involved. The first wreath had a ribbon on it which read: "In commemoration of the victims." It was a very simple wreath, made of natural materials, such as raffia. The second wreath, which had a light gray ribbon on it, read: "Forgive us our trespasses!" And the third wreath, made of raffia, green branches, and leaves, read: "Neither victims nor perpetrators!"

Lydia's densely concentrated narrative picked up so many threads of the issues we had been dealing with on individual and group levels, that day as well as several weekends before: participation in National Socialism and in Resistance movements, individual speechlessness and collective silence, and family secrets. The dream took on a special significance because the parents and grandparents of the group members (including the co-leader and myself) represented many of the possible roles in this historical period: unshakeable Nazi Party members, "fountain pen criminals", those unwilling to join the Nazis but unable to resist them, active Resistance fighters, Jews who had suffered interrogation by the Gestapo and gone into hiding, and Jews who were forced to emigrate once it was clear that their lives were at stake, as well as Jews who had emigrated at the end of the 19th century and whose European relatives were murdered during the National Socialist regime. The description was so concentrated that I asked Lydia to stop her dream narrative for the moment and suggested to the group that we enact the dream up till this point and see what emerged. We began with the catlike animals on the prowl, and everyone followed the original narrative until we came to the part about the delivery of the money, at which point Lydia reported an uncomfortable feeling that errors would be made. Suddenly a brook appeared in her memory of the dream, and something was swept up in the mud that transformed itself into riches. A group member was attributed this role with the sentence: "I am valuable; everyone wants me; and then I disappear." Following this, an airplane landed at the airport, and a scene ensued in which every participant was involved in his or her given role and extemporized freely, as if on cue. It was breathtaking for me to witness the different levels of action taking place simultaneously and observe the animation of "inanimate objects"! Every single group member was involved in portraying a part in this common endeavor and appeared highly concentrated. This atmosphere proved to be too much for Lydia, especially the dilemma about the money delivery. I noticed her distress and suggested that she intentionally step outside the "stage" and look at the actors in order to decide what her priority is here and now.

Lydia claimed that she was very attached to the wreaths and that she didn't want to forsake them: "I want to care for and protect them; I want to find a good place for them to stay." She gave me the impression that this theme was of overwhelming importance to her, and yet she hesitated to go further. I asked her if she had something more to say to the group, and she replied: "Choosing three people to represent the wreaths and deliver these weighty messages was like breaking a taboo! Can I dare burden these three individuals with such heavy messages?"

I reassured her that we would work these themes through in a collective effort, and I tried to restate what had just happened in her dream in the context of the group process. I couched her individual experience in the context of the entire group, giving her interpersonal support and solidarity: we need a suitable place to work through the individual sentences; when taboos are broken, fears arise that others will be overwhelmed; we appear to be dealing with the ambivalence of the second and third generation after the Shoah, and they are neither victims nor perpetrators.

Now the group members had the chance to describe what it was like to be in their respective roles and what meaning this had both for them personally and for the group process as a whole. Listening to their accounts, it was as if pieces were falling into a puzzle and we were close to finishing a particularly difficult one. The dream brought together many individual themes of the group members and presented them cogently as social and political issues on the group level. When asked what was new and valuable for her from the dream, Lydia said: "The warmth I felt in my responsibility for the wreaths! Now I can differentiate between being guilty and having responsibility, which means being part of continuing history. I feel that it is important and correct this way. And I'm astonished by the import of the dream for the group!" Our reflections on the individual and group levels considered the phrase "Neither victims nor perpetrators" to be *the* chance that those who were born after World War II have – as a checked force, as the potential to begin anew. Vigilance was deemed necessary and our focus was on collective *silence*, not on collective guilt! The political claim that psychotherapy should make was called for, not the usual polite restraint of failing to address political issues that are of obvious importance to patients, or refusing to take a stand on political developments that affect the psychotherapeutic profession. Lydia enabled us to deal with all these explosive issues by presenting her dream. The group expressed satisfaction and gratitude that the Nazi era was dealt with during our time together, since this brought the social aspect of our relational field to the fore. Several group members requested relevant literature from me (see Rosenthal, 1997; Bar On, 1989; Heimannsberg and Schmidt, 1993) and organized a study group on this subject. The entire group was still touched by the silence, taboos, and significance of this historical period for intergenerational conflicts within their own families as our session came to a close. I was in awe of what the group was capable of identifying with and amazed at their extempore portrayals and the way they discovered the meaning of the dream process within the context of their own lives.

VII. Unique Individuals and Unmistakable Styles

Practicing Gestalt therapy cannot be equated to using Gestalt therapy merely as a technique. What truly earns the name Gestalt therapy is the production of a gestalt, stemming from the historical awareness of the theoretical foundations of our method and an appropriate form of intervention. This connection of theory and practice should not be substituted by shortcuts, such as naming the founders of Gestalt therapy in one's list of references or trying to imitate them in one's work. As Gestalt therapists, we can only kindle the fire of Gestalt therapy by both applying our own unique backgrounds in therapeutic encounters with our patients and by treating our patients as unique individuals, which they obviously are. Laura Perls described psychotherapy to me as the encounter of two unique individuals. Every single encounter is thus unique. As Gestalt therapists, it behooves us to keep this in mind in our therapeutic interventions. In practice, this translates to one unmistakable style encountering another unmistakable style, and the involvement of these styles with each other forms a new relational field in which they can interact – hopefully productively.

VIII. Repeating vs. Innovating

Repeating overly accustomed interventions leaves me bored and mildly fearful of stagnating in my profession. Well-established yet rehearsed, amusing yet planned, these ready-to-wear therapeutic interventions are used widely in therapeutic practice and offer mixed blessings. On the one hand, they are known to have a remarkable impact on patients and may even trigger the expression of heart-felt emotions. Many patients may feel understood and well-supported by these familiar interventions. With time, they come to expect them, too. On the other hand, however, the repetition of these interventions spread an aura of staleness, tedium, and shallowness to the therapeutic atmosphere. While routine may work in the sense of being "good enough", it isn't facilitating the kind of doing and daring that earns the adjective "creative" to me. Well-tried interventions don't bring forth anything new and valuable; nothing novel and enriching is accessed; no insights become evident. Comfortable, routine interventions from the therapist lead to therapist-patient dynamics that have little "muscle tone"; that is, they are much slacker than the kind of dynamics stemming from unrehearsed, "custom-made" interventions. Non-routine interventions carry a slight risk and are inevitably exciting to those involved. During my work with patients, I yearn for the excitement of an insight I dare to articulate, the venture of a risk by sharing a fantasy, or my immediate emotional reaction to engagement with my patients, guided, of course, by process-oriented diagnosis and wise timing.

Viewing the process of creative expression within a therapeutic relationship attributes a different meaning to creativity; it is defined by novelty and value, and it emerges between two or more persons. It is the result of joint risk-taking, experimenting with the unknown, and leaving familiar territory behind. Thus, creativity is an aspect of relationship, a part of the relational field. It involves what happens between us!

IX. Creative Process Over Time

Considering the development of creative process over time, my flourishing imagination came up with a number of disquieting and, for the most part, unanswerable questions. For instance, does the creative process ripen with age? Does the ability to intervene creatively increase with years of experience? Is it foolish and idealistic to demand the constant co-creation of novel interventions? What strategy would counteract the common tendency to revert to comfortable, predictable patterns and practice our "favorite" and trusty interventions? How is the approach to practice of those colleagues – who haven't read recent theoretical literature on their specific method for decades – affected? Do all Gestalt therapists need constant connection to theory, to the current theoretical discourse – not only of our own method, but of psychotherapy theory in general – in order to have a good sense of professional identity and stimulation for our practice?

I am aware from experience that the pitfalls of the repetitive and indiscriminate use of overly familiar interventions and routine exercises are stagnation and general feelings of dissatisfaction. I personally become irritated if an intervention "doesn't work" with patients, discontent and perplexed at first, not understanding why "this" or "that" didn't work this time. Then, hopefully, I am able to attend to the vexation and realize that these are countertransference signals warranting attention! Lapsing into routine implies having taken a shortcut, looking for the easy answer or for the least strenuous intervention. The opposite pole, I believe, is to be disposed to be surprised, to take a risk, and to trust one's intuition in cooperation with one's theoretical foundation. Moreover, it involves the willingness to be perceived as clumsy or embarrassed, adjectives that psychotherapists do not like to attribute to themselves.

X. Daring to Risk Awkwardness and Embarrassment

Working in a creative mode necessitates relying less on habitual and more on emerging solutions. This implies the courage to be awkward and clumsy (see, for example, the excellent explication by Wilson-Sanford, 2001) as well as the willingness to be embarrassed, the advantages of which Laura Perls

(Kitzler et al., 1982, p. 17) has discussed. Not pretending or assuming that you know exactly what is happening, not constantly producing a patent answer to every question, and indeed showing that you are a learner, too, requires courage from a therapist. This approach also means being humble enough to share uncertainty and to undergo several unsuccessful attempts to access a disorder or symptom with a patient, risking the possibility that patients may become disappointed, because you do not immediately appear to know what is good for them. Some patients may be accustomed to a posture of high confidence when consulting medical doctors, who treat physical disorders with medication and give the impression that the cure to an ailment can be reduced to one drug (or a limited number of them). To me, the courage to be awkward appears a strong antidote to the tendency of certain therapists to behave narcissistically! Although it is a position that is sometimes uncomfortable and often disquieting, I am appreciative if patients or trainees criticize or challenge me, because this usually indicates an I-Thou relationship in which each treats the other as a subject and an equal.

XI. Conclusion

It was my intention to demonstrate how theory and practice productively connect by using examples of memorable moments from case studies. Lapsing into the familiarity of routine interventions or well-established exercises gives Gestalt therapists a pseudo-certainty and a false sense of confidence. In fact, this may even disguise insecurity or prevent therapists from realizing that they are stagnating professionally. Naturally, having to constantly produce fresh experiments and new perspectives in daily therapeutic work is challenging, risky, and strenuous. Yet it is precisely these risks and strains that are necessary if we want to experience the deep satisfaction and elation that can result from such an investment. In order to find good form, we will be best equipped with a solid theory from which to practice and, conversely, solid practice from which to derive theory! This prompts my appeal to colleagues to allow themselves to be fascinated by the individual lives of their patients and to feel passionate about their professional work. It is hardly possible to fulfill this request in each and every therapy session. All the same, such thoughts accompany me as silent, supportive reminders through the day and help me gain richer satisfaction in my work. I also find I am better able to concentrate on the needs of those individuals, couples, and groups who enter my office.

References

Amendt-Lyon N (1999): Kunst und Kreativität in der Gestalttherapie. In: Fuhr R et al. (eds) Handbuch der Gestalttherapie. Hogrefe, Göttingen, pp 857–877
Amendt-Lyon N (2001a) Art and creativity in Gestalt therapy. Gestalt Review 5(4): 225–248
Amendt-Lyon N (2001b) "No risk, no fun!" A reply to commentaries. Gestalt Review 5(4): 272–275

Bar-On D (1989) The legacy of silence. Encounters with children of the Third Reich. Harvard Univ Press, Cambridge

Heimannsberg B, Schmidt CJ (eds) (1993) The collective silence: German identity and the legacy of shame. Analytic Press, Mahwah, New Jersey

Kitzler R, Perls L, Stern EM (1982) Retrospects and prospects: A trialogue between Laura Perls, Richard Kitzler and E. Mark Stern. Voices 18(2): 5–22

Rosenthal G (ed)(1997) Der Holocaust im Leben von drei Generationen. Familien von Überlebenden der Shoah und von Nazi-Tätern. Psychosozial Verlag, Giessen

Wilson-Sanford J (2001) A call to courage – applying principles of art and creativity in organizational development in large systems. Commentary on article by Nancy Amendt-Lyon. Gestalt Review 5(4): 262–271

Part IV
A Taste of the Field in Practice

Creativity in Long-Term Intimate Relationships

Joseph Melnick and Sonia March Nevis[1]

I. Introduction

Most of us yearn to have a long-term relationship that is lively and stimulating, one that continues to grow and develop over time. The challenge is in keeping the relationship fresh, filled with unexpected elements and pleasant surprises. Creativity can play an important role in sustaining a vibrant and evolving relationship.

Needless to say, describing this activity in long-term relationships is not easy, since unlike most creative processes, there is no simple artistic medium, such as paint or clay, with which to create. It is much more akin to improvisational theater, where actors make contact with an audience and with each other, and where anything can happen. However, in intimate relationships, the emotional and psychological stakes are higher, and the consequences are riskier.

A couple's artistic materials include words, gestures, and touch, but the primary one is the experience of relationship, what happens between them. This is not to say that the larger field, which includes culture, religion, time, place, and world events, does not affect them. Nor do we mean to ignore the inner world of each individual that is filled with a range of creative potentials as well as limitations. However, while acknowledging the importance of the individual's internal experience and that of the larger environment in which we live, our primary focus in this chapter will be on what happens *between* two individuals, what we term the relational field.

Each creative process has a structure. In the arts, people are trained technically and aesthetically to know "good form". Potters, for example, are taught to perfect their artistic sense while mastering the skill of working at the wheel. Couples, on the other hand, are seldom taught the concept of good relational form. Usually their knowledge and skill base derives from a blend of unaware and unexamined introjects handed down from their parents and the wider culture.

[1] We would like to thank the participants of the East Coast Eaters and Writers Group as well as Bud Feder, Joseph Handlon, and Isabel Fredericson for their comments on an earlier draft, and especially Gloria Melnick for her insights and editorial help.

If this is the case, then how do we assess good form, especially since there are no designated experts or critics (other than therapists) to evaluate the product? It is hard enough to evaluate a good piece of art or a musical performance, even with some agreed upon criteria, but how does one determine a successful intimate relationship?

Throughout this chapter, good form will be described by articulating certain qualities that a couple must possess and exhibit for a long-term creative and intimate relationship to flourish. More specifically:

- *Creative Adjustment*: Are they able to adjust creatively to life and to each other? Are they able to stay with sensations and emotions long enough for integration to occur?
- *Experimental Attitude*: Do they have an experimental attitude toward their relationship? Do they have a healthy process for managing the difficulties, disappointments, disillusionments, hurts, and betrayals that go hand in hand with being together over time?
- *Hard Work and Discipline*: Do they have the capacity to work hard to create an agreed upon structure? Of equal importance, do they have the discipline to live out their agreements and to translate agreements into behavior over time?
- *Creative Stabilization*: Do they know when enough is enough? Do they know how to let go of old forms in a mutually respectful way?
- *Bearing Disappointment*: Are they able to bear both being disappointed and disappointing their significant other? Do they know when to address these hurts and when to let them pass?
- *Maintaining Interest*: Do they know how to generate and maintain interest in each other and the relationship?
- *Sense of Humor*: Are they able to, at times, take themselves and their relationship less seriously, so as to de-escalate and make conflict safer? Are they able to use humor and play?

Before beginning to take a closer look at these questions, the reader should be warned: despite the forthcoming discussion describing the hard work that relationships take and the difficulties and disappointment that couples must learn to manage, the perspective presented may appear overly optimistic. Although fully aware of the hurts, betrayals, and long impasses that are a part of every long-term relationship, we believe that this foundation of optimism is an essential ingredient for all creative experience.

II. Creativity from a Gestalt Perspective

"... fundamentally, an organism lives in its environment by maintaining its difference and, more importantly, by assimilating the environment to its difference; and it is at the boundary that dangers are rejected, obstacles are overcome, and the assimilable is selected and appropriated. Now what is selected and assimilated is always novel; the organism persists by assimilating the novel, by changing and growth" (Perls et al., 1951, p. 230).

The creative process has historically been viewed from an individual perspective (Martindale, 2001). Thus, creativity is thought of as a characteristic or a type of energy – tapped or untapped – that resides within. For example, we often think of people as having creative talents or personalities.

The Gestalt perspective views this concept in a different and important way. Rather than seeing creativity as a trait, property, or product of exclusively intrapsychic processes, it is, instead, conceptualized as an *aspect of relationship*, existing between the self and the environment. Thus, the focus of creativity is shifted from something that resides in the interior of the person, to the dynamic of the individual in relation to the environment. Creativity then becomes a process that happens outside one's skin, "where the self meets the other"[2].

A. Contact

"... in the process of assimilation the organism is in turn changed. Primarily, contact is the awareness of, and behavior toward the assimilable novelty; and the rejection of the unassimilable novelty. What is pervasive, always the same, or indifferent is not an object of contact" (Perls et al., 1951, p. 230).

Although there are many names for this meeting of self and other, the basic term used is contact. Contact by definition is creative, for with contact something novel and unique occurs. Therefore, all contact is transformative, in that two initially separate entities or aspects of self are, for a brief period of time, experienced as one. Contact can be with parts of oneself or of the environment, such as a tree in bloom or a beautiful sunset. This basic process of the transformation of the self through contact with the environment is termed creative adjustment. It is considered essential for psychological health and will be discussed further below.

B. Intimacy

"Long-term intimacy is the result of individuals experiencing a wide range of intimate moments over a significant period of time" (Melnick and Nevis, 1994, p. 297).

Viewing creativity from the vantage point of the individual, while useful, is insufficient to address it fully as it exists within intimate, long-term relationships. In order to understand this form of creative process, it is essential to go beyond the idea of a self and an other. What happens *between* these two individuals must also be addressed – how creativity develops, and how it is sustained. To do this, the concept of contact needs to be expanded to include an interpersonal perspective. When one is engaged in an intimate relationship, there are not just two people interacting. There is a third entity – a "we" that the creative couple is continuously shaping.

---

[2] An example is described by Fogel (1991). Rather than children responding to a mother's parenting, Fogel presents convincing research that demonstrates that mother and child are continuously influencing each other: they create the moments between them.

The term *intimate moment* (Melnick and Nevis, 1994) is used to describe a contact episode between two individuals, and it is the creative building block to intimacy. An intimate moment can occur when two people have the same degree of energy or interest in the same thing at the same time. These moments are characterized by the element of vitality and a sense of "boundarylessness", accompanied by feelings of connectedness and mutuality. Each individual does not experience the other as separate and differentiated from the self but, instead, experiences an openness to knowing and being known.

III. The Development of Intimate Relationships

In the beginning of an intimate relationship, nearly every moment is novel, because there is little shared experience and the awareness field is narrow. Most everything about the other person is new and, therefore, of interest. In fact, intimate moments seem to happen with little awareness or effort. As we have said elsewhere, it is the pure joy attached to this ongoing, effortless process of mutual discovery that we call infatuation or romantic love (cf. Melnick and Nevis, 2001).

At the beginning of a relationship, much of the couple's focus is on one another. As a result, a great deal of everyday life is often ignored. However, as the relationship develops over time, there is generally less to be discovered about the other. This "wearing off of newness" is often perceived as a great loss, and to some extent it is. However, the increased familiarity also brings with it some positive benefits. There is often a transition from learning about the other to learning about the relationship. Furthermore, much of the interest and energy that originally went into discovery becomes available for daily living. At its best, a type of balance ensues in which personal, relational, and wider needs get appropriate attention.

There is a safety embedded in predictability. There is so much uncertainty in the world and in our lives that we are often on the edge of anxiety. If lucky, increased familiarity allows for relaxation in the presence of another, establishing a safe haven from the tension that accompanies life's constant surprises. This safety often supports habitual ways of relating. Life is easier if the couple knows who will pay the bills, cook the meals, and clean the carpets. Some of the more important and formalized habits are called *rituals*. At their best, they are complex habits, developed to provide continuity by acknowledging important events, such as birthdays, promotions, marriages, and deaths. Meaningful ritual supports the structure and stability of relationships.

Most important, there is something inherently pleasant in knowing and being known. To be seen, understood, and acknowledged touches the core of what it is to be human. It is as if we are designed to be in relationship with another, without goals or agendas. Many have written about this experience, but none as elegantly as Buber (1958).

There is, however, also a downside to this increased knowing of the other. What is familiar, complex, and predictable can quickly become uninteresting and boring. Aspects and characteristics originally experienced as attractive and novel can unexpectedly take on a more negative hue and become problematic, defying resolution (Zinker, 1977). Let us briefly view a beginning relationship, that of John and Mary.

Like many couples, they became attracted to each other because of their differences. John loved Mary's spontaneity and playfulness; she loved his passion for work. As the relationship grew they began to experience the downside of this originally attractive polarity. Mary began to notice that John had difficulty relaxing and that work took him away from her. She found herself competing for his time. Rather than relaxed and playful, she was becoming resentful and tense. John, on the other hand, originally attracted to Mary's energy, began to notice that Mary never seemed to get things done. She was, to his surprise, "irresponsible". He began to resent the burden of planning their lives.

This vignette ends at a crucial point for Mary and John. For the relationship to succeed, they will need to learn to creatively manage their relationship. For example, they will need to learn to deal with the surprise and disappointment that comes with discovering that as time passes, what was originally attractive starts to fade and often even begins to repel us. This learning is not easy. Nor is the next step, learning to develop the "good form" to manage these disappointments.

IV. Creative Adjustment

"All contact is creative adjustment of the organism and environment" (Perls et al., 1951, p. 230).

Over time, there are not only sharp disappointments that need to be addressed, but also an oftentimes, gradual diminishment of interest in the other. To paraphrase Perls et al. (1951), the couple's "novelty" naturally lessens. As the relationship field becomes more and more familiar, energy for the other is less easily generated. The couple is left with a dilemma to resolve. They must learn to mutually create a process that is ongoing and unending, that infuses the relationship with vitality and positive newness, while at the same time develop habits and patterns that allow them to move freely about in other parts of their lives. Ultimately, they will have to find a rhythm that supports them in creatively adjusting to the relationship.

Creative adjustment, while often cited as an important cornerstone of the Gestalt approach, has been developed only minimally.[3] The concept, as used by Gestaltists, reflected a disagreement with Freudian theory, which postulated that individuals, in order to lead rich and fulfilling lives, need to repress their needs and conform to the environment. This "adjustment" was anything but creative.

---

[3] A notable exception is the recent article by Parlett (2000). Parlett defines five dimensions of creative adjustment: responding, inter-relating, self-recognizing, embodying, and experimenting.

Gestaltists believe, instead, that the environment and the individual mutually influence each other and that without novelty, there is no adjustment. Individuals, in order to adjust creatively, must have a wide range of skills. They must be able to live in the present and be aware of their own and the environment's constantly changing needs and patterns. Of equal importance, they must know about resolution and withdrawal, when and how to end, and how to make meaning out of their experience.[4]

Creative adjustment and contact, although reflective of a relational process, were originally used to describe change from the individual's perspective. As discussed, it is much more difficult to articulate what happens between people. When applied to couples, creative adjustment necessitates the development of an environment that is filled with available energy, so that people can grow. A more accurate term might be creative co-adjustment.

This need for continuous co-adjustment is necessary because, as John and Mary are beginning to discover, many important differences are simply not resolvable. In this sense "win-win" is just a myth. The work is to manage the energy generated by these ongoing and ordinary dilemmas in such a way that the relationship does not become stuck, frozen, or destructive.

This involves learning to accept the fact that seldom, even in the best of relationships, does anyone get their own way. As a result, individuals are constantly involved in a balancing act between their own desires, the wants of the other, and what is best for the relationship. To learn to manage these seemingly contradictory conditions is at the heart of creative adjustment. Management, at its core, requires not only a set of skills or conditions, but also a way of approaching the relationship. What is needed is an attitude, in this case, an experimental attitude.

V. Experimental Attitude and Methodology

"Here as everywhere the only solution of a human problem is experimental invention" (Perls et al., 1951, p. 233).

Experimental attitude involves a willingness to temporarily interrupt or transform one's ongoing life in order to "see" or perceive the other and the relationship in a new and different way. It is driven by the question: "What would happen, if..."(cf. Melnick, 1980).

An experimental attitude involves a commitment to try out new forms without an evaluative component. By this we mean that the couple does not have a heavy investment or interest in viewing the relationship through the lens of success/failure. Instead, each displays a willingness to explore the other's perspective. Rather than being interested in outcomes from the

---

[4] It must be understood that creative adjustment also incorporates the concept of "good form", growth, and development. Otherwise, one could argue that Hitler, bin Laden, etc., "creatively adjusted" to their environment.

stance of good/bad, the focus is on what is learned from the experience. An experimental attitude embraces the unknown and accepts the uncertainty of change (cf. Staemmler, 2000).

In order to translate these experimental values and beliefs into "living", the couple must have a methodology for creating novelty within the relationship. This methodology helps to define the shape and the form of the unique creative process. For example, they have to discover how much change and newness is "enough", and thus how much is too little or too much.

Let us use a metaphor to describe the experimental attitude and method – a long-term relationship as a work of art. Suppose you purchase a beautiful painting. Over time as the newness fades, it is easy to lose interest and succumb to being dulled and desensitized by it. For many, buying a new painting fills the need for novelty. But with an experimental attitude, a belief that even the most predictable of patterns contains novelty generates many creative options. For example, we can stay longer looking at the painting. We can look at it in different and fresh ways to capture the subtle nuances of the work. We can discuss it with others, asking their impressions. We can move its location, change the lighting, or group it with other paintings. Can we recover the feeling we had when we first saw and desired it? Probably not, for the first time comes only once. What we can do, however, is create novelty by expanding the ground and shifting our relationship with it.

Turning back to the couple, an experimental attitude and methodology incorporates a commitment and ability to look with freshness at old patterns, no matter how functional and effective they are. It further involves the skills to let go and change these patterns in order to remain involved in a process of continuous discovery of new ways of experiencing the self, the other, and the relationship.

VI. Hard Work and Discipline

"A considerable body of research highlights the role of hard work in creativity; this research suggests [that]creative eminence depends on the application of consistent effort over long periods of time" (Amabile, 2001, p. 334).

For most, new relationships just seem to happen without much effort. In fact, if one had to work hard in the beginning, most relationships would never develop. Few infatuated couples can ever imagine all that it will take to maintain and nurture the relationship. Not surprisingly, some believe that if a relationship takes so much hard work, there must be something wrong.[5] This common idea, that the creative process is a spontaneous, easy event, flies in the face of research on creativity and creative individuals. For example, ac-

---

[5] Unfortunately, the Gestalt culture has contributed to this misconception. It helped generate the belief that if one expresses his or her wishes and wants with passion and energy, change will occur. The context in which the want was expressed was largely ignored.

cording to Martindale (2001), the workday of geniuses is essentially seven days a week, 16 hours per day.

However, even if it is accepted that hard work is essential, it is not enough unless there is discipline. Discipline means a commitment to a structure that incorporates three elements: a *shared way of being together; an ability to live out the agreed-upon decisions;* and, *a willingness to seek novelty within a relational context.*

"A way of being together" incorporates a willingness to stay with the other person's process, despite the sometimes painful consequences. It also involves the capacity to affirm the other's existential validity (Zinker, 1977). What this means is a deeply-felt acknowledgment that the other's experience is as legitimate and "correct" as mine is for me.

"Living out the agreed-upon decisions" may be the most difficult of all. It is relatively easy to commit to do better in the heat of guilt, remorse, or reconciliation when energy is high. But translating these resolutions into day-to-day practices, when energy diminishes and where distractions abound, is at the heart of discipline. It is here that the skills involved in developing positive habits are of prime importance.

Last, there is a potential for disaster if the couple is unable to "seek novelty within the relational context". This "need for novelty", which we have termed seeking, is part of our human nature, present from birth until death. In fact, ill health is often correlated with seeking behavior that is contextually too small or great. We often confuse seeking with experimenting, as, for example, in experimenting with drugs. Yet seeking is different. It is without boundaries, without a highly developed sense of the other, without a full interest in consequences, and without an aesthetic form. It is experimenting without discipline.

At its worst, seeking can lead us down an endless road in which our appetite is sated for only a short time. To desire is an essential part of being human (Melnick et al., 1995). However, to let one's appetites run wild can result in negative consequences, not the least of which are our addictions – sex, substances, money, the Internet, exercise, etc. An experimental attitude, when applied to relationships, implies more than a love of novelty. It suggests a form, a bounded relational experience.

VII. Creative Destabilization

"Such destruction of the status quo may arouse fear, interruption and anxiety, the greater in proportion as one is neurotically inflexible; but the process is accompanied by the security of the new invention experimentally coming into being" (Perls et al., 1951, p. 233).

In order for the couple to generate novelty, they must have skills at letting go of old forms. This process is called creative destabilization. Sometimes this is easy – the old forms just do not work. For example, neither one enjoys going to concerts anymore. But what if the old forms still have some life in them? When is the right time to let go of the familiar so that the novel can emerge? When does an endearing term or a celebratory gift lose its creative potency? When are we hanging on a little too long? The creative couple must have the ability to break paradigms and repetitive patterns, promote unusual expectations and, thus, create fluidity, flexibility, originality, and novelty.

This is rarely easy and, for many, feels entirely undesirable. There are many legitimate reasons to hold on to stability and to embrace the practical and familiar. What if the new is less satisfying than the old and we end up rejecting what is valuable along with what is useless? We all have within us a fear of the unknown. Yet, it is just this "holding on" stance forged from our fears that stifles creativity.

Instead, the creative couple must be committed and willing to take the risk, break the rules, let go of old forms, and be willing to fail: in essence, to destabilize. How does it find the courage to do this? It involves practicing a major component of the experimental attitude, the ability to let go of outcomes – and even more importantly – to let go of critical judgment.

VIII. Bearing Disappointment

"But suffering and conflict are not meaningless or unnecessary; they indicate the destruction that occurs in all figure/background formation, in order that the new figure may emerge" (Perls et al., 1951, p. 249).

As discussed above, creative process in couples necessitates a deconstruction of old patterns, skills, and competencies. In doing this, what will emerge is unknown, or at least uncertain. Rarely will it be a mutually agreed-upon event. More often, one or the other will be one step ahead. Whereas one will want to hold on, the other will wish to let go. In order to shift, the intimate system must develop the capacity to disappoint and to be disappointed (Melnick and Nevis, "Being with another: The development and maintenance of intimacy", unpublished manuscript).

As discussed, disappointment seldom exists in a beginning relationship. At the start, what is new and different is rarely disappointing. In fact, most novelty is pleasant, and discoveries are usually positive and welcomed. However, as relationships mature and positive projections decline over time, disappointments naturally occur. They must be viewed as normal and ordinary, not as a sign that the relationship is bad.

A creative couple must discover a form for managing and living with them. It is easy to withdraw or repress these unpleasant sensations or feelings that accompany disappointments. On this track, a process of mutual isolation can develop. The "in-between" can become frozen and lifeless; the relationship field can become fixed and stuck with both individuals feeling hurt, angry, and defensive.

Instead, the couple must learn to bring their disappointments to one another. The one creating the disappointment must be able to reach across to the other, to ask, "Have I disappointed you? How? Tell me more." The one being disappointed must be able to move through the hurt to express feelings of pain and vulnerability. Furthermore, there must be an aesthetic that includes a highly developed sense of the other and the relationship. For example, each must know when the intensity is too high, and things must simmer down before meaningful contact can occur. It is through this mutual exploration that hurts are healed, a wider meaning emerges, and the relationship evolves and grows.

IX. Maintaining Interest in the Other

While mutual interest seems to just happen in a new relationship, it takes skill to maintain it after the initial novelty wears off and interest in the other often gets transferred into objects and activities such as children, cars, and vacations. These joint endeavors often become the vehicle for contact.

The creative couple needs to understand that these activities, as important as they are, are also focal points for structuring relationship and connectedness. Thus, when a couple in trouble enters therapy and is asked what is wrong, nine out of ten will mention sex, money, or children – and often all three. Seldom do they refer to the inability to join each other's interests without resentment.

In fact, they are often stingy, living in withdrawal, and holding back their interest and energy. What is lacking is a type of generosity. It involves an understanding that what interests the other is inherently neither less nor more interesting than what interests oneself. Generosity also incorporates a willingness to join what interests them.

Our case study continues: John and Mary were having a good Saturday. She was completing some housework – doing yard work. He had exercised. She started getting ready for her Saturday walk with a friend, when the phone rang, and the friend said that she had to cancel. After five minutes, Mary asked John if he would like to take a walk. Thinking of the amount of exercise he had already undertaken that day, he quickly said no. She silently turned away. Noticing this, he asked her if something was wrong. She replied in a hurt voice, "I wanted to take a walk with you." "Oh", he replied, "I didn't know. I thought you just wanted to exercise." (The reader can fill in the rest of the dialogue. Needless to say, if all intimacy dilemmas could be creatively resolved with just a few words there would be no need for this chapter.)

X. Sense of Humor

"Among those I like or admire, I can find no common denominator, but those whom I love, I can. All of them make me laugh" (Auden, source unknown).

Hard work and discipline need to be balanced with humor. Humor may, in fact, be the most important criterion for a successful long-term relationship. Without it, who can move through disappointments, hurts, broken promises, disillusionments, or times of painful disequilibrium?

By humor, we do not mean that these feelings and experiences are seen as funny. Humor allows the intimate couple to move to the larger awareness of all human frailties and frustrations and to smile at them. It combines negative and positive emotions at the same time and, therefore, supports the expression of negative feelings without being stuck. It allows each to stay in contact with the other when moments of conflict and anger have the potential for shattering the "we" and leading to withdrawal.

Ultimately, humor allows conflict to be safe, for it is a way of modulating energy and arousal. It is a way of letting off steam. In relationships, humor allows the couple to not take themselves so seriously. It lifts the weight, for embedded in it is support of the "we". Humor, when used sensitively and respectfully, provides a short cut from the negative to the positive. It allows us to move on.

XI. In Conclusion: The Creative Couple

How do we know when a couple is, in fact, creative? Foremost, their process is not seen as residing in one individual as opposed to the other. Neither can honestly say "I did it" or "I contributed more". They each understand and experience their relationship as a joint endeavor.

Creative process in a couple does not result in a product. Creating intimacy in a long-term relationship is an ever-changing development of the shared awareness of the couple. It leads to a joint, equal, and vital life. Maybe that is the product – the virtual, satisfactory life of a "we".

The creative couple finds ways to move through anger, rage, and withdrawal from the other. Instead, the partners know how to incorporates sadness, disappointment, and regret into their relationship, and they are committed to dialogue.

If the process of creating in long-term intimate relationships is so difficult and complex, why even attempt it? Maybe the simplest answer is that when couples learn to balance the need for change and stability, for the old and the new, and incorporate the right amount of experimentation within a context of discipline and structure, they develop a capacity to create a unique form of joy, the joy of doing it together.

References

Amabile TM (2001) Beyond talent: John Irving and the passionate craft of creativity. American Psychologist, Vol. 56, no. 4: 333–335

Buber M (1958) I and thou. Scribner, New York

Fogel A (1991) Developing through relationships. Univ of Chicago Press, Chicago

Martindale C (2001) Oscillations and analogies: Thomas Young, MD, FRS, Genius. American Psychologist, Vol. 56, no. 4: 342–345

Melnick J (1980) The use of therapist-imposed structure in Gestalt therapy. The Gestalt J 2: 4–20

Melnick J, Nevis SM (1994) Intimacy and power in long-term relationships: A Gestalt therapy-systems perspective. In: Wheeler G, Backman S (eds) On intimate ground. Jossey Bass, San Francisco, 291–308

Melnick J, Nevis SM (2001) Jealousy: The protection of intimacy, or caring gone wrong. The Australian Gestalt J 5: 49–60

Melnick J, Nevis SM, Melnick G (1995) Living with desire. British Gestalt J IV: 31–40
Parlett M (2000) Creative adjustment and the global field. British Gestalt J IX: 15–27
Perls F, Hefferline R, Goodman P (1951) Gestalt therapy: Excitement and growth in the human personality. Dell, New York
Staemmler F (2000) Like a fish in water: Gestalt therapy in times of uncertainty. Gestalt Review IV: 205–218
Zinker J (1977) The creative process in Gestalt therapy. Brunner/Mazel, New York

Creativity in Family Therapy

Edward and Barbara Lynch

The question frequently arises about the interface of Gestalt therapy and systemic family therapy. The answer is predicated on a thorough understanding of the basic concepts and practices of each theoretical model. Both the Gestalt therapist and the family therapist view the family as a unified whole, an entity existing within a field, and creators of a "family field" with unique characteristics inherited from and influenced by a larger context. The conceptual framework of both Gestalt and systemic family therapies lead the therapist to be essentially, and almost exclusively, concerned with the interactional *process* in the family, rather than the *content* as spoken by members. Both modalities are nonjudgmental; they work with interactions as they occur *in the present*; and they are attentive to nonverbal expressions and family members' responses and reactions. In addition, the hallmark of Gestalt therapy is the experiment, and in family therapy, the enactment is the same basic technique. The fundamental connection between Gestalt therapy and systemic family therapy emerges sharply when structural/systemic family therapy is performed by a therapist who is thoroughly grounded in Gestalt therapy and who brings this lens and internal process to the art and craft of therapy.

Creativity is an intricate and vital force in family therapy. The symptom, also called the fixed gestalt, serving as the motivator for the pursuit of family therapy, is the first piece of evidence that the creative forces are at work within the system. This fixed gestalt is an outward manifestation of the system's attempt to remediate some disturbance in the system: a creative attempt to balance internal processes. The unaware creative adjustment may be to repair a dysfunction or, in some instances, to form a protective cover for possibly more feral processes that interrupt the healthy flow of systemic life forces. Viewed in this light, the therapist must at once honor this heroic attempt and gently and creatively work to disentangle the misguided efforts that have resulted in the need for therapy. From this perspective, the therapist must both keep in mind that therapy represents the failure of a creative effort and, at the same time, understand that the system has the means and desire to engage in a creative process (see Lynch, 2000).

Since it is most commonly a child who is offered as a presented patient, it becomes important to recognize – and validate – the child or children as the most creative and confluent members of the system. They seem to be the ones who are most receptive to disturbances in the intimate dyadic system. With this awareness, and from a naive perspective, they unconsciously devise a "solution", a creative adjustment that, with some prescient knowledge, often temporarily eases systemic tension. The difficulty arises when the system does not utilize this temporary "quiet" period as a time to engage in some systemic repair, but instead compounds the initial disturbance with other similar tensions that cannot be relieved by normal processes. The creative child, having experienced success in a previous endeavor, tries again. When this does not succeed, efforts are often redoubled. For example, when marital tension erupts and the dyadic system can no longer contain it, a child will unerringly provide a deflection for the stress. The child will manifest behaviors that command the parents' attention, thereby providing them with a respite from their intra-systemic turmoil. The marital pair, in most cases, will rally their parental resources, allowing the marital system to become background in deference to the best interests of the family. And thus, the family system is stabilized. However, this remedy is short-lived. With this relative harmony, the marital stress slowly ascends to the foreground, almost in direct proportion to the degree of the larger system stability. The cycle repeats itself without deviation. The symptomatic child escalates deflection-beckoning behavior, and the marital tension decreases. Eventually, the symptom becomes entrenched in routine behavior, and the system requires the intervention of professionals.

The first task of the systemic family therapist is to invite the entire system to engage in the effort to re-structure the system. The goal of this endeavor is to allow the system to function without the inclusion of *entrenched* "creative" symptoms that cause pain in individuals or in marital, sibling, or extended family subsystems (Lynch, 2000, pp. 53–72). This must be accomplished while conveying respect for the system's right to preserve the symptom for future use, if necessary. As a vital part of the therapeutic invitation, joining must be the therapist's priority and a function of the therapist's creative process. Inherent in this function is the therapist's understanding that the family must be co-creators of therapy and that the joining will set the stage for the entire course of treatment.

The family offers the therapist the raw material. The therapist receives, holds, and offers something back to the family in a manner that connects the therapist to the family and begins to allow the formation of a new, therapeutic system that includes the therapist. This is the first "test" of the therapist's creativity – the ability to don, in chameleon fashion, the family's manner and style. Whatever has to be done to insure inclusion and retain the status of benevolent expert must be exercised. Salvador Minuchin would begin a session dressed in a suit and tie. Once observing the family's casual dress, he would shed the jacket, undo the tie, roll up his shirtsleeves, and casually sit down to initiate the process of change. Effective joiners modify their cadence, their language, and their body postures. The therapist is an expert on observing data. Small idiosyncratic tokens are noted and commented on. The therapist will notice the baseball cap worn by a child and inquire if that team is a particular favorite of the child. This casual piece of attire will become an invitation to find out about the family's interests and serve to initiate the therapist as someone interested in all aspects of this family's life, not just those that are dysfunctional. The therapist maintains the connection with the family by bridging the time between sessions. The family responds to the therapist remembering events that have taken place in the interim. For example, if a child reports that he had to take an important examination during the week, when the family returns to therapy, the therapist remembers to ask how that was for the child. If there has been no event of note, the therapist begins the session, compressing time, by recalling a statement or action from the previous session and beginning the current session at that point. For instance, a therapist might say at the beginning of a session, "I was thinking about this family during the week. I remember that one of the things that you all agreed upon was the sadness you all felt at not having positive time together." It is unimportant to delve into this subject more fully. Primarily, it serves to inform the family that they, and their concerns, are important to the therapist and that they occupy more than a single hour session in significance. Therapists who do not have a good memory should make careful post-session notes and prepare for a session by formulating their opening gambit. Eventually, the experienced therapist negotiates these aspects of joining and accommodation without conscious effort. Careful monitoring of the family's responses and reactions gives the therapist instant feedback on the success, or failure, of these attempts. The family may exercise token resistance; however, the skilled therapist accommodates this behavior, utilizing the resistance in the service of joining. An example of this type of resistance would be to negate the therapist's attempt to bridge by brushing off the therapist's statements, changing the subject, or simply not entering into the interaction at even the most superficial level. At this point, the therapist must accommodate, supporting the resistance, perhaps by a simple statement: "I guess that's my mistake. I need you to give me feedback on just how important things are with you, and you just did that. Thank you."

One of the most frequent forms of resistance is to block attempts to engage the entire system in treatment. Many families want the therapist to "fix" the presented patient without any effort on their part. Here, the therapist's creativity must rise to the forefront. The therapist may support the resistance, for example, by reminding the family that although family therapy, with all members present, may be the most effective form of therapy, it is possible that many families are unable to take advantage of this manner of treatment. Continuing in this vein, there may be some acknowledgement of this particular family's strengths, linking them to success in family therapy with the addition of reflective caveats that suggest that the therapist wonders about the family's ambivalence. The following dialogue between the therapist and family members illustrates this point:

Parent: Charles is the only person in the family who has ever been in trouble. Everyone else is fine and always has been.
Therapist: That's remarkable. Most families have more than one member who is suffering. Your family must have many strengths.

Oldest child: I don't know why I have to be here. He's the problem. The rest of us are do-
     ing fine.
Parent: We've treated all three of them the same way. There must be something wrong
     with Charles. He is always in trouble, in school, at home ...
Charles sulks and mutters under his breath.

The therapist resists focusing on Charles, despite his cue to the therapist
and the rest of the family's attempts to organize the therapist to reinforce
Charles as the only negative force in an otherwise perfect family. A careful
unifying statement of purpose must be devised, or the treatment of the family as a system will be lost. The therapist makes a statement that hopefully
respects the resistance and, at the same time, encourages the family to remain in treatment:

It sounds as if the family thinks that Charles should be in some form of treatment as
an individual. I hear that. I think at some point we might suggest to do just that. However,
first I want to be sure that I completely understand how all of you function with Charles a
part of your family. It also helps the therapy go more quickly and more successfully if I get
a picture of Charles in the family and the family with Charles. I'd like us all to work together for a very short time, and if there is no change in your feelings in three or four sessions, then we'll renegotiate. I know it's a sacrifice, but I hope it's a short one.

The therapist remembers that resistance represents movement and an invitation to change and exercises novel strategies to encourage compliance.
A family recently came to therapy with the presenting problem that the
mother's 8-year-old son would not clean his room, eat the meals that were
prepared and, in general, follow any of the rules of the family. This child was
the youngest of three; there were two older sisters. The eldest daughter had
left home at 16 to live with another family, because she couldn't get along
with her mother. The younger daughter, 14, had just left to go live with the
(divorced) father and his family in another state, following a minor run-in
with the law. The mother told the court that she couldn't control the daughter
and thought it better that she live with the father. The most recent event in the
mother's life was that as soon as the 14-year-old left, she married a man she
had been dating. He was assisting her in disciplining her son. Every attempt
the therapist made to join with the parents as a consultant met with failure.
The adults kept reiterating that they had tried everything and nothing
worked. They were at their "wit's end". The therapist, recognizing this resis-
tant stance, knew that something creative was called for. She decided to make
a bold move. In a grand drama staged for effect, the therapist called in a team
of experts – the family was impressed. The experts sat in the room and sol-
emnly proclaimed their findings. In essence, they said that Stephen, the son,
was testing the new family arrangement and that since he was so intelligent
(the parents' claim), he knew exactly what had to be done. If he thought the
couple needed time alone together, well then he would continue to act out
and disobey the adults, and eventually he would be placed in residential
treatment, which would give the couple the alone-time they needed to form
a strong couple system. If, however, he believed that the couple could accept
the role of parenting together, then he would slowly improve his behavior,
monitoring the adults' process as he went along.

Whatever form of resistance the family might engage in would result in some significant structural change. The impact of the unbalancing statement forced the family into new, uncharted territory. They strongly resisted the idea that their couple relationship was being tested. In "proving" that the therapist was incorrect, they began to co-parent in an effective manner, negotiating all the pitfalls of bringing a step-parent into an already enmeshed system. With dramatic evidence that the two adults in the family were united in their parenting, Stephen slowly became more conforming to the rules at home and at school. The experiment devised by the therapist and carried out with a cast of consultants acting with dramatic flair was sufficient to neutralize the resistance.

When the therapist is confident that engagement is secure, it is then possible to move on with the process of treatment. In an organized manner, the therapist views the course of treatment as a blank canvas waiting for delicate and bold strokes of brush and color to complete the masterpiece. However, different from the artist working alone, the therapist and the system work in concert to fill the canvas. From inception to completion, the process has an orderly progression:

joining	assessing	intervening	support change	termination

One factor that makes systemic family therapy distinct and inspires creativity is the freedom to engage in the steps of treatment from a perspective that varies with the individuality of *both* the therapist and the family.

The assessment phase, giving the therapist a picture of the family personality function disturbance, is realized with the family demonstrating their unique style. With questions, such as "How does the system support the symptom, *and* how does the symptom support the system?" unable to be answered in words, the therapist must devise an experiment to elucidate a meaningful response. The therapist obtains the necessary data to devise interventions that will bring about desired changes in the system by being creative enough to support the emergence of hierarchy, subsystem functioning, boundary maintenance, and limit-setting *without overt manipulation by the therapist.* A simple example comes to mind. When a family with young children comes to therapy, the therapist always makes sure that the room contains some toys, preferably in a container: large blocks in a canister, for instance. When there are just a few minutes of the session remaining, the therapist gently tells the parents that the toys need to be picked up and put away, so that another family can use the room. No further explanations are given. How the adults manage this task is an enactment of their systemic process. Do the parents take over and put the toys away? Is the child instructed, and perhaps helped, in the clean-up chore? Whatever happens is a *natural* assessment of how their system manages tasks. It is not contrived: it is consistent with the context.

The culmination of this phase results in the reframe, a creative statement linking the family's content and process in an understanding of the "problem" that includes all family members and is benevolent and acceptable to the family. The example of Stephen and the consultants' bold statements to the family represented a reframe that took into consideration the family's process and the presenting problem, rearranging "facts" in a creative way that allowed the family to expand their view of themselves.

Systemic family therapy from a Structural model has prescribed suggestions from which to devise intervention strategies. Boundary-making, unbalancing, heightening the intensity, supporting the hierarchy, searching for competencies, and enactment are the foundation for the engagement in change. However, with this proscription, the therapist is free to unleash creative forces, limited only by the willingness of the family to engage with the therapist in the process. Successful interventions, contacting, are the product of a conception that takes place between family and therapist. They are fertilized in the context begun in the joining process, nurtured in a climate of respect for the family's style of functioning, and are supported by the joint knowledge of the family's id function disturbance. Additionally, there is awareness that the family has an intense desire for survival of the system concomitant with equally intense fear of change.

Some creative boundary-making enactments have been used with props. For example, in an extremely enmeshed family, the therapist began to make a pile of pillows that were originally on the couch. Without saying a word, he built a wall of pillows, eventually becoming so high that the parent moved away from her son to a place across the room in order to be in sight of him. Once she was seated in a separate place, the therapist, again without words, began to remove this wall. This intervention was never spoken about, and it was repeated at least two more times before the mother said, "Okay, I got it. I know where I belong." Her subsequent interactions with her child were much more respectful of personal boundaries, and the symptoms began to abate (ibid., p. 107).

Along with creativity, the therapist must be able to take risks and to resist being "attached" to the outcome in order to devise and execute intervention strategies. There must be a willingness to suggest, without insisting, to take different steps, to step back from "mistakes" gracefully and with humor, to avoid coalitions, nurture functional alliances, and more. The therapist has to have an endless repertoire of ways to sustain emotion in the face of a system that is anxious about any but the most superficial expression. At the same time, the therapist must be able to draw from this well, respectfully halting family id and personality function emotional outbursts. This is all overshadowed by the therapist's wisdom to know when to do which! One "brave" therapist who had continued to fail at interrupting a dysfunctional process in a family system took a risk. When the system began to go into their routine, she slid off her chair and sat on the floor. The family instantly stopped and just looked at her. She stood up, brushed herself off, and changed the subject. The process was clearly interrupted, and from that point on she just had to begin to inch toward the edge of her chair to get the family to turn their attention from attacking each other to worrying about her ending up on the floor. Not every therapist should attempt such dramatic and risky moves; however, when a supervisor strongly suggests that a therapist "make something happen", some therapists will attempt anything!

Tantamount to success in systemic family therapy is the therapist's ability to take a therapeutic and respectful position in the structure of the system that now includes the therapist as part of the system. The family enters therapy with a preferred structural arrangement that has *both* served the system well *and* contributed to the entrenchment of the difficulty, the symptom. Most common in families that are referred for therapy is a significant disturbance in the executive subsystem. This usually takes one of three forms, illustrated by the static structural maps below.[1]

(empty)	one parent	child or children
a.	b.	c. ....
children & parent(s)	children & other parent	parent and other children

The therapist must determine an effective position from which to intervene and also one that is accepted by the family system. There also needs to be an awareness of the impact on the system of the therapist taking any hierarchical position that may usurp a parent's domain while, at the same time, accepting the family's view of therapist-as-expert. The question, for example, in schema "a" above, is how does the therapist maneuver to be expert and parent's peer with the larger question of how to engage the parent as co-executive of the system, together *with* the therapist. The successful answers are dependent only on the accuracy with which the therapist has assessed the family's style of functioning and on the creativity with which the move is approached. In each of the schematic representations, similar questions are present. In each of the structural representations, the therapist must align with the adults in the system. With an empty executive subsystem, the parents (inappropriately) in the child, or subordinate, subsystem, it is extremely difficult for the therapist to avoid becoming the executive, either alone or in concert with another executive system outside the family, either Child Protective Services, the judicial system, school personnel, or some other outside agency that has usurped the parental functioning in an effort to protect the children. The therapist must ally with the parent(s) in their positions in the subordinate system. At first, the therapist/parent alliance is that of older siblings – still in the "child" system, but functioning from a wiser, more concerned position. The therapist does this in a variety of manners, limited only by the range of creativity employed. The initial move would be to physically create a separation between the parents and the children with the therapist in the pivotal position between adults and children. A skilled therapist will find a way to move slightly, so that her back is more toward the children than the adults: a subtle boundary. When this, and other, physical moves are accepted by the system, the therapist can proceed toward making verbal demarcations. Choice of words becomes consistent with reality. The therapist uses every opportunity to proclaim for example, "As *adults,* we know how *children* react in these situations". Or "Our 20-plus more years of

---

[1] This boundary designation does not necessarily represent the actual interactions.

living and learning must count for something with these *young* kids". When the therapist intuits or learns that there is a weak or empty executive system, it may even be important to begin with boundary definitions by referring to the parent, and him or herself, as Mr. or Mrs., formal titles, while at the same time referring to the children by their first names. Of course, the parent may invite the therapist to call her by a first name also, but the therapist can "forget" conveniently until other boundaries are well-established. Further, inclusion words – we, our, and other similar ones – should only be used to delineated the adults from the children. Once the boundaries are clearer, the therapist can go on to other phases of the therapeutic process; however, these boundary-making interventions are powerful therapeutic moves that are crucial to re-structuring the family and may represent the whole process of treatment.

Not only does the therapist need to be creative; there also must be a high degree of flexibility. Families who find themselves in therapy have usually limited "amounts" of both creativity and flexibility. They have met all sorts of minor and more major crises with the same or similar strategies. When one attempt fails, the family usually does more of the same, remembering a time (albeit under different conditions) when this strategy succeeded. Therefore, while the therapist is concerned with the mechanics of the therapeutic process, and assessing and intervening, there must also be a thrust to expand the family's ability to be both creative and flexible. This function is vital when the goal is more than alleviating the current dysfunction – that is, when it extends to the expectation that as an outcome of therapy, the family will have incorporated new ways of meeting ongoing developmental and environmental crises.

In this context, there is no better "teaching" strategy than modeling followed by an invitation to "mimic". By taking risks that are sometimes followed by "failures", then demonstrating, by actions, that this is both acceptable and a form of learning, the therapist teaches the family that these failures are valuable feedback devices – to be welcomed, not punished. The therapist who is willing to adopt the family's style makes an undeniable statement to the family that their resources are valid and valuable. The therapist should be unlimited in ways to show the family that they are respected and, as a byproduct, the family will be strengthened, better able to co-create viable solutions to their difficulties.

For example, the therapist introduces an experiment/enactment with a statement, such as "I have an idea. It might work with your family, but it involves all of us taking a risk". With this statement, the therapist has included herself in the system, *all of us* and introduced the element of risk: *it might work with your family, we're taking a risk*. Then the therapist waits for some family member to accept the invitation. If a child responds, the therapist comments on the process to the parent with attention to the hierarchy: "It looks like there might be a family spokesperson. (She turns to the parent.) Do we (*marking a boundary between adults and children*) respond to him or wait until we (*continuing boundary making and establishing hierarchy*) discuss it in more detail?" Whatever the parent decides, it is settled from an executive system that includes adults only. The parent makes the decision! In carrying out the experiment, the therapist engages the parent in the design, at times intentionally leaving space for the parent to add, subtract, or veto an idea. In this way, the system witnesses the parent in control with the therapist in a more distant position and the children ensconced in their system. Boundaries are clear, and hierarchy has been established.

There is no limit to the evidence that the effective family therapist needs to be a creative individual. There is some foundation for the belief that the family is "helped" most by a combination of therapist creativity supported by a sound theoretical foundation, liberally interspersed with demonstrable respect for the family. It might even be said that the more creative a therapist is, the more likely the family is to realize successful and desirable change.

How, then, does a therapist maximize creativity to maximize success? In looking at the lives of therapists who are recognized as successes, interesting facts emerge. They seem to be engaged in creative endeavors that extend beyond their profession. There are artists, poets, musicians, dancers, storytellers, crafters, jewelry designers, and beaders, among the legions of highly successful therapists. Their lives extend beyond the world of therapy to cooking, knitting, embroidery, sewing, baking, sports, and other nonrelated activities. They shed their therapeutic posture and *practice* being creative, enhancing the creativity of their practice. They refresh, re-create, and enliven themselves with behaviors that seemingly have little or nothing to do with therapy, but they draw strongly on this respite to continue to bring life and humor to their work. Therapists who actively and intentionally maintain a creative life rarely burn out. They are able to approach some of life's tragedies that come along with the families they treat with faith in the human spirit and a realistic optimism that allows them to continue to assist families in their quest for health and satisfaction.

Creativity is the hallmark of outstanding therapists and their supervisors. It is a character trait and an acquired skill that must be recognized, supported, and revered by the therapists themselves, their supervisors, and their teachers. With a focus on creativity underlying teaching, supervision, practice, and living, there will be an outpouring of successful and rewarding therapy.

References

Lynch E, Lynch B (2000) The principles and practices of structural family therapy. Gestalt Journal Press, Highland New York

Creative Processes in Gestalt Group Therapy

Carl Hodges

> Creare: (Latin) To make, to bring into existence.

> "... all contact is creative and dynamic. It cannot be routine, stereotyped, or merely conservative because it must cope with the novel, for only the novel is nourishing (...) *All contact is creative adjustment of the organism and environment*"
> (Perls et al., 1994, p. 6).

> "Contact is awareness of the field or motor response in the field"
> (ibid., p. 5).

Gestalt therapy *is* creativity. Awareness is the creation of figures and grounds. Our contacting (re)organizes our experience, creating new possibilities. Experiencing is gestalt formation/destruction.

> "The achievement of a strong gestalt is itself the cure, for the figure of contact is not a sign of, but is itself the creative integration of experience" (ibid., p. 8).

A group is a gestalt! At the New York Institute for Gestalt Therapy, through the re-examination of our foundations initiated by our senior Fellow Richard Kitzler and others, and through attending to our process as a learning community, this notion has emerged and profoundly shaped our direction. A group can be conceived, not as a "system", not as a collection of "interactions" between individuals, not as a portable "hot-seat", but as a *gestalt* with figure and ground, wholes and parts, processes and events, forces and constraints, gestalt formation and destruction. These concepts come from Gestalt field theory.

I. Gestalt Field Theory

Our foundations are in field theory, which revolutionized 20th-century thought, perspective, and existence: in physics (Faraday, Mack, Einstein, Heisenberg), in art (Picasso, Braque, Léger), in psychology (Wertheimer, Köhler, Koffka, Goldstein, and later Lewin, Bion) in biology (von Bertalanffy), in ecology (Osama), in music (Stravinsky, Berg, Parker), and in literature (Joyce, Musil). As the art critic John Berger (Dyer, 2002, pp. 71–92) has written, in a brilliant essay called "The Moment of Cubism", we became aware for the first time in history of a global whole of which we are all a part, created by it and creating it, changing our vision of time and space, rhythm and tempo, connection and relation. Picasso invites us to see a whole that shows many sides at once, challenges our previous sense of reality, and involves us in new relations to space, awareness, and memory. A whole that is not complete without us making figures and grounds, traveling in and out and over, and bringing our experience and history into this here and now event (ibid.).

We come from a rich heritage! Wertheimer and Einstein were friends and musicians together, Köhler studied with Max Planck, and Lore Perls studied with Wertheimer and Gelb and was greatly influenced by Goldstein, while Fritz worked with Goldstein and Gelb.

There are many field theories. I use the field theory of the Gestalt psychologists Wertheimer, Koffka and, particularly, Köhler:

"[W]e are inevitably led to the concepts of field physics. In this part of science the consideration of what might be called 'processes-in-extension' is regarded as a matter of course. The term which I have just used is simply another name for the self-distributed processes to which I referred in Chapter IV ['Dynamics As Opposed to Machine Theory']. In such processes, it will be remembered, local events occur, as they occur, only within the distribution as a whole" (Köhler, 1975, p. 124).

This is different from the later field theory of Kurt Lewin, which tends more toward systems: structure and space, boundary between, and goals.

The field theory of the Gestalt psychologists is concerned with:

– figure and ground,
– wholes and parts,
– process and events,
– forces and constraints,
– gestalt formation and destruction.

A field is the dynamic interplay of forces and constraints. When these *forces* interact without constraint, a *dynamic equilibrium* is reached. This equilibrium has form, shape, structure, and organization. This organization, this creation of a figure against a ground we call a *gestalt*.

A gestalt may be strong – clear, bright, energetic, flowing – or weak, less of each of the above. A gestalt can only be as strong as the field conditions (interaction of forces and *constraints*) allow. The forces in a field may be organized around the field's constraints: i.e., a locomotive or other machine, a TV picture, organic psychosis, and so on.

A field is a *process*, not a thing: "processes in extension", as Köhler says. Field theory substitutes events for things-having-fixed-properties. Part-processes are themselves determined by the intrinsic nature of the whole (Köhler, 1975, pp. 60–79).

The familiar example is the "rock". In this place, at this time, this temperature, at this atmospheric pressure, at this gravity, we have an event that we call a rock. If we were to change this equilibrium, for instance the temperature a few hundred degrees up or down, or change the atmospheric pressure, etc., then we may no longer have the same event, the same "rock". Notice that the "observer" is part of this event, this figure-making.

II. The Gestalt Group

What if we take seriously these concepts from Gestalt field theory – figure/ground, wholes/parts, process/events, forces/constraints, and gestalt formation/destruction – and apply them to group. What are the implications for "treatment", learning, leadership, authority, experiment, creativity, and our Gestalt theory itself? What does such a group look like?

A. Some Examples

Any example, two-dimensional, verbal, and abstracted must seem stilted. Three come to mind anyway, from different kinds of groups.

1. This was a practicum. I was asked to "demonstrate" a Gestalt therapy session. A young woman and I, the leader, sat in the middle of a group that had been meeting for about six months and that was at that time in or near a configuration that could be called "intimacy". The power struggles and competition had waned; there was a feeling of working together, of sharing support, even of "family".

We sat down on the carpeted floor about two feet from each other. I felt the pressure to "do" something, to make something happen, but let it pass and noticed her eyes, her face, her body. The room disappeared, and I saw a father, a mother, siblings in and out, a childhood, difficult relationships, having to be strong, "abusive hurt", tears, profound sadness, acceptance, yearning: feelings were evoked in me, and our seeing her seeing me seeing her – figure into figure and, like shifting sand, ground forming, shaping, re-shaping, shared in us. I felt tears and could see hers. The "session" lasted eight minutes. I said five words. She smiled, and I knew she knew they were five words too many. We paused (there is no "end" to what was touched and built). We paused, breathed, and sat back, inviting the rest of the group, deeply moved, in. They, too, were participants in what had happened, with their resonance, harmonies, emotions, the succession of figures and grounds evoked in them, not through our words, but through our/their visions, connections, touching. Later, as a practicum again, we could talk about figure/ground, about the importance of the nonverbal communication, about awareness of what your body is sensing, experiencing without the words. On a cognitive level, we could talk about body position, breathing, eyes, facial expression, energy level. And yet, what happened was more than all these, because field is more than stimulus-response, more than cycles, more than linear: it is apprehensive, total; it is presence in the "wholes of experience".

2. A therapy group that had gone on for some months and was in what could be called a power-and-control configuration: competitiveness and unexpressed fears of being vulnerable. A woman client, D, who had early abuse issues, was finding me, despite my best efforts, to be unsupportive: when I tried to "explain" myself, she felt even more unsupported, not understood, not heard, and "abused". I was feeling misunderstood; I was beginning to feel "helpless" as our attempts to communicate with each other seemed to be driving us further apart and making each of us feel more alienated and isolated. I felt on the spot, vulnerable, and stuffed with something that seemed to make it hard to think, or even breathe. I wondered if D and I were in the same subgroup, and if we were "holding" something for the whole group. I did breathe, and I noticed that all the interaction in the group was now between D and myself, and that the other group members were sitting back quietly. D and I had become figure against the ground of the group. I made a "field statement" to that effect: I said what I was experiencing in my part of the field, and I described what I was noticing in the field as a whole. An experiment then occurred to me, and I proposed it to D and the group: that we invert the figure/ground relationship and that we, the pair, keep silent and become ground for the rest of the group as figure. D and I would observe our own experiencing in our bodies and notice if or when we began to feel "un-stuffed". We sat, as other group members talked, eventually, about their own vulnerability, their frustration in finding their own voice and being heard, and their irritation with the leader, who was going too fast and demanding too much. D and I began to smile at each other, as we noticed the "stuffed" feelings begin to drain and as the group began to take up their own aggression, vulnerability, and needs, as figure.

3. In a conjoint therapy session with a husband and wife: the wife was depressed and had what the husband called "addictive behaviors", namely an obsession with telephone (sex) chatlines. Her obsession enabled her to "avoid" her husband, children, and household chores. The husband, feeling abandoned, chose to be in rage rather than in vulnerability and hurt, and ultimately felt helpless, since his ranting carried with it no consequences (he threatened many times to leave). The wife had a history of depression since pre-adolescence and was overweight, with body-image issues: she appeared washed out, defeated, and limp. He appeared angry, demanding, constantly defining her in his terms and speaking for her. Conversation between them in the session was remarkably one-sided, and she retreated more and more into the woodwork, looking increasingly beaten down. She seemed powerless, with no options, and she grew quieter. "Where are you?" the other therapist asked gently.

Eventually, the patient says she wants to "get away". Her husband derides her more. "Where would you like to go?" I ask. "Can you imagine where you'd like to go?" Eventually, she says she can imagine someplace by the sea. "Can you describe it?" It is a rough, powerful sea, smashing against huge, rough rocks and boulders, and behind that there is a quiet, off-season deserted village. "Can you be the sea?" Eventually, at last, she is able to feel her own power, energy, and excitement. "I'm a changing sea!" she says. I ask her husband if he could join her fantasy – as the rocks and boulders. "I am strong and hard and tall. I meet your strength with my strength, I feel my energy with you." In my mind a tune appears: Perry Como singing, "... it's just impossible, like the shoreline and the sea, it's just impossible". We talk about "paradigms" and the shoreline as a paradigm: it is the place where the sea and the land meet, the product not of one or the other, but of both, a very alive, changing, active boundary where the two meet in their differences. We talk about making room for that difference in each other and being able to allow it: at times in its strength, and at times in its gentleness.

B. Creativity in the Gestalt Group

In the Gestalt group, we are working with the organism/environment *field*, and we are looking for *figures* and the *grounds* from which they emerge, wholes and parts, process and events, forces and constraints, gestalt formation and destruction.

The Gestalt group can be three members or three hundred. The prototype is not the family, with parent and child (or teacher/student, doctor/patient, leader/follower). The prototype for the Gestalt group is the *polis*, as members take up their "citizenship" (de Mare et al., 1991, pp. 1–74), their flexible, transient roles in a community of equals, and take up their creativity as well: "[The self] is the artist of life" (Perls et al., 1994, p. 11).

The group members are engaged in an ongoing forming, discovering, creating, and re-creating of that artwork we call "group" (or "couple", "family", "community", or "organization").

In that forming, discovering, creating, we are looking for what is figure, and also for where the energy is – or is not! Is the interaction bright, lively, energetic, graceful, fluid, in contacting?

"*Contact, the work that results in assimilation and growth, is the forming of a figure of interest against a ground or context of the organism/environment field* (...) The figure (gestalt) in awareness is a clear, vivid perception, image, or insight; in motor behavior, it is the graceful energetic movement that has rhythm, follows through, etc." (ibid., p. 7).

"The process of figure/background formation is a dynamic one in which the urgencies and resources of the field progressively lend their powers to the interest, brightness and force of the dominant figure (...) [which is specifically psychological and] has specific observable properties of brightness, clarity, unity, fascination, grace, vigor, release (...)" (ibid., pp. 7–8)

This is our *autonomous criterion*, and it is vital here, for it gives an indication of "the depth and reality" of the experience and whether "the need and energy of the organism, and the likely possibilities of the environment are incorporated and unified in the figure" (ibid., p. 7).

Where are the forces (needs, excitements, feelings, fears) and where are the constraints (the holding back) that affect the clarity and brightness of the figure (*prägnanz*)? What is the whole and its parts (as in Example II.A.2)?

In the organism/environment/field we may speak of whole-processes and part-processes. Everything that occurs in the group/field – thoughts, feelings, interactions, behavior, musings, daydreams, songs, images, metaphors – emerges from the ground of the group and tells everything about what is going on – or not going on! – in the group. Every behavior emerges from the ground of the group, is event in the group's process: every part has to do with the whole.

The implications of this are many. First, there are no "individual" issues, there are *only* group issues: there is no individual or "identified" patient; there is no pathologizing. Introjection, confluence, projection, retroflection, egotism are all seen as *group* issues, which interrupt and affect the group's flow, energy, aliveness. (They act as constraints.)

Second, whatever comes up as figure for a group member or members "internally" or "externally", in their bodies, in their emotions, or as issues or concerns, is now seen as figure emerging out of the ground of the group. Whatever you're feeling in a group, given the shared ground, chances are that at least one other person is feeling or experiencing something similar. If you "voice" your feeling, issue, difficulty, you may be a voice for a part of the whole. If others *join* you in stating similar feelings and experience, and together you all begin to voice, share, *and explore* your experience, that is what Yvonne Agazarian, in a brilliant conceptualization, calls *"subgrouping"* (1997, pp. 41–62). These mini-groupings emerge as figure out of the process of the whole group: they explore their part of the field, bring into contact and context, then dissolve back into the process of the whole, their work becoming ground for the next figure.

This exploring and sharing together of your experience here and now is the definition of *work* in the Gestalt group. The subgroups allow the exploration of conflicting parts and splits and enable us to see many sides at once. Splits can then be explored, not in the individual in isolation, but in the group as a whole, which holds and contains all sides of the splits, in diverse subgroupings: compliance and defiance, yearning to be closer and wanting to maintain distance, wanting to aggress and the fear of aggressing, the desire to compete openly and the fear of it. The subgrouping is ongoing experiment: there is opportunity for experiencing "flexibly various" standpoints, "travelling in and out and over", exploring the diverse parts of oneself and of the field, and the opportunity to go "to the thing itself", to explore feelings, impulses, and concerns *as processes* here and now, finding words, voice, meaning. One's grounds and possibilities become larger and livelier. Members can explore in subgroups *all* parts of themselves, including the unfamiliar, the uncomfortable, the fearful. Distinction is made between impulse and action. Feelings, impulses, issues, concerns are *experienced and explored* rather than acted out or discharged, or even necessarily "expressed" to their object.

This is a slightly different style of contacting – more middle mode, more id-oriented, being open to voicing the *experience*. Voicing makes more of the background foreground, which creates a different figure and a different dialogue. A member may be angry (at X). It is the *experience* of her anger here and now that is explored, and she may be joined by others, who are also experiencing anger, though not necessarily at X. If X is experiencing anger also, he is in the *same* subgroup – one which is together exploring, digesting, and integrating anger and its meanings in this context, at this time, for this (whole) group.

This voicing together and exploring of experience in the group here and now *transforms* the experience as it is happening and builds a new context, re-configuring old issues and giving them new and deeply-shared meanings. *This is the essence and definition of creativity in the Gestalt group.*

C. Leadership

In this model, leadership is seen not as a role, but as a process which anyone can enter. Your vulnerability expressed is your leadership. Your vulnerability is your statement of where you are in the field. If expressed, it is also a statement about the field and your relation to it, and in the expression the field is *changed*: more of the background becomes foreground; more of the structure of the actual situation becomes known. The identification, articulation, and expression of your vulnerability is an act of leadership in the Gestalt group.

The designated leader or worker is an imposed structure, a role which, like all roles, with contact and gestalt destruction/formation, over time dissolves into the fluidity of the group.

The role of the designated leader changes according to what is required and what configuration the group seems to be in. A two-way process, the group also leads the leader. At various times the leader may be: a holding environment, "authority", a target, a steady course, a conductor, an interpreter, a model, a guide, a clarifier, an advisor, a vital member, the repository of the group's energy, faith, playfulness, or history.

D. Words, Words, Words!

A vast amount of what goes on in a field is nonverbal, preverbal, "a-verbal". We are creating a new, shared space – a "transitional space" in Winnicott's sense: a space of projection and discovery, of play and exploration, which is transforming.

Our tools in this creating are ourselves, particularly our bodies, our images, sensations, feelings, our style of contacting and experiencing ourselves and our "other" – our ability to make a kind of poetry and dance in, with, and of our contacting. Our language must be the language of ap-prehension and delight, symbol and metaphor, poetry and description. Pedestrian language cannot catch the field.

> Canst thou draw out Leviathan with a hook?
> Will he speak soft words unto thee?
> Lay Thine hand upon him,
> Remember the battle
> Do no more
> (Job 41: 1, 3, 8)

Kurt Goldstein, writing about applying Gestalt theory to the organism/ environment field, spoke of the need for symbols and images in thinking about field (Goldstein, 1975, pp. 3–33), that the old constructs do not give us adequate knowledge. Metaphor and poetry evoke a "contemplative, pre-logical mode of knowing, exhibited so forcefully in art, the knowing that terminates in recognitions and not 'conclusions'" (Cox and Theilgard, 1987, p. *ix*): "The image has touched the depths before it stirs the surface" (ibid., p. 195).

In the Gestalt group, we take time to breathe, to pause, to find our metaphors for the present actuality (as in Example II.A.3), and to let them lead us. We, too: "Attend. Witness. Wait." (ibid., p. *xxix*). The metaphors are shared, we apprehend the field and connect, rather than the usual analyzing, dissecting, and distancing.

In the Gestalt group, as the frame of reference or the context changes, so do the meaning of words and "existing categorizations"(ibid., p. 196). We begin to create new shared language and new shared meanings.

E. Group Gestalten

A group is a gestalt. With contacting, over time, the group's gestalt or configuration changes. It may organize into millions of configurations but, heuristically, I like five. The five-stage model (Garland et al., 1973, pp. 17–47) I use is not normative, not a blueprint, but a map. It does not tell you where you must go or how you must go, but it does orient you as to where you might be. These group gestalten or configurations are: I. Orientation; II. Power and Control; III. Intimacy; IV. Differentiation; V. Termination.

1. Orientation

When members begin a group, they first "check it out". They are orienting themselves before making any commitment, and their behavior is approach/ avoidance. Their frame of reference and their norms (about "men", "women", "good", and "bad") are from society, their culture, and previous groups they have been in. The designated leader's task is to clarify and support the approaching and avoiding, normalizing it, helping members to put it into words and into subgroups, rather than acting it out. It is no longer an individual issue if members are able to subgroup and explore together the impulse to invest more in the group or the impulse to flee or be skeptical. The leader helps the members to experiment and connect in a new way.

2. Power and Control (Authority)

Once members do invest in the group, there is then concern about where one "fits in" with the other members and with the leader. What behavior is valued: openness? intelligence? emotionality? defiance? Who does the leader seem to like? Much behavior is leader-centered, and there are competitive feelings among the members.

There is a tremendous demand for creativity from the designated leader in this configuration. Anger and frustration, fight and flight, fears about being vulnerable come up in various disguises in this configuration and must be recognized, named, experienced, explored, and understood in the context of this group here and now. Feelings and the fear of feelings have to be recognized and expressed clearly and cleanly, and part of this is their being explored in subgroups. Most groups, even therapy groups, stop in this configuration of authority/dependence, and the relationship to authority is never examined as a *group* issue. In this model, if the members are to go on and to create their own space, this authority/dependence must also be explored and worked, exploring both the compliance and defiance as group issues (and as ways of avoiding going deeper).

If the leader is good, there will be a rebellion, what Bennis and Shepard call a "barometric event"(Bennis and Shepard, 1957), a challenging and unpredictable time for the leader-as-authority who may feel as if "the storm is up, and all is in the hazard" (W. Shakespeare, Julius Caesar, Act V). Yet, this "storm" is vital and essential for the group's growth and further development. The leader has to steer a steady course, not deflecting or defending or explaining away, but listening. He must also support the expression of the anger, disappointment, hurt, or betrayal aimed at himself and help clarify what the *issues* are. He has to be fully present and let the members know they have affected him. Arnold Mindell calls this "sitting in the fire" (1995, pp. 17–47). The leader acknowledges their issues and, with them, sees what needs to be changed. Was there a misunderstanding? Is there something they want to change in the group, some change in behavior, structure, time, or method?

At the other end of this process, there will be a new norm, a change in structure; the leader will do something differently, and the members will have taken on more responsibility for how the group is organized and develops. The group is no longer so leader-centered: the member's empowerment has begun. The frame of reference is no longer society, but is *this* group at this time, what we can co-create and who we can be within it.

3. Intimacy

The group, after the rebellion against the authority of the leader, now turns to issues of authority and intimacy with each other. The group begins to feel more like a "family", and members "remind me of my mother, brother, sister", and so forth. The leader's task is to clarify what belongs to the family "then", and what to the group now; what is similar, and what is novel here and now: "for only the novel is nourishing" (Perls et al., 1994, p. 6).

The leader supports the deeper levels of exploration, intimacy, and sharing now possible in the subgroups. Shame issues and early trauma can now be explored in a different way, in a different context. The frame of reference is family, but in *this* group, and who we can be for one another.

4. Differentiation

Having created a deeper level of trust, cohesion, clarity, and empowerment, members are ready to bring in parts of themselves not yet explored, perhaps the unaccepted parts that make them feel existentially "different". The group is seen as *a space we have created*, where we can more fully be ourselves, in all aspects, where we can explore ourselves with others "in the same boat", where we can connect on all levels. Where my selfing is an integral part of our "grouping", and where we can experiment with new behaviors. The leader's task is to support this, but more and more as a resource, a consultant, as she encourages members to take on more leadership and supports the group in running itself.

5. Termination

> "Parting is such sweet sorrow ..."
> (W. Shakespeare, *Romeo and Juliet*)

> "Do not go gentle into that good night ...
> Rage, rage against the dying of the light"
> (Dylan Thomas)

Termination is the final configuration. Members know that the group will be ending; there may be sadness, hurt, anger, and feelings of abandonment. These must be named and worked out in our subgroups together. There may be a "return" to earlier forms of behavior – avoidance, defiance – or denial that the group "was that important." There may be: "I'll leave the group before the group leaves me." The leader's task is to help the group make the feelings clear, to help reaffirm the skills that have been learned, to hold the history and the ground of what has been created, and to aid the creative integration of experience, including the letting go, in this new context. She makes room for members' taking back projections and group roles, for appreciations and recognitions, and for goodbyes. Her frame of reference is this group and what has been gained in this special creation, now as a ground for the next steps in the journey:

"What we call the beginning is often the end and to make an end is to make a beginning. The end is where we start from" (T.S. Elliot, *Little Giddings*).

Notice the enormous possibilities for new creative adjustments, for "selfing" and exploring our issues in each configuration – dependency, authority, intimacy, shame, loss – and the tremendous support given by the subgrouping together, to "hold" those issues as they are explored. Notice also that the stereotypical social scripts – "woman", "man", "black", "white", "old", "young" – will have different meanings, will be different processes in each configuration. As the frame of reference changes, these scripts will dissolve and reappear as increasingly novel events: "... *the self is not the figure it creates but the creating of the figure*" ... (Perls et al., 1994, pp. 191). "... anxiety as an emotion is the dread of one's own daring" (ibid., p. 192).

References

Agazarian Y (1997) Systems-centered therapy for groups. Guilford Press, New York

Bennis WG, Shepard HA (1957) A theory of group development. Human Relations 9(4): 415–437

Cox M, Theilgard A (1987) Mutative metaphors in psychotherapy. Tavistock Publications, London

de Mare P, Piper R, Thompson S (1991) Koinonia: From hate, through dialogue, to culture in the large group. Karnap Books, London

Dyer G (ed) (2002) John Berger selected essays. Pantheon Books, New York

Garland J, Jones H, Kolodny R (1973) A five-stage model for social work groups. In: Bernstein S (ed) Explorations in social group work. Milford House, New York, pp 17–47

Goldstein K (1975) Human nature in the light of psychopathology. New American Library, New York

Köhler W (1975) Gestalt psychology. New American Library, New York

Mindell A (1995) Sitting in the fire: Large group transformation using conflict and diversity. Lao Tse Press, Portland, Oregon

Perls F, Hefferline R, Goodman P (1994) Gestalt therapy: Excitement and growth in the human personality. The Gestalt J Press, Highland, New York

Creative Adjustment in Madness: A Gestalt Therapy Model for Seriously Disturbed Patients[1]

Margherita Spagnuolo Lobb

I. How Can We Understand Creative Adjustment in Serious Disturbances?

The lamented increase in serious disturbances in our society has become a stimulus to improve the language of psychotherapy. Today, the treatment of seriously disturbed patients constitutes a challenge for all psychotherapies: "We all know that if psychotherapy is to fulfill its function, it must be based on a theory of psychological maturity which is, of course, in debt to the social, historical-cultural, sometimes even political context, in which it happens to arise and operate" (Spagnuolo Lobb et al., 1996, p. 45). There has been an evolution in psychological disturbances in these last decades; certainly there has been a series of changes since Gestalt therapy was founded.

A crucial challenge for Gestalt therapy with regard to madness is whether psychotics' behavior should be considered creative or not. On the one hand, the oddity of psychotic behavior astounds us with the originality of the solutions the patients adopt (e.g. wearing three pairs of pants in order not to be invaded by other people's sperm); on the other hand, we realize that this creativity neither leads the person to growth, nor to satisfaction in relationships, but rather it brings about a dramatic limitation of the person's opportunities for contact. And so we wonder in what sense we can speak of "creative adjustment" in psychosis. Far from naively admiring the presumed creativity inherent in the eccentricity of madness (an attitude characteristic of humanistic psychotherapies until the 1980s, and one whose logic was the evaluation of the individual's potential in the face of the "normalization" imposed by society), today we accept the relational limit inherent in the psychotic behavior and experience, and we differentiate it from the creative adjustment that characterizes the original choice of that behavior, as the best solution possible in a difficult field. The creativity that pertains to that primary adjustment is

[1] This work develops a previous one published in the *British Gestalt Journal* (Spagnuolo Lobb, 2002). I thank the editor, Malcolm Parlett, for the trust with which he welcomed this study and for his inspiring editorial notes.

not, then, supported at a relational level: the anxiety that the "odd" behavior aims to avoid and solve is neither seen, worked through, nor approached in any way by the environment, so that the "odd" behavior remains for years like a dress on a hanger, which is of no use to anybody. We can say that with repetition the original creativity is reduced, is lost; the attempt to solve a problem is always there, like a broken record, and the old solution, out of the present context, does not create an evolution of perceptions in the field.

It is in this sense that we can speak of creative adjustment in madness: an attempt to solve a field problem that has never been successful and never interrupted, never revealed in its most profound intentionality within the relationship to which it refers.

The present contribution to the relationship between creativity and madness will start from an analysis of psychotic language in evolutionary terms and from a phenomenological-relational viewpoint; I then proceed to a proposal for the application of Gestalt therapy hermeneutics in the treatment of serious disturbances, both in a private setting and in psychiatric institutions.

II. Developmental Approach and Phenomenology of Psychotic Experience

Although we know that nobody can guarantee that there will not be an earthquake in the next five seconds, we live as if the unexpected is not going to happen. In our development, we have to forget this possibility in order to focus on what we want and do not want, on what we identify with and what we alienate from. Normally, we do not attend to our basic safety, or again, consider that our very existence is in doubt.

An old Sardinian folk tale relates that an angel kisses newborn babies on the brow to make them forget that one day they will die. Using this story as a metaphor, we may say that in psychotic experience, this kiss is wanting: seriously disturbed people in fact live in a constant state of emergency, since they are unable to make use of those basic certainties that would permit them to forget their perception of living in situations of extreme difficulty, situations that threaten their very existence.

The most recent psychological theories of child development establish a connection between babies' earliest relationships and the structure of experience of seriously disturbed patients. This structure is no longer explained in terms of a worsening – a mental involution experienced at the moment the psychosis is generated – but in terms of evolutionary experiential competences for contact-making and withdrawal. In this context, the seriously disturbed patient has not had the chance to develop a perception of the self, one which is integrated and clearly differentiated from the non-self, from the environment: "The experience of self has not reached that perceptive and relational competence that Fairbairn (1970) calls mature dependence, that Mahler et al. (1993) call the ability to separate/individualize, that Stern (1989) calls the narrative self, that Gestalt psychotherapy calls competence for full contact and withdrawal" (Salonia, 1992, p. 33).

For Gestalt therapy, our basic security derives from the ground of acquired contacts, which constitute that structure of experiences called the id-function. In other words, it constitutes our ability to make contact with the environment through our bodily experience and all that is perceived as if "inside the skin" (Spagnuolo Lobb, 2001b). Little by little, as the child experiences the world, she assimilates contacts that she can take for granted, and she no longer needs to learn the consequences of these contacts. For example, when the child is ready to stand up, she has already acquired a whole series of sensory-motor and proprioceptive notions that enable her to feel safe in standing up. The child learns a whole series of relational and emotive certainties in the same way. As she gradually learns to deal with her archaic fears, which are often catastrophic in early childhood (Winnicott, 1970), she feels protected and supported by her environment (the adult caregiver does not abandon her, for example), and she is able to draw on a series of acquired contacts, which allow her to form an integrated experience of "self", distinguished from what is "not self", and hence is capable of facing the world as a differentiated self.

Speaking in terms of the phenomenology of psychotic experience, three aspects seem to characterize it:

1. Psychotic patients lack the confidence born from this *ground of acquired contacts*. Still occupied in the attempt to emerge from their archaic fears, they cannot clearly define themselves in relation to the world. Because of this lack of differentiation between the experience of "self" and of "non-self", the seriously disturbed patient has no defenses against those environmental stimulations a neurotic patient considers normal or banal. He notes, for example, that a member of the therapeutic team sits on a different chair or that she has a cross expression, and he attributes these circumstances to himself: "Has she changed her seat because of me?" "Is she looking cross because she is angry with me?" "How did I make her change seats?" The experience of one-self is not differentiated in the relationship and is therefore extremely "permeable" in relation to all that happens. In this context, normal daily social activities become highly stressful; moreover, they are not particularly interesting for these patients.

2. As Object Relational theorists (Greenberg and Mitchell, 1986) have made clear, the experience of self of a seriously disturbed patient is *qualitatively different* from that of a neurotic one. For psychotic patients, it is not a matter of being less able than the neurotic to accomplish social requirements or be with someone else. Their experience has a different quality, since it is focused on the possibilities offered by the field to remain "alive", to cope with the intense anxiety they constantly live with. In the experience of seriously disturbed patients, existential certainties are in question. An example quoted by Resnick (1970) may be useful in this regard: during a session, the electric current failed, and the light went out; in the dark, the therapist asked the patient whether he would prefer to postpone the session until the following week. The patient replied that since he did not know whether he would be alive or dead by then, he preferred to carry on in the dark. The

lack of light was nothing compared to the real anguish that made his treatment necessary. The therapeutic intervention must therefore be aimed at a form of anguish that is qualitatively different from what neurotic patients experience, because it is connected to the person's existential certainty: "In a few minutes will I be alive or dead?" "Will I be smashed to pieces by the therapist's anger (or the nurse's)?" "Will I destroy him with my anger?" "Whom will I kill or annihilate with my emotions – which sometimes seem to be on the point of exploding." Taking this aspect of psychotic experience into consideration is crucial for any psychotherapeutic intervention: a great deal of treatment, especially in the case of chronic disturbances, is in fact normally based on the acquisition of "social skills", with behavioral instruments, as if what is needed is to behave.

3. Since the reassuring perception that a boundary exists between one's self and the external world does not form part of a psychotic's experience, any experience perceived as "inside the skin" overflows toward the outside, just as every external event can penetrate uncontrollably the inside. This quality of psychotic experience *makes useless for the other any attempt to hide*. A social lie, as a form of differentiation of the self from the environment, even a healthy one, belongs to neurotic experience. Only a neurotic patient who has experience of boundaries can believe another's lie, thus desensitizing herself from the series of phenomenological facts to which a psychotic patient remains sensitive. As a consequence of this particular permeability of the boundary between the self and the world perceived by a psychotic individual, every element of experience, of the self or of the other, is visible. It is as though both therapist and patient are engaged in a sort of "transparent" relationship: the psychotic can see parts of the experience of the therapist that are usually not seen (or the therapist has learned to hide to become a "social" person), and similarly he will tend to consider anything the therapist says to be true or pertinent or possible, since he has been unable to learn to experience a boundary capable of hiding parts of his experience (he has not learned to lie).

A Gestalt Therapy Concept of Creativity in Madness

To summarize these differences in Gestalt therapy terms, in neurosis, what seems new is defined as "not for me", via the ego function; the support of *personality function of self* is lacking in this case. The self cannot adjust creatively to the changes in social relationships, on account of a split between the definition of "who I am", as assimilated from previous contacts, and the new social requirement.

In psychosis, because the ground of security arising from assimilated contacts is missing (*id function of self*), the ego cannot exercise its ability to deliberate on this ground. Contacting is thus dominated in the psychotic by sensations that invade a self with "no skin", and so invade the world (Spagnuolo Lobb, 2001c, p. 63). Creativity, a human quality exercised freely in situations when spontaneous contacting is possible, is limited: it cannot be relaxed, and what could appear to us an artistic eccentricity is in effect a hard-won solution, charged with anxiety, which attempts to hold a catastrophe in check. I do not mean that there is no creativity in the experience and behavior of psychotics, but rather that theirs is a creativity that does not resolve a grave existential anxiety, at least until such time as it is recognized within a meaningful relationship.

III. Consequences for Therapeutic Praxis

There are basic aspects to be considered in the treatment of what we call psychotic experience. Although the model I present here has been made for psychiatric structures, the following basic aspects must also be taken into consideration in the private context, since they provide a diagnostic/therapeutic key for treating psychotic experience.

From the premises cited above, it follows that to apply Gestalt therapy in the treatment of seriously disturbed patients, we need first of all to accommodate a change in perspective from that adopted when dealing with neurotic patients. With psychotic patients, treatment must start from the background so as to construct the figure, whilst with neurotic patients the opposite is true. In fact, for neurotics, the learning process is built on the dialogue between therapist and patient, on the history/figure which, in its evolution, also causes a "re-shaping" of the background. In psychotherapy with seriously disturbed patients, the starting point is in building the background, and the figure emerges later, in the post-contact phase, as the therapeutic result (Spagnuolo Lobb, 2001a).

The creativity that such patients have used to cope with an emergency should be modulated into a more relaxed capacity to play. The difficult field must become a welcoming field.

Hence, a fundamental difference for the treatment of seriously disturbed patients is the balance of the attention to be paid to the figure and to the background of experience. Everything that constitutes the ground where the intervention is carried out (such as the armchairs we sit in and the pictures on the walls, or even a thought which may momentarily distract us), while in neurotic experience it is normally taken for granted, in psychotics' experience becomes the first code of access to their experience.

Second, it is important to approach the basic existential anxiety in treatment, and to possibly use behavioral tools or rehabilitation techniques (such as training patients to keep themselves clean and behave – social abilities that they are less interested in) in a way that must be pertinent to the therapeutic relationship. A psychotic patient is, for instance, ready to shower every day or stop cutting her wrists only if she feels that this is important for the therapist and that the therapist is in touch with her "real" anxiety.

Third, more than upon an analysis of archaic experiences or in support of unexplored potentiality, the therapeutic relationship must be focused on the coherence between the *what* and the *how* things are communicated, a coherence in all that Stern et al. (1998) mean by "implicit knowledge". In fact, the perceived permeability of boundaries, the quality of the relational "transparence" with which the patient feels that he is on the one hand "read" by the therapist and on the other hand capable of "reading" the therapist, is the basic condition from which the patient must construct a background of existential security on which to base himself. If he is to emerge as an individual capable of knowingly choosing between what he identifies with and what he alienates from, he must first experience that what happens at the boundary is not threatening. Every time a seriously disturbed patient tells us anything about our relationship, which seems untrue to us, like a delusion, such as, for instance, if he says that we are angry or in love, it is always very informative, instead of labeling these utterances simplistically as paranoia, to consider what might be true along the lines – "In what way is this patient right? How am I expressing anger or love at this moment?" – rather than to look at what is untrue. The ability of the therapist to answer these questions largely determines the success of the treatment.

IV. A Gestalt Therapy Model for Addressing Psychosis in Psychiatric Institutions

Gestalt therapy, given the importance it attaches to group processes and relationships, is well-suited to psychiatric settings. Beginning with Buber's concept of "betweenness", it supplies an analysis of the here and now of the relationship (the process of contact), which makes it possible to trace and understand aspects of pathology and their treatment, via a dialectic between the individual and society. According to Gestalt psychotherapy, we need not refer to inner (e.g. the superego) or external (e.g. society) elements to resolve Freud's supposed irreconcilability of the relationship between the individual and the community. There is no need to create a dichotomy between the individual and society (Spagnuolo Lobb et al., 1996). Today, it is possible to consider psychotherapy – even in the case of seriously disturbed patients – as a way of integrating individual needs and perceptions, and social requirements. Both "needs" and "social adaptation" are the fruit of relationships and are, therefore, achievable through contact. The humanistic emphasis on the self-regulation of the organism needs to be rethought in terms of self-regulation of the relationship (Salonia et al., 1997).

Paul Goodman's idea of creating a community made up of individuals who are fully themselves, one that is rich and harmonious like a Greek chorus, which is not rendered uniform by the imposition of external rules, but rather discovers harmony through spontaneous social self-government, is the guideline for the application of Gestalt therapy in a psychiatric structure. Nowadays, we tend to consider that the therapeutic approach for seriously disturbed patients treated in psychiatric settings needs to be directed toward fostering the *relational potential* that is being expressed, in its own language, through the pathological behavior.

There are aspects that are peculiar to the treatment in psychiatric institutions, which deal with two separate, important elements: the chronic nature of the disturbance (in effect, acquiring a social role that is defined as "disturbed") and the context of treatment (which is not a single figure, but an interdisciplinary team of workers and the physical structure where the treatment occurs).

In-patients in psychiatry often lose ordinary personal and social skills, on different levels, depending on the individual process of involution. One person is incapable of making her own bed and has to be helped by another to do it; another person is incapable of "tuning in" to the normalized language of the world around him. As a result of a long history of failures in their attempts to solve a situation perceived as threatening their own existence, sometimes caused by a long history of institutionalization that has merely dramatically reinforced their sense of personal failure and dependence on a doctor or on drugs, such people cannot easily operate within normal social modes of behavior.

With regard to the second peculiar aspect, the psychiatric team, the new perspective of working on the ground should correspond to a multi-modal and interdisciplinary treatment, in which various levels are integrated (clinical, psychotherapeutic, pharmacological, personal, and family/social) as well as various professional figures (psychiatrists, psychologists, social workers, educators, nurses, and psychotherapists).

Paradoxically, though active treatments are often of a transient nature, what seriously disturbed patients particularly need from therapy is long term consistency. How is it possible, then, to help guests of psychiatric institutions build a sense of security, something that only a physically and emotionally stable context can provide. The answer given to this question is fundamental for any psychotherapeutic model applied to chronic patients in residential psychiatric settings.

Success in creating a therapeutic context for severely disturbed patients, not only in a specific psychiatric setting but in the wider context of the mental health culture with which they have to deal, requires, as a first step, that we acknowledge the depth and nature of their individual experience. That is, we must develop a uniform therapeutic intent (obtained through the necessary group process among the staff) and hence provide a sense of security that is derived from a stable relationship. It is important, here, to accept the idea that it is the setting that treats the patient, and not one particular member of staff. Even an excellent psychiatrist in isolation can only have a limited effect in the long run on a therapeutic level, compared to a setting which, in its human and structural dimensions, communicates treatment. The role of the psychotherapist in a psychiatric setting should be defined as that of promoter of a ground condition. It is therefore necessary to create a healthy perceptive background – a "cradle" or mother's arms: a series of learning experiences that constitute the ground; a background of security that can be taken for granted. Obviously, it is not possible to give these patients the security they lacked in their infancy; but we can give them a new experience of security that can help them to balance an interest in the present and anxieties connected with their past.

The Problem of Diagnosis

The phenomenology of psychotic experience that I have described in section II. is based on experiential and relational codes, a different perspective from the usual psychiatric diagnosis. We refer to experience of boundaries and of ground support in contact-making, while they refer to behavioral and statistical categories. Nevertheless, once we are aware of the different "glasses" we put on when we look at the same reality, diagnostic results do not seem so different, and a dialogue is possible.

As we know, the diagnosis is a map that the therapist needs in order to orient himself in the therapeutic relationship with the patient. In the Gestalt therapy perspective – as in recent research by Stern and the Process of Change Study Group (1998) – the map (the diagnosis) is never actually defined a priori, but is co-created by therapist and patient in the therapeutic relationship, and thus comes to coincide with the therapeutic process itself.

We may therefore speak of lines of inquiry in which the therapist is interested: the result being, not a univocal answer from the therapist, but a co-creation that cannot ignore the specific nature of the particular encounter, between those two (or more) specific individuals, at a specific time.

Here are a few research paths that exemplify what I am curious about when I activate myself in the complexity of the therapeutic situation:

1. What Language – or Experiential Code – Does the Person Use in Contacting the Therapeutic Environment?

There is no psychotherapeutic intervention without creative adjustment to the patient's language, because language is the expression of the patient's experience; it is the code of access through which we can contact her. A patient who says "ants are walking in my veins", has an entirely different way of expressing herself than one who says "I'm a failure, I'll never do anything right." The former expresses herself using the language of the id-function, whilst the latter uses that of the personality function. With the first patient we need to use a form of language that springs from bodily experience and archaic fears that cannot be defined; the second patient requires a language that springs from role experience, unrealized ideals, and a desire to be appreciated for the good she has achieved.

Language tells us about many other aspects of the experience of the speaker: for instance, his capacity to interconnect experiences (the grammar of his experience) and to differentiate "me" from "not me", as well as aspects concerning the kind of contact abilities he is using and even of implicit messages to the person the speaker is talking to.

The following example illustrates what I mean:

If a patient says that "the air is heavy", he is speaking from the experience of his body (or id function of the self, according to Gestalt psychotherapy). He is using his concrete intelligence, connected to concrete thought, and so also a sort of magic/animistic form of conceptualization (things have a soul). All this provides us with very useful information about the experience of the patient, to whom our therapeutic language must be adapted if we want to access to his experience. First of all, this patient is speaking of the balance between the air (heavy) and his body's ability to breathe heavy air without feeling that he is smashed or poisoned by it. We could reply to this patient, for example, that it is true that the air is heavy, but that it is also true that his body has the capacity to inhale and exhale, to take what it needs for nourishment and then get rid of the heavy air. Second, we should ask ourselves which part of the relationship at that moment can be considered "heavy". We could, for example, ask the patient: "How do I make your air heavy at this moment?" Every experience, in fact, finds its significance in the here and now of a specific contact. Nothing occurs by chance, not even the most incomprehensible "word-salad" of a schizophrenic. Language is always the expression of our present experience, and our present experience is always a contact experience. Only in cases where there is a compulsion to repeat – for example, a patient who *always* says "the air is heavy" – can we say that it constitutes a block in experience, something incomplete, in the same way a broken record interrupts a melody.

2. Which Evolutionary Phase is the Person Living in?

The stage of the patient's life cycle places her behavior and experience in a context of meanings and needs that make her sense of being in the world, the continuum of her existence. It is necessary to consider a whole range of experiences connected to the existential moment being lived by the patient. A boy of twenty has a different way of looking at life and different needs than a woman of fifty facing menopause.

Thus, treatment is placed in the evolutionary moment of the patient's individual "biography".

Here is an example:

A woman of thirty-five with intermittent hospital stays from the age of about twenty, who gave birth to two daughters without really realizing what was happening, abandoned her children before her first stay in hospital. Since this time, she has always had a marginal relationship with her daughters, who were subsequently brought up by their paternal grandmother. She has never wanted to be with them for more than a couple of hours, but, in her confused way, she loves them. Now she is obsessed by a desire to see her daughters – and she is devastated when rejected by them. She has attempted suicide more than once and, on occasion, she has locked herself indoors and starved herself. To address this self-isolating and self-destructive behavior, she has been admitted into our psychiatric community. Treatment must take her life cycle into account: she is a mother of adolescents – i.e., she must come to terms with the end of her children's childhood. What the patient needs to know in order to accept her daughters' adolescence and the rebellious behavior typical of their age, without being destroyed by it, is whether she has been a good mother up till now and has done all she could for them. Saying "yes" to her means allowing her to move on to the next stage of her life cycle, to be a mother of adolescents. Of course, her daughters now refuse to see their mother. The psychiatric team decided that to avoid upsetting the balance created by the grandmother and the daughters, it would be better for the woman not to see her children. "What good would it do, anyway?

It would only destroy a delicate balance, on one hand, while creating false affective bonds on the other." The woman makes a suicide attempt. The team decides to change strategy and to explain to the daughters what their mother has gone through. Despite the anger and pain caused by discussing their mother's absence, the daughters manage to meet their mother and ask her things such as: "Did you want us or were we an accident?" Surprisingly, with a kind of simplicity, the mother is able to answer many of these questions. After a few conversations, neither the mother nor the daughters ask for further dialogue. The feeling all three seem to share is that a common pain has finally been faced, and there is now greater serenity about it. The daughters continue to live with their grandmother; they no longer express anger toward their mother and, in a certain sense, they have regained a sense of being daughters; the woman has regained her sense of being a mother and no longer tries to commit suicide.

3. What Specific Support is Needed in Order to Spontaneously Make Contact?

Within the experience of existential anguish that characterizes them, these patients have various ways of dealing with it in contacting the environment and giving up the spontaneity of their being. Our job is to help them do better what they already do with anguish. The Gestalt therapy diagnostic tool, the contact-withdrawal cycle, allows us to pinpoint the specific support that is required at the boundary of their contact-making by both therapist and client (Spagnuolo Lobb, 1992), in terms of the missing ego-function and the disturbed self-function (Perls et al., 1994, pp. 149–161).

This is an example to explain the concept:

Giorgio has lost his father and has a troubled, insane mother. When she comes to visit him, she entraps him with flattery – but then betrays him: for example, she remarries without telling him. The history of the families of these patients often conceals betrayals, madness that has confused the patient, making it impossible for them to differentiate. As Bateson et al. (1956) point out with their concept of "double bind", whatever these patients do, they are losers. Giorgio transfers the relational pattern with his mother that causes him distress (and for which he has found no solution) to today's important relationships. Not by chance, he feels invaded by sperm during the night, and he declares that the other patients introduce it into his body during sleep. He cannot sleep, and he says he has nightmares. Giorgio's symptom reminds me of the invasion/betrayal of his mother; the sperm appears to be perceived in a pre-personal mode (in Giorgio's experience, there is still no clear distinction between the sexes). The sperm seems in fact similar to the mother's power, capable of invasively penetrating his body, inside the skin/self-boundary, and Giorgio strenuously tries to defend himself (normally wearing two or three pairs of trousers at the same time). We observe that he is particularly afraid when he is asleep, a time when he loses control and is rendered most vulnerable. Creating a structural and honest communicative context is vital in preventing Giorgio from reliving the experience of being deeply betrayed but, conversely, he needs to build up a ground of security in relationships. His drugs are therefore explained to him and his sleeping space is clearly defined, as are his daily activities. Any message that leaves too much open to interpretation agitates him, and his symptoms become paroxysm. Giorgio, however, cannot relax. He continues to be unable to sleep and complains of his nightmares. At this point, I come up with a specific supporting strategy that does him far more good than drugs. I remembered the "dream-catchers" that American Indians use: a little net with a hole in the middle that they hang on the entrance of their tents when they sleep. For them, this object has the power to net the nightmares, which are then destroyed by the morning light, while good dreams can pass through the hole and float in the air. Bad dreams therefore cannot disturb us. The explanation of the use of the "dream-catcher", and his constructing one to hang on the wall behind his bed, convinces Giorgio, who finally manages to rest at night. The following morning – and for many successive nights – he happily greets me saying that he has not had nightmares. A concrete and animistic thought that justifies the use of "dream-catchers" is the appropriate language for Giorgio, who does not respond to explanations based on abstract thought ("try to relax") or on the perception of boundaries ("sperm cannot invade you"). Giorgio needs an environmental support which makes it possible for him to do better what he already does (protect his privacy with three pairs of pants), so that he can rest. As a matter of fact, he doesn't need to rely on ego function ("try to relax"); he rather needs to trust the environment (with the positive relaxing consequences of id functioning).

V. Therapeutic Goals of the Model

How is the healing environment evolving in the perception of the patient and of the therapist? If this line of inquiry is fundamental in the treatment of any kind of disorder, in the case of the treatment of psychotics it becomes, as I have said, the figure of the therapeutic intervention.

The first goal is to create a therapeutic environment capable of fostering in the whole community the experience of a healthy ground. As an environmental aspect, the setting becomes a most important focus of treatment, especially insofar as it affects the relationship. In this context, the group relationship that is created in the psychiatric structure involved is likewise a primary place of treatment.

From attention given to the ground in the form of the therapeutic setting and climate (the first goal and an indispensable premise for any future progress in the relationship), it is possible to foster other important experiences for the harmonious differentiation of the self, such as creative differentiation (second goal), the perception of time and space as categories that orient and give a rhythm to the self (third goal), and the clear and distinct perception of one's own needs (fourth goal). These four goals constitute the therapeutic journey for residents in a psychiatric setting. They are evolutionary phases in building a well-grounded experience of one-self. Since they are holistic acquisitions, they also integrate with each other. Each phase represents a gestalt of new contact capabilities that are added to the gestalt of the previous acquisitions, just as new notes follow each other in a melody, creating a new melody.

1. Goal 1 – The Therapeutic Environment

To create a therapeutic environment means to arrange a welcoming, reassuring, and flexible setting in relation to the patient's needs for separation and fusion: "closed" enough to transmit a sense of security, "open" enough to give the necessary support to independence, but also "flexible" enough to adapt itself to the patient's attempts to integrate her inner and outer needs. This is a fundamental requirement, a platform to reach further goals. It concerns two fundamental aspects: the physical structure in which community life is lived and the communicative attitude adopted by the staff.

As far as the physical structure is concerned, it must be capable of fulfilling the basic psychological functions of any home (Giordano, 1997): holding, supporting, integrating. Studies of environmental psychology (Fisher et al., 1984; Bonnes and Secchiaroli, 1992) highlight other structural characteristics that should be taken into account. For instance, the staff's overall communicative attitude must be considered, such as their ability to convey empathy, unconditional acceptance, esteem, and congruence (Franta and Salonia, 1981). They represent necessary and specific competences for communicating with seriously disturbed patients. Important "relationship guarantees" are, for example, *clarity* (the opposite of confusion), *encouragement* (seen as faith in the organism during anxiety crises), and *absolute respect for the rules* (the rules are like a containing wall, and to leap over them would mean losing a significant sense of security). In this context, verbal communication by the staff must be empathetic and at the same time normative, making the resident feel that she is accepted as a person – as a unique being with individual thoughts and needs – who is nevertheless able to respect the rules of the community.

Nonverbal communication on the staff's part must express *welcome* (a smile is always more relaxing than an angry face), *being there* (these residents have a special sensitivity in perceiving if a person is "absent"), and respect for boundaries (communicating familiarity beyond what the role calls for is always confusing for these patients, given that roles, like rules, protect them from "invasion" by external elements). Particular attention must also be paid to physical contact, which is obviously necessary in a health context. It is also important to remember one is touching a person who has "no skin" and that any physical contact has fusional reverberations.

The imprinting of the therapeutic atmosphere is transmitted to the person from the moment of admission. A new resident's arrival is pre-announced to the community, and preparations to welcome the new "guest" follow. On arrival, the newcomer is introduced to the community in a group setting, whilst drinking a cup of coffee and eating a biscuit. A warm round of applause greets the new in-patient. Then he is introduced to the group by a member of staff; an open sharing follows, where the new resident is invited, if he wishes to do so, to tell the group what hopes and fears he has about this new experience. Thanks to this welcoming moment, the newcomer knows that he is considered as a person in the community and not simply as a case-record.

Here is an example:

> Once a newcomer said, at the end of this introduction – referring to the chaotic manner of the patients' participation during the meeting: "This is the best possible organization of total disorganization." The Gestalt therapy leader said: "Each of you has felt the need to distinguish yourself from all the others. In fact, nobody has continued to talk about a point raised by anybody else. You have reacted against your fear of being wiped out by taking refuge in individual chaos! This chaos is the community group's life-blood" (Argentino, 2001).

This is a good example of how the Gestalt therapy leader can organize the various remarks, the climate, and the group process into a single "gestalt", a global, harmonious, and meaningful configuration with which both the individual and the group can identify.

2. Goal 2 – The Sense of Creative Differentiation

For these patients to feel positively different from the others, as unique human beings, it is necessary for them to feel integrated with the environment. In other words, once the person experiences being accepted, she can begin to focus on herself and recognize her own uniqueness. Many activities can support this discovery, an example of which follows:

I was in a group, running a drawing activity. I had asked participants to concentrate on themselves, on their breathing (a very delicate thing to ask of this kind of patients, since it connects the person immediately with her strongest anxieties). I then asked them to draw a figure on a sheet of paper, whatever in that precise moment they wanted to draw. One person drew an old lion walking alone in a desolate field; another drew a beautiful sea in a storm, full of rough waves, with no evident boats, and a very small line that might represent a distant boat. One person drew a tree, with very weak lines; it gave a sense of loneliness. I told him that I could feel that drawing, that it said much of him. I also told him that he could play this tree if he wanted to. So he did: he played the tree. He was so much inside the experience that the whole atmosphere changed. The rest of the group remained looking at him as if at something magical. At the end, he said: "That's me", and the group spontaneously applauded. He felt so much himself, and after this experience, he changed; he participated more in the activities of the group; his face was more open, especially when he was in front of some of the people who were with him in this experience.

If you consider that psychotic patients are usually desensitized and do not distinguish how the person who is in front of them is different from another person, because they are wholly taken up by their anxieties, this experience shows how it is possible for them to see others more clearly when they can experience "their being", themselves as unique human beings.

Giving residents space and time to concentrate (as far as possible) on themselves, to discover the spontaneous movement of themselves toward the environment, is the therapeutic goal at this stage. All the while, therapists are providing them with adequate support to complete interrupted spontaneous contacts (in this example, the patient's wish to express his loneliness, to say it to someone).

Activities connected with the care of the environment, like cleaning one's room or looking after common areas with others, are perceived by residents as a necessity that regulates life together. Perhaps this behavior also acts as a concrete duty that leads to an experience alternative to anxiety (since it contains and confines anxiety). It is important to help patients to overcome their sense of inadequacy or failure, through productive or socialized activity, so guaranteeing them a point of reference that, although normative, calms their anxiety.

3. Goal 3 – Time and Space: The Rhythm of Self

Once a person is able to experience his own unique being, to experience the "I", he is ready to dance, that is, to orient himself in time and space. When the baby acquires a sense of "I am hungry, I can wait for mom", her sense of herself can be placed in time and space. The voice of the mother, who calms a crying baby from another room, acts as a container for the anxiety of the child. It fills the void in space and fosters a trust in "time". The experiential dimensions of time and space, and how we handle them, frame that feeling of "stable continuity" we attach to the self. Because of the experience of time and space, we acquire the certainty that we continue to be ourselves, although things change, both inside and outside. (I remember when my daughter was three, and she used to look at herself in the mirror with my glasses on and say "I'm Mommy", then wear my husband's T-shirt and say "I'm Daddy". She laughed a lot at this very interesting discovery: the possibility of changing outside while remaining the same person inside.)

This goal consists in favoring the perception of space and time as experiential containers, capable of directing the patient's multiple sensations and perceptions in the sense of rhythm (time) and spatial placing (distant/close, etc.). This helps in calming anxiety, since in seriously disturbed patients, sensations, emotions, and general perceptions are experienced in a confused manner (without I-Thou boundaries, now-then boundaries, here-there boundaries) and with much anxiety.

The patient who represented himself as a lonely tree was taking part in a daily group with other patients and staff members. All the participants were saying, in turn, something of their experience. When he was ready to speak, he said: "It's sunny today." The Gestalt therapy leader asked herself what the relational meaning of this sentence could be: what the sunny day had to do with his actual being in the group. Up till then he had proposed himself to the group as the sad, lonely tree, and the group had accepted him. She said: "What are the trees like when it's sunny?" He answered: "They stretch out toward the sun. I'm an oak today, not a weeping willow." The Gestalt leader said supportively: "There are many more oaks in our Mediterranean area than weeping willows." The patient stood up and opened his raised arms; he continued to look around; he did not close his eyes. He was experiencing himself as a new tree, with great courage, trusting the environment to overcome the "normal" anxiety he so often connected with novelty.

Many activities conducted in psychiatric settings mark a periodical rhythm, such as meals, medications, a Christmas party, going to the beach in summertime, and so on. These help residents to get a sense of continuity and of the passage of one moment to another. But it is important that caregivers notice a person's readiness to use these categories to contain experiences and thus calm psychotic anxiety.

4. Goal 4 – The Differentiated Perception of One's Own Needs

Once a person has acquired the sense of continuity of himself in a changing field, he has conquered an important step in building a sense of self-integrity. This ability will lead him to differentiate his own needs from others' needs, to emerge from the symbiotic confusion in which the self and the environment were previously perceived.

A group of residents were busy preparing lunch for themselves. To decide "what to cook" implies, first of all, a capacity to define what one wants to eat (second goal); it then presupposes a consideration of space and time in choosing ingredients and knowing cooking times (third goal). It also means knowing how independently to define and try to satisfy one's individual needs, given what the environment offers (fourth goal). A staff member was assisting them, and she wanted to cook something appetizing for them. In the group there were people with different developmental needs. Those who were in the first phase of needing to be welcomed by the environment, accepted gladly "being fed" by her (a piping hot dish of spaghetti with tomato sauce can be irresistible). Some were wondering whether they wanted spaghetti or something else (phase of creative differentiation), while others were curious about where to buy spaghetti and how long does it takes to cook (phase of the rhythm of self). One of the group, who was already well ahead on his therapeutic journey, said he wanted a scrambled egg, which he wanted to cook himself. This was a beautiful example of becoming autonomous. The Gestalt leader said how much she appreciated both his clarity in declaring what he wanted and his ability to resist being swallowed up by the desires of others. Notice that she did not appreciate his will or determination, which is more a neurotic stance, but his ability to experience boundaries between himself and the rest of the group, which is more part of the psychotic experience.

Readiness to look after themselves (personal hygiene, care of possessions) as well as to respect nature by not throwing their litter on the ground (bad habits often acquired in institutions), to be involved with the staff in doing the cleaning, and to respect those who are different are all important signs of the residents' ability to belong to the community in a differentiated and integrated way, without giving up their individuality or running away from the rules of society.

VI. Conclusions: The Existential Meaning of Meeting the Psychotic Experience (to Remain Alive in our Madness)

Given forty or more years of international endeavor to include knowledge from psychotherapy in our work with patients in psychiatric settings, mental health professionals still need to ask themselves whether and how psychotherapy methods can be used in psychiatric settings.

What seems to be missing in relevant previous experience (see, for instance, the experiences – first in the United Kingdom and then in other countries, like Italy – in the field of community care, during and after World War II, in Spagnuolo Lobb, 2002) is a well-defined method able to take care of the individual and of the group at the same time. For instance, the therapeutic power of the group does not solve the need to see each person individually, as in the case of seriously disturbed patients. The need to address the individual remains ever present in contemporary society, with its generation of ever new pathologies connected with modern living (note the continued emergence of the borderline structure of experience, baby-killers, and children who kill their parents).

It is not easy to work with seriously disturbed patients. I have seen young staff members psychologically destroyed after a few months' work in such settings, and I have met older workers who become cynical when faced with the impossibility of reacting to the pain they witness every day. The present model proposes a method of working with these highly demanding patients, which does not overlook the tragic nature of their existence, but rather tries to integrate it through human contact with staff and other patients.

An implication of this method is that workers in this field cannot be effective unless they recognize and come to terms with their own "madness". Working with seriously disturbed patients demands that you develop a great capacity to contain painful experiences and tragedy. For this, it is necessary for you bravely to maintain an awareness, both of the anguish that is part of our own experience of distress and of the ways you have learned to support yourself through it. Only then will you be able to enter deeper and "growthful" contact with another's pain and personal tragedy. Being unaware of the most distressing and archaic perceptions of himself leaves the psychiatric worker powerless when faced with the patient's own madness. Failure here will lead carers to either turn once again to the normalizing perspective of old-fashioned psychiatry (assuming a one-up position), or to suffer daily anguish (one-down position), from which only a new job or retirement can save them.

An effective healing community needs to provide support for the staff, so that they are not alone in bearing that world of pain and anguish that characterizes patients suffering from serious relational disturbances. These patients live eternally in a tragic dimension, even though they may have learned how to numb it. However, this anaesthetic reaction only puts their pain in hibernation – while leaving it intact, which, in turn, frustrates their growth toward a more mature existential position. It is therefore important that staff, in addition to being adequately trained in helpful relational competence with seriously disturbed patients, do not hibernate as well, but remain aware of the magical quality of existence as a moment of balance between life and death, so that they can support the emergence of this feeling, experienced tragically in psychotics, as soon as they start to awake from their hibernation state. Such an existential position as this gives them an added strength to face their own lives.

The application of this Gestalt psychotherapy model to psychiatric settings and their structures has, in my own experience and that of my colleagues, proved highly effective. Indeed, research has shown evidence that this model improves the quality of life of residents in psychiatric structures (Argentino, 1997), while at the same time fosters a pleasant and interesting working environment for staff. In this respect, creating spaces for and moments of significant human contact provides valuable learning for both, enriching the experience of staff and patients alike.

References

Argentino P (1997) Efficacia del modello gestaltico nelle comunità terapeutiche. Quaderni di Gestalt 24/25: 39–48
Argentino P (2001) La psicoterapia della Gestalt come terapia di comunità. In Spagnuolo Lobb M (ed) Psicoterapia della Gestalt. Ermeneutica e clinica. Angeli, Milano, pp 120–138
Bateson G, Jackson D, Haley J, Weakland J (1956) Toward a theory of schizophrenia. Behavioral Sci 4: 251
Bonnes M, Secchiaroli G (1992) Psicologia ambientale. La Nuova Italia Scientifica, Roma

Fairbairn WRD (1970) Studi psicoanalitici sulla personalità. Boringhieri, Torino
Fisher JD, Bell PA, Baum A (1984) Environmental psychology. Holt, Rinehart and Winston, New York
Franta H, Salonia G (1981) Comunicazione interpersonale. LAS, Roma
Giordano G (1997) La cassa vissuta. Percorsi e dinamiche dell'abitare. Giuffré, Milano
Greenberg JR, Mitchell SA (1986) Le relazioni oggettuali nella teoria psicoanalitica. Il Mulino, Bologna
Mahler MS, Pine F, Bergman A (1993) La nascita psicologica del bambino. Boringhieri, Torino
Perls FS, Hefferline R, Goodman P (1994) Gestalt therapy: Excitement and growth in the human personality. The Gestalt J Press, Highland, New York
Resnik S (1970) Spazio mentale. Sette lezioni alla Sorbona. Bollati Boringhieri, Torino
Salonia G (1992) From we to I-Thou. A contribution to an evolutive theory of contact. Studies in Gestalt Therapy 1: 31–41
Salonia G, Spagnuolo Lobb M, Sichera A (1997) Postfazione. In Perls FS, Hefferline R, Goodman P (1994) Teoria e pratica della terapia della Gestalt. Vitalità e accrescimento nella personalità umana. Astrolabio, Roma, pp 497–500
Spagnuolo Lobb M (1992) Specific support in the interruptions of contact. Studies in Gestalt Therapy 1: 43–51
Spagnuolo Lobb M (2001a) Linee programmatiche di un modello gestaltico nelle comunità terapeutiche. In Spagnuolo Lobb M (ed) Psicoterapia della Gestalt. Ermeneutica e clinica. Angeli, Milano, pp 139–158
Spagnuolo Lobb M (2001b) La teoria del sé in psicoterapia della Gestalt. In Spagnuolo Lobb M (ed) Psicoterapia della Gestalt. Ermeneutica e clinica. Angeli, Milano, pp 86–110
Spagnuolo Lobb M (2001c) From the epistemology of self to clinical specificity of Gestalt therapy. In Robine JM (ed) Contact and relationship in a field perspective. L'Exprimerie, Bordeaux, pp 49–65
Spagnuolo Lobb M (2002) A Gestalt therapy model for addressing psychosis. British Gestalt Journal 1: 5–15
Spagnuolo Lobb M, Salonia G, Sichera A (1996) From the discomfort of civilization to creative adjustment: The relationship between individual and community in psychotherapy in the third millennium. International J of Psychotherapy 1: 45–53
Stern D (1989) La nascita del sé. In Ammanniti M (ed) La nascita del sé. Laterza, Bari, pp 117–128
Stern D, Bruschweiler-Stern N, Harrison A, Lyons-Ruth K, Morgan A, Nahum J, Sander L, Tronick E (1998) The process of therapeutic change involving implicit knowledge: Some implications of developmental observations for adult psychotherapy. Infant Mental Health J 3: 300–308
Winnicott D W (1970) Sviluppo affettivo e ambiente. Armando, Roma

The Psychoportrait: A Technique for Working Creatively in Psychiatric Institutions

Giuseppe Sampognaro *

Using art therapy to work with a seriously disturbed patient is by now a universally recognized practice, which seems to rest on the romantic stereotype according to which there is a touch of madness in every artist (as the lives of such figures as Caravaggio, Vincent Van Gogh, Edvard Munch, and others seem to confirm). If the language of art is congenial to those whose control of reality is uncertain, why not use it in the context of therapy?

Gestalt therapy has risked sharing this simplistic, narrow view of the application of art to the treatment of seriously disturbed patients. Excessively conditioned by the concept of experience, our therapeutic model failed for a long time to go more deeply into the importance of creativity, which is fundamental to a true understanding of the course and finalities of any art therapy technique. It was taken for granted that the Gestalt therapist was *creative* in the sense of being *free of preconceived patterns*, and that the patient's creativity (which is evident in the "choice" of symptom and in the personal and original way she or he avoids contact) was to be exploited as a tool of emotional catharsis or as a recovery of spontaneity. It is only relatively recently that the background has become figure and increasing attention has been paid to individual artistic creativity as a potential quality to be better known and used. Furthermore, there has been an enrichment of the meaning of the choice of applying creative techniques to the treatment of psychotics: this is not because the seriously disturbed patient is a virtual artist, but because the expressive channel of creativity is perhaps the only one that permits such a patient to set up a bridge to the surrounding universe.

The course I intend to develop is the following: starting from the Gestalt concept of creativity, I will then delineate the principles on which the art therapy treatment of seriously disturbed patients is based, and end by discussing one of the most effective techniques, the psychoportrait.

---

* Translated from the Italian by Ruth Anne Henderson.

I. Creativity According to Gestalt Therapy

The application in a Gestalt therapy sense of art therapy techniques is based on a fundamental principle: every creative act expresses the search for a contact with the other. This contact sometimes actually came about; it was then transformed into intrapsychic contact and is now recalled; it is sometimes unfulfilled, denied in reality, but in any case greatly desired by the individual (Sampognaro, 1992).

Non-Gestaltists had already attributed the origins of creativity to the unappeased desire for the loved object. In the face of the offense of a denied or betrayed desire, the human individual takes refuge in the merely hallucinatory satisfaction of dream, imagination, and art, creating those fantasies whose content satisfies the desires frustrated by reality (Freud, 1969). The loss of the object and the development of mourning represent the fulcrum of the theory of Melanie Klein (1978), later taken up and enriched by Hanna Segal (see Ricci Bitti, 1998), so that creating is equivalent to repairing the loved and then destroyed object, subsequent to the passage from the schizo-paranoid to the depressive state.

Donald Winnicott (1971), the writer of the psychoanalytic matrix who comes closest to a Gestalt conception of the theory of creativity, sees the creative act as the attempt to maintain contact by means of the transitional object. Winnicott also defines creativity as the search for the self, but he does not mythicize it – from the therapeutic point of view – as accomplished self-fulfillment: to produce a work of art is not always to find oneself, or in his words: "The creativity that concerns me here is a universal. It belongs to being alive. (...) [It] belongs to the approach of the individual to external reality" (pp. 67–68). To create, then, is to make contact:

"In a search for the self the person concerned may have produced something valuable in terms of art, but a successful artist may be universally acclaimed and yet have failed to find the self that he or she is looking for. The self is not really to be found in what is made out of products of body or mind, however valuable these constructs may be in terms of beauty, skill, and impact. If the artist (in whatever medium) is searching for the self, then it can be said that in all probability there is already some failure for that artist in the field of general creative living. The finished creation never heals the underlying lack of sense of self" (ibid., pp. 54–55).

Artistic creativity and life creativity do not always coincide. If the creative aspect is not balanced by adaptation to reality, there is neither growth nor authentic contact. This principle had already been expressed by Perls and his colleagues through the concept of creative adjustment between organism and environment, so that the self is defined as "a creative contacting" (Perls et al., 1994, 24): "The 'mystery' of the creative for psychoanalysts comes from their not looking for it in the obvious place, in the ordinary health of contact" (ibid., p. 175).

Perls et al. (1994) also indicate two fundamental motivations for the creativity of the organism: the need to close unresolved situations and tension toward change:

"... first is the safe expression of unaware unfinished situations – these are the garru-
lous plans, busy-making enterprises, substitute activities, etc.; but also there is the expression of dissatisfaction with one's circumscribed self, the desire to change without
knowing how, and hence the reckless adventure, which in fact is often perfectly reason-
able and integrative, but felt as reckless only by the neurotic" (ibid., p. 184).

What is the meaning of this "gratuitous act", this "flight from reality"
(ibid.)?

"... the self seem hardly responsive at all to organic excitations and environmental
stimuli, but acts as if, hallucinating a goal and flexing its technique, it were spontaneously making a problem for itself in order to force growth" (ibid.).

Wheeler (1991, p. 62) also draws an analogy between contact and problem-solving. Many other non-Gestalt psychologists (Getzel and Jackson,
1962; Guilford, 1967; Powell, 1974) have stressed the parallelism between
creativity and problem-solving ability.

But what is the problem to be solved, which makes an individual turn to
the world of art, writing a poem or doing a sketch – as Perls and his colleagues say – apparently gratuitously?

Their example about poetry is enlightening:

"... the problem is to solve an 'inner conflict' (...) The poet is concentrating on some
unfinished subvocal speech and its subsequent thoughts; by freely playing with his
present words, he at last finishes an unfinished verbal scene, he in fact utters the complaint, the denunciation, the declaration of love, the self-reproach, that he should have
uttered; now at last he freely draws on the underlying organic need and he finds the
words (...) His Thou, his audience, is not some visible person nor the general public, but
an 'ideal audience': that is, it is nothing but assuming the appropriate attitude and character (choosing a genre and diction) that let the unfinished speech flow with precision
and force. His content is not a present truth of experience to be conveyed, but he finds in
experience or memory or fancy a symbol that in fact excites him without his (or our) needing to know its later content" (Perls et al., 1994, p. 102).

There are two kinds of contact: one is supplementary, conclusive, and
complete; the other lacks authentic satisfaction of the original need, but satisfies the current need for communication and elucidation of, as well as recalling, *that* contact. It is this that becomes concrete in the creative act (Sampognaro, 1992, p. 15).

Contact is creativity. And the creative act for Gestalt therapy in the strict
sense expresses the search for a contact. But in that sense, the Gestalt creative
act does not refer only to the experience of physical encounter between organism and environment. "... contact extends into interaction with inanimate
as well as animate objects; to see a tree or a sunset or to hear a waterfall or a
cave's silence is contact. Contact can also be made with memories and images, experiencing them sharply and fully" (Polster and Polster, 1973, p. 102).

Contact through imagination allows us to recover unconcluded relationships with people who are not presently available or who for some reason
are unreachable:

"... fantasy is often the only route back to a generic situation. A parent may be dead,
an old flame gone to another city, or a childhood friend no longer important enough for
actual contact. Even when a situation is available in terms of time or space, it may still be

either too frightening or too impolitic to go to it directly. Fantasy becomes invaluable then because it recreates what is close to reality yet is relatively safe, while going beyond gossip, strategy or ruminative speculation" (ibid., p. 258).

The contact fulfilled in the creative act is therefore an interior contact with a memory or a part of the self. It always originates in an interpersonal contact, with the environment, but it is experienced in the present in hallucinatory form. In addition, it has a specific characteristic as compared with the original contact: it has communicative value toward the audience, the "Thou" being addressed (Sampognaro, 1992, p. 17). Perls et al. (1994) grasped the importance of this element constituted by the "ideal audience", whom the artist addresses through her or his works, and of whom she or he asks attention, understanding, and recognition.

II. Art as an Expressive Channel for the Seriously Disturbed Patient

If it is true that the creative act implies a real or desired contact, it is equally true that seriously disturbed patients cannot command use of the same capability as psychically healthy individuals: the fragmented self hinders them from a fitting, relaxed competence of contact:

"In terms of the development of the experience of self, the seriously disturbed patient has not been able to perceive an integrated self, clearly differentiated from the not-self, from the environment or context" (Spagnuolo Lobb, 1997, p. 25).

And:

"The experience of self has not reached that perceptive and relational competence which Fairbairn (...) calls mature dependence, Mahler (...) calls separation/individualization ability, Stern (...) calls the narrative self, and Gestalt therapy calls *contact-withdrawal competence*" (Salonia, 1992, p. 33).

In contacting their environment, psychotics show a disturbance of the id function. The "taken-for-granted" contacts, which are an integral part of the id function, are minimized in the seriously disturbed patient. In the same way, bodily experience is so charged with anguish that we are led to believe that the filters between external and internal have entirely failed:

"The psychotic cannot enjoy the lightness given by the perception of the boundary, so that all that is outside is also inside, penetrates the skin and reaches the intimate, the heart, the stomach, the brain. (...) Everything that happens outside also happens inside; the self moves without the clear perception of the boundaries with the environment (confluence), without a solution of continuity, in a state in which everything is anxiety-inducing novelty (...) and nothing can, in effect, be assimilated (because nothing can be really recognized as different, as new" (Spagnuolo Lobb, 2001, pp. 96, 105).

The task of therapy with seriously disturbed patients is thus made even more difficult by the lack of integration of the organism, which very often makes it impossible to use a shared communicative code. "The psychiatric patient presents fundamental problems of identity, of perception of the body and of incommunicability" (Cipriani, 1998, p. 86). If people are shut into

their own chaos, from which it will be difficult to draw a necessarily individualized communicative medium, how can an authentic contact be achieved?
On what can the interpersonal relationship be based?

Difficulty in communicating is, however, secondary compared to the lack
of awareness: there is neither an I-Thou nor a We. The seriously disturbed
patient has no sense of belonging because everything, in such a patient, is
confused and disintegrated. Interpersonal contacts seem to be functional
only to the satisfaction of material needs (eating, drinking, getting dressed,
etc.). "One of the most dramatic aspects of the experience of illness is the
desocialization which derives from the loss of a series of elements of 'share-
ability' and the sense of belonging" (Ferrara, 1990, p. 45). It is at this point
that the expressive power of artistic creativity is inserted:

"The creative process, inasmuch as it is a phenomenon of transformation and change,
may stimulate and activate in the individual mechanisms similar to those that come into
play in the therapeutic situation. But where the word seems dumb, the expression may all
the more communicate something of that world which is often a thing apart, entirely
closed into itself and, as such, functioning perfectly. In fact, expression enables the opening of an opportunity, the establishment of a contact to help the individual to understand
something about her [or] his manner of functioning" (Mariotti and Peduzzi, 1998–99, p.
97).

In art therapy, graphic-iconic language takes on special expressive value.
The narrative power of the image is great. In the psychotic person, this
power becomes still greater, as the only means of uttering what cannot be
said in words (words, that is, which presuppose an integrated link among
the experiences), given the loss of the personality function.[1]

Compared with other expressive media, art responds optimally to the demand for visibility that the seriously disturbed patient expresses through
symptoms and crises (Sampognaro, 2001). The projection of "parts" of the
self onto paper or into modeled material is the ideal place to make one's own
experiences coexist outside any spatial and temporal logic:

"Simultaneity, in other words, the ability to present several objects in a single perceptive space (in contrast with music, which by its very nature must be sequential) and the
substantial timelessness of the figurative product are the features which in a certain sense
distinguish this form of therapy from other art therapies and which contribute to the creation of an area of 'illusion'" (Caterina and Ricci Bitti, 1998, p. 65).

The illusions Winnicott speaks of become the creative fulfillment of the
creative act which, as with a kaleidoscope, reflects every form and color with
which the fragmented psyche has entered into contact during the experience of life.

Art therapy, in this context, seems to be the most suitable approach to increase the levels of awareness that have been zeroed by the poor function-

---

[1] As is known, the personality function is "the system of attitudes assumed interpersonal relations, is the assumption of what one is, serving as the ground on which one
could explain one's behavior ..." (Perls et al., 160). When this function is disordered, the
individual finds it difficult to answer the question "Who am I?", loses her or his social role
and can no longer set up nourishing contacts with the environment.

ing of the self: "When awareness is not functioning, the organism cannot exactly identify its own needs and use suitable instruments to meet them; it thus loses contact with itself and with reality" (Argentino, 2001, p. 130). Taking possession of the responsibility for tracing a mark, constructing a figure, or modeling a shape in a personal, original manner, is the first step toward awareness of one's own power over things. It is *I* who do this, and others can see it and appreciate or criticize it.

The drawing space, with its boundaries and intrinsic rules of balance between forms and dimensions, imposes a restraint on the individual, which mitigates the internal chaos that harnesses and channels tensions. This regulatory effect counterbalances the typical narcissism of those who create and permits the patient to appear at the boundaries of the self:

"Learning the *limits* inherent in the figures, or more generally in the artistic products [she or] he makes, leads her [or] him by analogy to cognition and perception of the *limits* of the self. (...) It may happen that, once the cognition of *being-there* is re-owned, the patient will go on (...) to the development of analogous communications relative to her [or] his (...) deeper needs" (Cipriani 1998, p. 86).

The use of art therapy with seriously disturbed patients thus makes it possible to attain another fundamental objective: sharing emotions as an antidote to the withdrawal and rumination typical of the psychotic. The studies carried out by Rimé et al. (1992) pinpointed the importance of emotional sharing – by means of various techniques of narration – as a criterion of mental health:

"Rimé (...) describes the diachronic elements of the emotional process typical of the emotional experience in his model regarding the *social sharing of emotions*. (...) Recalling (...) has as its end the establishment of a social contact with specific individuals. (...) The recalling of emotions is, however, to be distinguished from a mere ruminating on what has happened. Rimé defines as *rumination* the memory of an emotional experience unsupported by any processing and not directed toward the communication to others of what one has experienced and felt" (Ricci Bitti, 1998, pp. 23–24).

Emotional sharing, relational competence, and awareness: these objectives, which in their turn become the instruments of change, interweave and are integrated into the art-therapy activity, above all when it is carried out in a group setting. Because awareness is always in function of the relationship, in the therapeutic community it is precisely through the relational space that the facilitator can help patients to be in contact with themselves, with their needs (see Argentino, 2001, p. 130).

Briefly, Cipriani offers this view of "some opportunities offered by art therapy" (Ricci-Bitti, 1998, p. 80), as follows:

1. Support for the creative act as an attitude antithetic to chaotic psychic situations
2. Reinforcement of the ego thanks to the acquisition of greater technical ability
3. Deeper self-knowledge
4. Increased learning of one's own sense of identity
5. The opportunity for the user to experience new, varied styles

6. Lessening of tension
7. Satisfaction of narcissistic needs, offering the user the opportunity to approve her/his own artistic production
8. Attainment of self-individuation and of progressive stages of development of autonomy

To these eight opportunities I would add a ninth: art therapy offers an internal spur to the integration of the experiences and emotions connected to it.

III. Art Therapy and Gestalt Therapy: The Psychoportrait

The traditional path within the art-therapy studio usually comprises certain standardized phases: free drawing, thematic drawing, exploration of alternative materials and instruments and, lastly, refinement of a specific technique that becomes the privileged tool for the expression of the patient's existential theme.

However, this pattern does not always work. Above all, it seems preferable to propose to seriously disturbed patients specific, structured activities that offer them emotional containment and save them from the ever-present risk of fragmentation. These activities are uncomplicated, pleasurable, and they have a clear pictorial aim: activities which "oblige" the patient to bring a little order to the chaos within, to recognize and set up communication among various parts of one's self, to interact with others, but not to tear "the veil that covers what still needs to be hidden" (Mariotti and Peduzzi, 1998–99, p. 93).

In the art therapy studio of a psychiatric, therapeutic community in Syracuse, Sicily,[2] a specific methodology was developed, arising from the need to: 1) offer the patients the opportunity to establish – or re-establish – a minimum level of relationship 2) permit the group to experience itself as a harmonic, lively whole, collaborative, and vibrant; 3) provide the individual with the chance to become a figure against the background of the group.

The technique is a matter of inviting the group to produce a psychoportrait of one of the participants, by means of a collective collage. This is created with a mixture of techniques: the patients may use photographs, newspaper cuttings, and collage paper; they may write important sentences or key words on strips of paper, which are then glued on; they may simply make colored marks (with oil paints, tempera, watercolors, etc.) directly on the placard which forms the background, or on the surface of a pre-sketched collage; or they may gather various materials (bits of cloth, wisps of straw, leaves, buttons, etc.) or fragments of play dough, producing a kind of bas-relief. All these are things which, when they have been glued on to the large

---

[2] The Assisted Therapeutic Community is a State Mental Health Service in Syracuse. At that time, the staff was composed of Paola Argentino (psychiatric director), Margherita Spagnuolo Lobb and Giuseppe Sampognaro (psychologists), Maria Concetta Zisa and Anna Monte (social workers), and Franco Leone (rehabilitation therapist), along with several psychiatric nurses.

placard which is the basis of the psychoportrait, may prove useful in telling the story of the protagonist.

The choice of collage is dictated by the need to facilitate the task, to make it accessible to all, including those with no specific artistic skills: in order to cut out and glue on, no special drawing ability or easy familiarity with pencils and brushes is needed. There is a sense in which the material is prefabricated: advertising images from the papers, photographs, already printed words, etc.; it need only be discovered and selected. It is how and in what context they are re-used that defines their creative significance:

"Collage may be regarded as a facilitating technique as compared with drawing, painting or clay modeling, activities which impose the 'recreation' of an internal image starting from a blank sheet or unshaped matter. Magazine images, by contrast, (...) are already a 'form' in that they are bearers of meanings which are immediately available and have (...) a certain degree of malleability to be adapted to the expression even of new [meanings]" (Gallorini, 1998, p. 24).

The psychoportrait should be understood diachronically (work in its development) and structurally (the completed work, with its unique, unrepeatable characteristics). From the diachronic point of view, the psychoportrait arises from a genuinely collective movement that may be schematized graphically as a Gaussian curve (see Fig. 1), which imitates the representation of the contact-withdrawal cycle (Spagnuolo Lobb, 1992, p. 45). Energy increases, reaches its peak, and then declines, until it is dissolved. At first, the participants, more or less unwillingly, focus their attention on their companion who is the "model" for the psychoportrait: they riffle through magazines, review the material as they wait for a sensation, an image, a stimulus to emerge which, by analogy, can recall the experience each one has of the subject (*orientation phase*). It is in this phase that the intrapsychic contact, typical of the creative act, takes place with the recollection of important encounters between the self and the other. The person asks her- or himself: "What is my experience of her or him?" From the formless mass of confused sensations emerges the memory of an event, an interaction, and an emotion, all of which is organized into a meaningful figure: "I always see him smoking ... She's kind, she lends me things ... He likes to wear white ... She's always talking about her son ..."

Energy increases: some start cutting out, others make a sketch or compose a short sentence, thus beginning to offer a personal contribution to the task of collective narration (*manipulation phase*). Ideas are translated and congeal into concrete, visible pictures. It is the language of analogy that uses that particular image or word, charging it with personal meanings. Once sufficient material has been accumulated, they move on to the *assembly phase*: each participant glues her or his own product on to the placard, which acts as a platform for the psychoportrait, as if it were the affective container of the individual identifications and projections (*contact phase*). It is here that the group's movement reaches its climax (the peak of the curve); each member fights strenuously to place her or his own products, driven by the desire to make themselves, their own being-there, visible and to participate in the definition of the companion portrayed by the group.

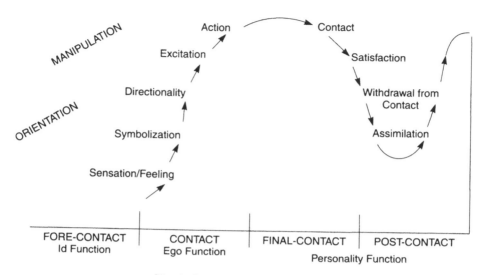

Fig. 1. Contact-Withdrawal Cycle

The *phase* of *full contact* is usually marked by the "great silence" that suddenly falls. Everyone has stuck on their own piece, and with hands still sticky with glue and stained with paint, they step back to look at the whole. This pause is necessary to the assimilation of the experience. The group observes the completed work, whereupon, finally, an outline of the sense of the We manifested by this pleased astonishment emerges, and they congratulate themselves and each other. What immediately follows (*post-contact phase*) is an interweaving of comments, criticisms, objections. The protagonist asks the others for explanations: one detail may strike her or him as difficult to understand, another as frankly unpleasant and unacceptable (learning/assimilation moment). The protagonist usually has a sense of fullness and pride at having catalyzed the attention of the group but needs time to assimilate and integrate in the deepest layers of her or his personality the new information, the new input coming from outside and shrinking the blind area of self.

In the structural analysis of the psychoportrait as a creative product, it is possible to use the same tools of interpretation as in the psycho-graphic approach. What is striking – and makes this technique a valid instrument of knowledge – is the degree to which the psychoportrait *really* represents the person in question. Beyond the will and ability of the single participants there always emerges a "truthfulness" in how the group has iconically narrated the subject.

For an effective reading of a psychoportrait, the revelatory elements are:

– The amount of material used and how it is arranged on the placard. The more the portrait is "matter-bound", the denser the superimposition and stratification of the elements and the "stronger" the status of the individual within the group. Catalyzation of so many energies is an index of popularity.

- The choice of colors. The chromatic range of any psychoportrait can be analyzed in the light of Lüscher's (1976) theory of the psychology of colors: thus a prevalence of cold shades is supposed to indicate a personality that tends toward depression, whereas warm, bright tones express a lively, little-restrained drive.
- Analysis of the content. Messages conveyed in the form of images, single words, poems, etc., represent the many micro-contacts that each component of the group has experienced with the protagonist of the psychoportrait. The range is vast: from superficial information (physical appearance, age, likes and dislikes, etc.) to metaphorical expressions, which unexpectedly plumb the depths of her or his personality and catch, at times, an outdated aspect. It may happen that the individual borrows from the "official" artistic world not only single images or phrases taken from various contexts, but even entire components that fit the circumstances, thus creatively solving the problem of finding "the words to express it".

IV. A Clinical Case: The Psychoportrait of Fabrizio

Fabrizio was a 20-year-old youth suffering from a schizoaffective disorder. At the time he was invited to take part in the art therapy laboratory, he had already been in the Community for two years, and it seemed that the right moment for his return to society had come. The fact is that after a positive phase of integration in the group of in-patients and of critical revision of his life choices (drug addiction and alcoholism), Fabrizio had found the strength to try to change, with the help of the staff and a community environment that gave him fellow-feeling and friendship. In the period before he began art therapy, however, he had gone back to his old disturbed behavior. It was not easy to convince him to take part in the psychoportrait group because of his rebellious spirit and the worsening of his delirious symptomatology. It was typical of his difficulties to be-there-and-not-be-there and to remain on the fringes of any group activity because he was afraid of bonding.

Looking at Fabrizio's psychoportrait (see Fig. 2) is like holding him up to the light. What is immediately apparent is the quantity, the wealth of material on the placard, testifying to Fabrizio's ability to provoke in others an overwhelming wave of emotions and creative production. Similarly, the liveliness of the colors (red predominating) and the cheerful chaos with which elements overlap are signs of Fabrizio's personality, which is thrusting and explosive. There are evident ironic hints at the factors and behavior that characterize him: his precarious financial condition ("Non ho una lira, *I don't have a cent*"), his laziness (two arms stretching in the morning), the objects and substances to which he is addicted (the packet of Marlboros, the glass of liquor, the mug of beer). In addition, there are references to his hobbies (a painter's palette, a pool table) and to his most noticeable physical detail (two big blue eyes). Prominent in the center are the words "Un amico vero (*A real friend)*". witnessing the degree of acceptance he has found in the group.

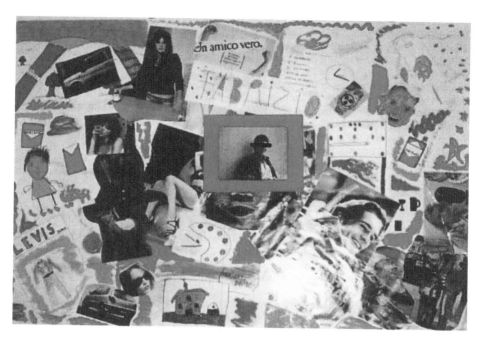

Fig. 2. Psychoportrait of Fabrizio

There is also a drawing of a country cottage by Luca, another young in-patient of the Community. When a member of the staff asked him what this meant, Luca answered: "What Fabrizio really misses is a home: I'd like for him to live here." It is in that sketch of a cottage, complete with a well and chimney, that the encounter between Luca and Fabrizio takes place: a contact missing in reality (the two were not friends), always remaining in the background, never fulfilled but, evidently, wished for and possible.

Several years have passed. Fabrizio, no longer in the Community, has sunk into his delirium and his vagabond loneliness. But somewhere, in a corner of his mind, he keeps that instant when Luca *saw* him and was concerned for him. I like to think that that knowledge, together with the few other nourishing experiences in his life, may yet bring him to the light of contact.

References

Argentino P (2001) La psicoterapia della Gestalt come terapia di comunità. In: Spagnuolo Lobb M (ed) Psicoterapia della Gestalt. Franco Angeli, Milano, pp 120–128

Caterina R, Ricci Bitti PE (1998) Arti-terapie e regolazione delle emozioni. In: Ricci Bitti PE (ed) Regolazione delle emozioni e arti-terapie. Carocci, Roma, pp 51–67

Cipriani W (1998) Esperienza estetica e cura in arte-terapia. In: Ricci Bitti PE (ed) Regolazione delle emozioni e arti-terapie. Carocci, Roma, pp 71–95

Ferrara M (1990) Manuale della riabilitazione psichiatrica. Il Pensiero Scientifico, Roma

Freud S (1969) Il poeta e la fantasia. Boringhieri, Torino

Gallorini T (1998) Collage: l'arte di "tenere insieme". QuArTer, 1: 24–25

Getzel JW, Jackson PW (1962) Creativity and intelligence. Wiley, New York

Guilford JP (1967) The nature of human intelligence. McGraw-Hill, New York

Klein M (1978) Scritti 1921–1958. Boringhieri, Torino

Lüscher M (1976) Il test dei colori. Astrolabio, Roma

Mariotti V, Peduzzi M (1998–99) La parola muta. Quaderni di Gestalt 26/29: 92–98

Perls F, Hefferline RF, Goodman P (1994) Gestalt therapy: Excitement and growth in the human personality. The Gestalt J Press, Highland, New York

Polster E, Polster M (1973) Gestalt therapy integrated. Vintage Books, New York

Powell TJ (1974) L'apprendimento creativo. Giunti-Barbera, Firenze

Ricci Bitti E (ed) (1998) Regolazione delle emozioni e arti-terapie. Carocci, Roma

Rimé B, Philippot P, Boca S, Mesquita B (1992) Long-lasting cognitive and social consequences of emotion: Social sharing and rumination. European Review of Social Psychology 3: 175–183

Salonia G (1992) From We to I-Thou. A contribution to an evolutive theory of contact. Studies in Gestalt Therapy 1: 31–41

Sampognaro G (1992) La creatività in Gestalt, tesi di specializzazione in psicoterapia della Gestalt, IV Training 1988–92. Istituto di Gestalt, Ragusa

Sampognaro G (2001) Lo psicoritratto in arteterapia. Quaderni di Gestalt 32/33: 80–89

Spagnuolo Lobb M (1992) Specific support in the interruptions of contact. Studies in Gestalt Therapy 1: 43–51

Spagnuolo Lobb M (1997) Linee programmatiche di un modello gestaltico nelle comunità terapeutiche. Quaderni di Gestalt 24/25: 19–37

Spagnuolo Lobb M (ed) (2001) Psicoterapia della Gestalt. Ermeneutica e clinica. Franco Angeli, Milano

Wheeler G (1991) Gestalt reconsidered. Gardner Press, Cleveland

Winnicott DW (1971) Playing and reality. Tavistock, London

Blocks to Creativity in Organizations

Edwin C. Nevis

I. Introduction

The study of creativity has fascinated psychologists, artists and writers, and others who have been intrigued, amazed, or shocked by an unusual concept, act, or product. What is creative? Whom do we call a "creative person"? What are the qualities of the creative person, or of someone to whom we apply the term genius? How does creativity differ or stand out from the ordinary or "non-creative"? What criteria shall we use to distinguish between "creative organizations" and "non-creative" ones? And, does the designation of creativity apply only to the truly unusual – a discontinuous paradigm shift – or is it possible to work within the boundaries of an accepted, current paradigm? These questions, and others like them, have been looked at, analyzed, and written about for hundreds of years. Yet to this day, creativity remains something of a mystery that does not readily yield its secrets to rational or intellectual understanding. Thousands of words have been written about the likes of Mozart, Shakespeare, Picasso, and Einstein, and yet we are still left in awe and possibly resigned to the conclusion that certain aspects in the creative process are unknowable.

Likewise, theorists have pondered about organizational innovation. How did the creators of Federal Express arrive at the ingenious notion to first ship all parcels to a central location and then send them on to their final destination? What allowed Microsoft to achieve pre-eminence in computer software by building on the opportunity given to them by IBM to develop DOS? How did Canon develop a handful of core competencies that enabled them to take commanding positions in camera and copier manufacturing? Were these the inventions of single individuals? If so, would they have been made possible without an organizational culture that was flexible and adaptable in providing resources and that supported "out-of-the-box" thinking and risk-taking? Much has been written about organizational innovation, and we can describe some of the factors at work in these situations. However, creativity in organizations remains enigmatic.

II. Toward a Pragmatic Perspective

Thirty years ago, Nevis et al. (1970) addressed the above issues and came to the conclusion that the dilemma of creativity was compounded by fixation upon the highly unique, novel outcome at the expense of looking at creativity in extending the known and the "tried-and-true". We postulated that an individual or group could develop something creative within a known paradigm or model. This is the new and different that emerges out of repeated application of what is known and accepted and what is sometimes referred to as "continuous improvement". A jazz musician can be creative within a given style – such as New Orleans Dixieland jazz – without having to create be-bop or to use unusual time signatures. An automobile company can develop a new, clever model of its car, yet it can remain powered by a combustion engine. The adoption by the European Union of the euro as a common currency may be seen as uniquely creative in that it challenges the assumption that each member nation should have its own currency. But it also can be considered as "business as usual" in its reliance upon paper and coin currency.

This line of reasoning is supported by the work of Nevis et al. (1993, 1995) on organization learning. Our research indicated that all organizations demonstrate some quantity and form of learning, and that the nature of this learning conformed to the culture of the organization. We formulated a two-factor theory of learning: *facilitating factors* and *learning orientations*. The first factor has to do with aspects of culture that support learning; the second deals with stylistic variations on what is learned in a given organization. This thinking further supports the notion that there are all kinds of creative outcomes, and it challenges the concept of creativity as an unusually unique, paradigm-breaking outcome.

With the above in mind, I define creativity as: *using one's competence and energy to extend the boundary of what is possible in any walk of life and at any level of complexity.* This definition means that any individual or group has the potential to be creative within the realm of what is possible. Almost 100 years ago, William James concluded that most people are able to actualize only a fraction of this potential. Organization theorists have concluded the same with reference to the ability to harness competence and energy in organizations. We are all capable of creative acts within the boundaries of our individual and collective human nature. The challenge is to find ways to allow this potential to flourish.

III. Contribution of Gestalt Therapy

A basic principle of Gestalt psychology is that of *prägnanz*, which states that every experience tends to become as "good" as prevailing conditions make possible. Psychological development moves in a compelling direction – that is, it is neither random nor unstable – and people use their energy in an attempt to reach outcomes that satisfy individual or group needs. One property of *prägnanz* is closure, which is defined as completion of a striving, or the reaching of the best possible outcome under existing conditions.

Gestalt therapy was created as a means of helping people increase their awareness of their *process*. That is to say, the aim is to teach people how to be aware of the way in which they function, and thus to release energy that enables them to better understand what they need at a given time and to have a more effective way of achieving it. Though it is not a value-free therapy, attention is largely focused on how people stop or prevent themselves from getting what they want or need, and on how they interrupt an essentially natural human *process*. Applying the principle of *prägnanz* to this process is to see every individual, group, or organization as doing the best possible at any given moment. This is perhaps the main cornerstone of the Gestalt approach, in that it assumes we all have the potential to do more, do better, or to be creative. It is only the obstacles or blocks inside us or in the external environment that prevent us from doing so.

The methods of Gestalt therapy were developed to help people heighten their awareness of the way in which obstacles prevented them from leading a fulfilling life. Emphasis upon working at the boundary is a major contribution in this regard, in that it asks people to pay attention to where they are stuck and to what prevents them from moving further.

What I remember most from my early studies with Fritz Perls, Laura Perls, and Isadore From is the almost relentless way they pushed me to look at my objections to considering a thought, an action, or an insight. Fritz kept asking: "And what are your objections ...?" "And what are your objections ...?", on and on. It was not required that I change my attitude or behavior; but it was imperative that I achieved enriched awareness of the potential to be different, if I so desired.

If we return to the earlier definition of creativity, we can now see that a major contribution of the Gestalt approach is its focus on the obstacles that prevent or limit it from unfolding in any individual or organization. Sonia Nevis, Elliott Danzig, and I refer to these as "Blocks to Creativity" (1970). (See also my "Blocks to Innovation in Organizations", 1972, unpublished manuscript.) The remainder of this chapter is devoted to identifying major *blocks to creativity in organizations* and to providing some suggestions for dealing with them.

IV. Blocks to Creativity in Organizations

Table 1 lists and defines the six most prominent obstacles to creativity in organizations. These blocks were derived from years of research by others and from the work of Nevis et al. (1970) and Nevis (1972, unpublished manuscript) in applying an earlier list of 12 individual blocks to many organizations. While they do not account for a full explanation of what stops the creative process, they are observed in almost every situation where change is attempted. In traditional theory and language, they might be referred to as manifestations of resistance to change. I prefer to look at them as different ways in which energy is managed as groups of people attempt to function as best as they can. (See Nevis et al., 1996, for a discussion of "multiple realities".)

Table 1. Major Blocks to Creativity in Organizations

Block	Definition
Fear of Failure	Avoidance or risk; giving up quickly when obstacles appear; overemphasis on short-term "easy" results; considering it shameful to experience failure; avoiding painful actions.
Reluctance to Play	Overly serious problem-solving style; avoid "playing around" with stuff; mistrusting fantasies; avoiding experiments or provisional tries (pilot projects); fear of appearing foolish or silly by indulging in the unusual; difficulty in doing "let's pretend".
Excessive Need for Order	Over-reliance on rules and control mechanisms; fear of confusion and ambiguity; annoyed at the unexpected; efficiency is the highest value.
Resource Myopia	Lack of trust in human capacities and in values or styles that are different from yours; failure to see resources in your environment; difficulty in asking for help; failure to see one's own strengths.
Overcertainty	Persistence in behavior that is no longer functional; rigidity of problem-solving approaches; not checking our assumptions; polarizing things into opposites rather than integrating the best of both positions.
Reluctance to Exert Influence	Fear of being seen as too aggressive or pushy in influencing others; hesitancy to stand up for beliefs; conflict-avoidant; ineffective in having your voice heard.

Another way to look at these blocks is to see them as *objections* to looking at the psychological boundaries they create when people are under pressure to change. Our job as consultants is to help bring these objections into awareness and to provide a forum in which they can be looked at and discussed.

A. Fear of Failure

In all entrepreneurial settings, it is customary to think of risk-reward equations: the higher the risk, the greater the expectation of a more than ordinary gain. Much creativity has come out of investments in new ventures that deal with more improbable ideas. But once organizations begin to reach a stage of maturity, there is a tendency toward preservation of what has been achieved. Leaders are rewarded in terms of their ability to make the most of what is; that is why one chief executive referred to a major change effort in his organization as undertaking a "revolution against ourselves". Most of us would agree that the odds against revolutions turning out to be what is first envisioned are great. Therefore, why take the chance to fail?

This block appears mostly in the setting of moderate or safe goals, a natural reaction to the fact that failure tends to be punished. As a result, many organizational leaders are reluctant to invest in something new, or to engage in an experiment in order to learn something. There is a failure to distinguish between "small" and "grand" failures. If something is tried and "fails", but the organization learns something that it can apply in another approach, is it correct to label it as "failure"?

Another aspect of *fear of failure* derives from the values of Western culture, in which outcomes are more important than process and winning is sometimes seen as "the only thing" that counts. There are many manifestations of this, including canceling of expenditures on projects if success does not come rapidly, and emphasis on short-term results. In addition, there is the issue of the shame that is often experienced when failure occurs. The irony of this is that sports heroes and accomplished business leaders of the Western world often have far from perfect performance scores. Teams lose some games, and CEOs have years in which their firm loses money.

In Gestalt terms, fear of failure may be seen as failure to internalize an understanding that destruction of the old is necessary before something new can be created. In the organizational world as well as in the individual world, the progressive formation and destruction of powerful figures is a scary business.

B. Reluctance to Play

Creativity requires playfulness. To innovate we must play with things, words, ideas, and people. In organizations that pride themselves in being innovative, it is sometimes hard to distinguish work from play, and to find people so engrossed in their work that they lose track of time and place. Highly-accomplished scientists, businesspeople, and artists often think of the work activities as games. Though they play the game with great seriousness of purpose, they are able to maintain a sense of humor and to see the contradictions in life as exciting challenges. Without this, leadership takes on a somewhat mechanical, distant quality.

Almost everyone is capable of using his or her imagination. We continually dream and fantasize about our existence. Yet in the organizational world, the focus tends to be highly directed to so-called objective reality, and dreamers are devalued – unless they are seen as inventors or "our creative people". Even organizations that engage in the development of an organizational vision generally do so with little imagination, which results in a credo that has little effect on most members of the organization.

Fundamental to *reluctance to play* is a fear of appearing emotional, out of control, or silly. Many managers, who are fully capable of occasionally looking foolish or of expressing emotion in their private lives, avoid this experience in the organizational setting. The result is that employees also tend to keep their playfulness hidden. On the other hand, if leaders are willing to model playful behavior, this can have a far-reaching effect in their organizations.

This block poses an interesting dilemma for the Gestalt-oriented practitioner, who is taught that projections are "bad" and that our job is to help undo them. However, all art and any kind of vision is impossible without the ability to project, that is, to visualize that which is not immediately present. If we want to support imagination, we need to teach people to engage in projections based on openness and to value engagement in "what if" exploration. People who are reluctant to play need to develop more of a sense of positive projection. One of the most useful ways of helping leaders be more playful is in the experiential exercises used by many consultants in retreat meetings. Another is in the highly successful Synectics Program, which takes actual organizational problems and asks participants to use fantasy in looking for solutions.

C. Excessive Need for Order

This block is a close cousin to *reluctance to play*. It deals with the potentially restricting aspect of an important ability: the capacity both to make order out of a confusing world and to learn the skills for surviving in a complex world. To help us with this, society provides rules, laws, and guidelines for maximizing efficient use of our energy. There is no question that society would fall apart without order; but we also know that to create new things requires the ability to tolerate confusion and ambiguity. Making the most out of existing conditions works *for* stability and *against* novelty or change, and mobilizing energy to handle the present situation reduces visioning a possibly new future.

The organizational world functions because people develop shared expectations. We accept that accountants provide financial information, and that salesmen have a manager who is accountable for their performance. That is why we often see tightly-defined job descriptions in which responsibilities are spelled out in minute detail, and personnel policies that are applied to everyone regardless of individual circumstances. Yet one of the most creative ideas of the last part of the 20th century is flexible work hours, in which individuals are allowed to select when they want to work, based on integration of their needs and the organization's requirements. Another creative development is the growth in working at home. Both of these practices test the ability of the organization to give up something with regard to orderly control.

The clinically-minded reader will inevitably begin to think of this as an organizational manifestation of obsessive-compulsive behavior. Yet, it provides a very important ingredient to an organization. Managers with well-applied, strong compulsive behavior are frequently found and often well-rewarded. Indeed, organizations function efficiently because of this. The problem is that it tends to restrict the range of behavior that is possible and to block people from seeing new possibilities. Fundamentally, fear of ambiguity and excessive avoidance of confusion contribute to this block.

D. Resource Myopia

A major ingredient of this block is the failure to appreciate the potential of people, both self and other. It is supported by a pessimistic view of human nature and a focus on what people may not be able to do, rather than upon what they might be capable of doing. In a sense, it is a lack of trust and a lowered expectation of how human beings may behave. It frequently results in managers doing things that can be delegated to subordinate employees. The organizational world is full of people who feel underutilized, often the consequence of failure to give them a chance to show what they are capable of achieving.

One of the great accomplishments in the last half of the 20th century is the growing appreciation of this phenomenon. There is greater awareness of the inhibiting nature of this block, and we see numerous examples where it has been overcome. These range from children in a poor neighborhood being treated as having intelligence and, hence, becoming national high school champions in chess, for example, to young people being given larger responsibilities at work. Champion sports teams often exhibit an internal attitude that they "expect" to win. Yet even so, most organizations continue to have policies, procedures, and managers that restrict the range of opportunities for their staff.

Another aspect of this block is manifested in the inability to ask for and use help from others. Many leaders and their organizations believe in what has been called "hero management". In these settings, there is a strong tendency to want to solve problems on one's own. Also, "blindness" to what may be useful prevents people from seeing what is often obvious to others. In one particular situation, I could not convince my client to hire higher caliber commercial sales and marketing people, even though senior management admitted that they were lacking such skilled workers. There was an underlying stubbornness in adhering to the view that the problem could eventually be solved without additional resources.

The Gestalt practitioner will recognize these organizations as having a strong component of retroflection. (For a discussion of the role of retroflection and other classical Gestalt "resistances", see Merry and Brown, 1987.) Even in those cases where there is great use of external consultants, the organization, through its basic inability to trust that others can truly be helpful, resists accepting the advice or the solutions provided.

E. Overcertainty

One of the paradoxical outcomes of successful experiences in organizations is that they reinforce old behavior that may no longer be effective when the external environment has changed and calls for new behavior. It is a natural tendency to repeat problem-solving approaches that have worked in the past. But creativity calls for a new way of seeing things, and requires freedom from customary approaches. Every great advance in science, art, and technology has come about because someone was able to give up a traditional perspective. The early paintings of Picasso, completed when he was a teen-ager, followed classical lines of 19th-century painting and showed his enormous talent for painting. At the age of 13 he showed a high level of creativity in working within a traditional form. When he began to experiment with new modes, including cubism, he broke free of the traditional and manifested creativity of another kind.

In simple terms, this block is based on rigidity. I prefer to label it as *overcertainty*, to convey the point that blocking behavior can develop out of unquestioned reliance upon what works. This inhibits our ability to look at more than one side of an issue. *Overcertainty* defies the systems theory principle of equafinality, which states that "more than one road leads to Rome". It focuses energy on proving that there is a "best" way, and it rejects other ways. It is a nagging problem for specialists, who run the risk that their substantial past experience will be applied in a unique setting that calls for something new.

The antidote to *overcertainty* is naïveté, the ability to position oneself as unknowing or as being in awe of something. The naïve stance implies that there is always something to be learned and that the presently workable is not set in concrete. To function from this perspective requires a robust experience of being centered as well as confident that engaging in a flexible process will sooner or later produce something new and valuable. It calls for courage to consider alternatives. In recent years, some firms have come to recognize the value of strategic scenario-planning, in which several scenarios are developed simultaneously in order to anticipate the probability that one approach will not be adequate and that they will need to shift direction rapidly.

The Gestalt practitioner will recognize the similarity of *overcertainty* to the concept of the fixed Gestalt, in which a strong figure becomes frozen and prevents flexible behavior from taking place.

F. Reluctance to Exert Influence

Creativity requires actions that not only produce something new, but also make possible other actions that would not otherwise take place. It involves manipulation of one's environment, in which an internal vision is imposed on the external world. Creative people often seem very single-minded in their purpose and stubborn and persistent in their response to critics or disbelievers. On a less intense level, we can say that all human interaction involves a desire to have an impact on others. In the organizational world, effective managers and specialists are rewarded for their ability to exert influence on others. With the flattening of work structures and the emphasis on non-hierarchical relationships, effective performance often depends upon the ability to have others pay attention to you.

From the above, we might conclude that effective individuals or groups have good skills for being influential. However, in studies of managers, this block is the one most often identified as an area for self-development. This suggests that they may sometimes feel unable to make an impact on an intransigent world.

What prevents people, individually or collectively, from being more effective in exerting influence? One of the answers to the question is that those who attempt to exert influence are often seen as "too aggressive", "too pushy", or "too egotistical". People who are uncomfortable about behaving this way tend to confuse healthy assertiveness with "aggression", which has negative connotations. They also define influence as power, another concept that carries negative connotations for many people. Others are very uncomfortable with conflict of any kind. Whether it is fear of being disliked or anxiety when in emotionally charged situations, maintaining a smooth interaction is highly preferred. For example, I consulted with a company headed by five brothers who were constantly stuck in indecision, because no one would express disagreement with the others. Having a "civilized" atmosphere was more important than developing creative solutions to their problems. In an academic setting, in which I was a member of the faculty, there was great difficulty in discussing a money-losing program. There was no way to find a creative solution, and the program died a slow death, which included losing money for several years. By contrast, in another academic setting where confrontation about an unproductive program took place, a new, very successful program was created.

Another factor that reinforces *reluctance to exert influence* is the inability to distinguish between standing up for what you want and having your voice considered, and imposing your will on others. Many people lose sight of the fact that just stating one's position clearly can be an act of influence; it is not necessary to dominate others to get their attention.

Yet another factor is the failure to recognize that there are different strategies for attempting to exert influence:

- Influence through use of power and status
- Influence through use of knowledge and ideas
- Influence through involving people in your endeavor
- Influence through appeal to conscience, morality, and basic values
- Influence through being helpful to another
- Influence through serving as a model

If an important goal of organizations is to be creative in carrying out their mission, these strategies need to be applied. But there is no rule that says one is better than the other.

The Gestalt principle that is most associated with *reluctance to exert influence* is that of *presence*, and the use of self as instrument. This is easy to see when we think at the individual level. In an organization, however, there are many "presences" and strong feelings about which one is the most desirable. Our work in helping organizations be more creative must involve teaching people to appreciate their own style and the style of others. The more our own presence conveys a range of attitudes and behaviors for exerting influence, the better others will be able to learn.

V. Reducing Blocks to Creativity: Several Case Studies

The Gestalt-oriented practitioner is very well-positioned to help organizations reduce their blocks to creativity. With our focus on process, our values in meeting clients where they are, and our push for having people examine the assumptions behind their behavior, we are able to deal with objections to new behavior. The founders of Gestalt therapy taught us to heighten "what is" at the moment and to help clients become deeply immersed in what they do – good or bad. They also taught that this tactic should always precede any attempt to influence them to change. This is exactly what we mean by increasing awareness about objections. The questioning of "what is your objection" is as useful at the organizational level as it is at the level of the individual. The challenge is to find ways to do this with people who did not hire you to do therapy.

The following case examples will show how this might be done. After several years of consulting with a highly specialized technical consulting firm of 1000 employees, I found that the top executives very much disliked their performance incentive (bonus) program. When it got close to the time for deciding the awards, these executives would grumble and make jokes about wanting to do anything but attend the two-day meeting devoted to this purpose. As we approached this for the third time in my experience with them, I decided to intervene – even though my assignment had nothing to do with compensation matters. I asked the top 14 executives to meet with me, and 11 did so. I spoke only a few minutes, telling them that as individuals they all complained to me about the compensation system. I then asked: "What is your collective objection to giving up the present system and building a new one?" In terms of our six Blocks, the objections seemed to center around *overcertainty* – persistence in behavior that is no longer functional. There was also a reluctance to experiment with something new – an aspect of *reluctance to play*.

Time does not permit a detailed description of these executives' reactions to my intervention, and of a subsequent two-year process in which – with the help of a compensation specialist – I facilitated the development of a new program. It is enough to say that it took several meetings with small groups of these executives to surface the objections, some of which reappeared during the time needed to develop the new system. The new program, though far from perfect, was created by the executives, and it has been fully embraced by the managers of this firm, resulting in higher, more equitable rewards for top performers.

In another case, the owner as well as founder and president of a very successful company asked for assistance in building a new management team. The task was to respond to the requirements of a rapidly growing business that had run into serious difficulties at a time when he wanted to work less. My task was to get to know him, his family, the managers of the firm, and the nature of the business, as a prelude to a new organization design. It soon became very apparent that he had a great deal of ambivalence about changing the company and sharing authority with anyone else. At frequent intervals, when he said that he would make these changes, I said that I was not convinced that he really wanted to do this and that I was not sure that I could help him. This led to an extensive examination of all the reasons why the proposed changes might not work (surfacing the objections). As an outgrowth of this process, my client became very interested in my recommendation for recruiting a new president, which has been accomplished as I write. I am not totally convinced that this will work, but at least we reframed the problem and created a structure different from that which existed in the past. The solution that emerged was different from that envisioned by the client when we started the process.

A third case shows the power of the combination of *resource myopia, excessive need for order,* and *overcertainty.* In this example, senior management of the company had great difficulty in delegating responsibility to the level of managers under them. In particular, they were reluctant to assign two part-time female managers to challenging management positions, even though they were the most qualified for these positions. The major objections were about ability to handle the jobs part-time, that coordination problems are greater when people are not available full-time, and the fact that it had never been done before in this organization. It required months of encouraging the senior managers to articulate their objections over and over again. It had appeared that the objections would win out, until one of the women sold a big project. Finally, the group agreed to appoint her on a trial basis. To their amazement, she accomplished more than many full-time managers and sold another big project. Today, there are several part-time managers in high positions in that organization.

Other examples of this approach may be found in Nevis (1987, 2001).

VI. Conclusion

Successful organizations are capable of finding creative solutions to their problems. This capability is often restricted, however, because of blocks that inhibit full functioning of organization members. Gestalt therapy provides a perspective and a method for dealing with these blocks, which are supported by unaware and aware objections. By focusing our work on the articulation, examination, and acceptance of these objections, we can help organizations release the energy and the imagination to be creative. But the work is far from easy; it requires trust in the process of staying with the objections while under pressure for results and quick solutions.

References

Merry U, Brown G (1987, 2001) The neurotic behavior of organizations. GestaltPress, Cambridge, Mass

Nevis, EC (1987, 2001) Organizational consulting: A Gestalt approach. GestaltPress, Cambridge, Mass

Nevis E, DiBella A, Gould J (1993) Organizations as learning systems: Research report 93–01. International Consortium for Executive Development Research, Lexington

Nevis E, DiBella A, Gould J (1995) Understanding organizations as learning systems. Sloan Management Review 36(2) pp 73–85

Nevis E, Lancourt J, Vassallo H (1996) Intentional revolutions: A seven-point strategy for transforming organizations. Jossey-Bass Pfeiffer, San Francisco

Nevis E, Nevis S, Danzig E (1970) Blocks to creativity. Danzig Nevis, Intl., Cleveland

Biographical Notes

Nancy Amendt-Lyon, Dr. phil., M.A., born in New York, studied psychology in New York, Geneva, and Graz. In private practice in Vienna as a psychotherapist and supervisor, senior teaching faculty of the Depts. of Int. Gestalt Therapy, Group Analysis, and Supervision (ÖAGG). Publications on Gestalt therapy (creativity, supervision, diagnosis, psychotherapeutic efficacy). Chair of the Extended Board of the EAGT, on the board of *Gestalt Review*, and associate of the board of *Gestalttherapie*. Channels her creative energy into writing and performing cabarets on Gestalt therapy.

Daniel J. Bloom is a psychotherapist in private practice as well as a supervisor and teacher of Gestalt therapy in New York City. He received a master's in social work and a juris doctor from New York University. He includes Laura Perls, Isadore From, Richard Kitzler, and Patrick Kelley as his teachers. He is a full member of the New York Institute for Gestalt Therapy and is its current president.

Todd Burley, Ph.D., ABPP, is currently professor of psychology at Loma Linda University, where he teaches courses in Gestalt therapy, cortical functions, neuropsychological assessment, and research and treatment of schizophrenia. He is a member of the Core Faculty at GATLA, a Post-Graduate Institute in Los Angeles that has trained Gestalt therapists internationally for 32 years. In addition to maintaining a private practice, he is an Action Editor for *Gestalt Review*. He is perhaps the only psychologist today combining a teaching career in Gestalt therapy and cognitive neuroscience.

Sandra Cardoso-Zinker, M.S., Lic.Psych., lived in Brazil, where she taught Gestalt therapy in work with children and the arts for 15 years. She has written articles about Gestalt therapy in relation to human development and attachment theory. At present, she lives in Massachusetts and teaches Gestalt Couples and Child Therapy in the USA as well as in Europe and South America. She recently published an article on couples therapy and *The Story of Daniel: Gestalt Therapy Principles and Value*. She is affiliated with The Gestalt International Study Center and is a faculty member of The Gestalt Institute of São Paulo.

Ludwig Frambach, Th. D., born 1954, Lutheran pastor and psychotherapist, director of The Spirituality Project in Nuremberg, Germany, Gestalt training

Symbolon Institute, and Fritz Perls Institute, Germany. He has many years of practice in Zen and Christian contemplation, and several publications in the field of psychotherapy, spirituality, and ecology.

Ruella Frank has a master's degree in movement education and a doctorate in somatic psychology. She practices psychotherapy in New York City, where she is the director of the Center for Somatic Studies, member of training faculty at the Gestalt Associates for Psychotherapy, and full member of the New York Institute for Gestalt Therapy. She also teaches at institutes and universities throughout the United States and Europe. Ruella authored the book *Body of Awareness: A Somatic and Developmental Approach to Psychotherapy* (Gestalt Press, 2001).

Carl Hodges has an abiding interest in Gestalt psychology and Gestalt field theory, and in the application of Gestalt field theory concepts to the varieties of social organization – self, groups, associations, community. He has taught at Hunter College in New York and is a trainer at the New York Institute for Gestalt Therapy, and a visiting trainer at the Gestalt Centre London and the Istituto di Gestalt – H.C.C., Italy. He was the second president of the New York Institute for Gestalt Therapy, and the third president of the Association for the Advancement of Gestalt Therapy.

Richard Kitzler has been a member of the New York Institute for Gestalt therapy since 1952 and is a fellow of the Institute. He is the author of innumerable articles, papers, and conference programs. He teaches, supervises, and maintains a private practice of psychotherapy in New York City. His interest has been a restatement of current Gestalt therapy theory and is working on a reconstruction of Gestalt Therapy theory. He is also interested in large group process and its effect on the polis.

Edward J. Lynch is an associate professor in the Department of Marriage & Family Therapy at Southern Connecticut State University, specializing in Gestalt therapy training. His background includes training and supervision with Isadore From, Erv and Miriam Polster, Joseph Zinker, and Michael Vincent Miller. He is a member of the New York Institute for Gestalt Therapy and workshop leader throughout Europe and the USA. He also studied family therapy with Salvador Minuchin at the Philadelphia Child Guidance Clinic.

Barbara Lynch is a professor in the Department of Marriage & Family Therapy at Southern Connecticut State University. Her training with Jay Haley and Salvador Minuchin forms the background for her specialization in systemic couple and family therapy. She is an AAMFT clinical member and approved supervisor and a frequent presenter at national conferences on issues relating to couples, youth, and families.

Joseph Melnick, Ph.D., is a clinical and organizational psychologist. He is a member of the professional staff of the Gestalt Institute of Cleveland and the Gestalt International Study Center, where he teaches in the Center for Intimate Systems. He is the editor-in-chief of *Gestalt Review*, an international journal devoted to contemporary Gestalt therapy. The author of numerous articles on Gestalt therapy, he teaches and trains internationally.

Michael Vincent Miller, Ph.D., clinical psychologist, practices Gestalt therapy in New York City and Cambridge, Mass. He taught at Stanford University and MIT, and directed the Boston Gestalt Institute from 1972 until recently. Consulting editor of the *International Gestalt Journal*, he has been a frequent reviewer for the *New York Times Book Review*. His book *Intimate Terrorism: The Crisis of Love in an Age of Disillusion* has been translated into seven languages, and a collection of his writings, *La Poetique de la Gestalt-therapie*, was published in France (2002).

Bertram Müller, Dipl.-Psych., clinical Gestalt therapist, trainer, supervisor, president of the German Otto-Rank-Association (DORG), founding director of the international cultural center Tanzhaus nrw/Düsseldorf, executive director of World Dance Alliance Europe, cultural expert at the European Commission (94/95). Award: Chevalier des Arts et des Lettres, Ministry for Culture, France. Publications on Otto Rank, diagnostic in Gestalt therapy, dance art and cultural management.

Sonia March Nevis, Ph.D., is director of the Center for the Study of Intimate Systems at the Gestalt International Study Center on Cape Cod, Massachusetts in the United States. She has a private practice working with individuals, couples, and families. She also does supervision.

Edwin C. Nevis has been a pioneer in applying the Gestalt therapy model to consultation with organizations. He is currently president of Gestalt International Study Center, which he started together with Sonia M. Nevis in 1979. He was a founder of the Gestalt Institute of Cleveland, and also developed the Gestalt Press. In addition, he spent 17 years as an adjunct professor, researcher, and administrator at the MIT Slogan School of Management. Author of several books and numerous articles, he currently sees his mission as creating a worldwide learning community of Gestalt practitioners.

Malcolm Parlett, Ph.D., has a background in academic psychology and research in education. A chartered psychologist and a Gestalt psychotherapist registered with the UK Council for Psychotherapy, he is visiting professor of Gestalt Psychotherapy at the Univ. of Derby, and has his own organisation consulting company. He studied at the Gestalt Institute of Cleveland, Ohio in the late 1970s, subsequently co-founding the Gestalt Psychotherapy and Training Institute in the United Kingdom. He is editor of the *British Gestalt Journal*, a member of the Human Strengths Research Group, and has written extensively on Gestalt themes.

Antonio Sichera was born in Modica, Sicily. He has a doctorate in lexicography and semantics, and is a professor of modern and contemporary Italian literature at Catania University. His research on hermeneutics from a literary and philosophical point of view resulted in books on U. Foscolo, L. Pirandello, C. Pavese, P. Pasolini, and E. Montale. After training in Gestalt therapy with Spagnuolo Lobb and Salonia at the Istituto di Gestalt, where he now teaches epistemology of Gestalt therapy, he wrote essays on the relationship between hermeneutics and Gestalt therapy.

Giuseppe Sampognaro, Psych. Dr., was born in Catania, Sicily. He trained in Gestalt therapy with Salonia and Spagnuolo Lobb. As a psychotherapist in a State Mental Health Service in Siracusa, he promotes art therapy with psychiatric patients. As a journalist, he writes on psychological issues for various magazines and edits a specialized teletext page for the R.A.I. (Radio Televisione Italiana). After publishing the novel *Mille mondi. Un romanzo terapeutico* (2000), he focused on the application of creative techniques to psychotherapy, above all the use of images and writing.

Margherita Spagnuolo Lobb, Psych. Dr., Director of the Istituto di Gestalt (Venice, Rome, Palermo, Ragusa, Siracusa), international trainer and visiting professor at various universities in Italy and abroad. Full member of the NYIGT. President of Ital. Federation of Assoc. of Psychotherapy, past president of European Assoc. for Gestalt Therapy (1996–2002). Editor of the journals *Quaderni di Gestalt* and *Studies in Gestalt Therapy*. She authored many articles, chapters, and books, some of which have been translated into other languages. She has organized a few important conferences of Gestalt therapy.

Daniel N. Stern, M.D., Prof. Hon. Faculté de Psychologie, Université de Genève; Adj. Prof. in the Dept. of Psychiatry, Cornell Univ. Med. School, New York; Lect. at Columbia Univ. Center for Psychoanal.; Hon. Doct. at Copenhagen Univ, and the Univ. of Mons Hinault, Belgium. For more than thirty years, he has worked at the interface between developmental psychology and psychodynamic psychotherapy. He authored several hundred articles, chapters, and six books, most of which have been translated into more than ten languages. The most recent is titled: *The Present Moment in Psychotherapy and Everyday Life.*

Gordon Wheeler, Ph.D., teaches Gestalt therapy in training programs around the world. Trained in clinical and developmental psychology, he authored a number of books and articles on: self theory, relationship and intimacy, child therapy, developmental and gender issues, and working with shame. He focuses on using the Gestalt therapy model to develop an intersubjective approach to psychoth. and relationship. A senior faculty member of the Gestalt Institute of Cleveland, he is editor and co-director of Gestalt Press. He and his wife have 8 children, and divide their time between Cambridge, Massachusetts and Big Sur, California.

Joseph C. Zinker, Ph.D., co-founder of the Gestalt Institute of Cleveland, trained with F. Perls in the 60s, and has been influential in the development of the Gestalt therapy approach for over three decades. Author of numerous articles and books (the most recent is *Sketches: An Anthology of Essays, Art and Poetry*, 2001), he served on the editorial board of several journals (*Voices, The Gestalt Journal, Gestalt Review* and *The Journal of Couples Therapy*). Affiliated with the Gestalt Int. Study Center, he is a faculty member of the Center for the Study of Intimate Systems and of many Gestalt Institutes around the world.

Subject Index

SpringerMedicine

Annette Schaub (ed.)

New Family Interventions and Associated Research in Psychiatric Disorders

Gedenkschrift in Honor of Michael J. Goldstein

2002. VI, 281 pages. 16 figures.

Softcover **EUR 39,–**

(Recommended retail price) Net-price subject to local VAT.

ISBN 3-211-83700-0

This book is dedicated to the memory of Michael J. Goldstein, one of the pioneers in psychosocial interventions in psychiatry. The structure of this book follows Goldstein's footsteps in this domain and is subdivided into family factors as well as intervention strategies for severe mental illness. Recent research on high expressed emotion (HEE) in schizophrenia (e.g., early psychosis) and borderline disorder, patients' perspectives of HEE as well as other variables predictive for relapse in recent-onset schizophrenia are covered in this book. ´

Family treatment strategies in schizophrenia, depression, bipolar disorder, substance use disorders and illness management programs as well as pharmacological treatment strategies are illustrated and current studies presented.

The book brings together basic research and therapeutic applications stimulating further research on the complex interactional components that influence the course of psychiatric illness and on treatment designed to ameliorate the symptoms, stigma, and disability experienced by patients with severe mental illness.

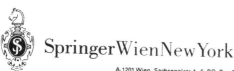

SpringerWienNewYork

A-1201 Wien, Sachsenplatz 4–6, P.O. Box 89, Fax +43.1.330 24 26, e-mail: books@springer.at, Internet: **www.springer.at**
D-69126 Heidelberg, Haberstraße 7, Fax +49.6221.345-4229, e-mail: orders@springer.de
USA, Secaucus, NJ 07096-2485, P.O. Box 2485, Fax +1.201.348-4505, e-mail: orders@springer-ny.com
Eastern Book Service, Japan, Tokyo 113, 3–13, Hongo 3-chome, Bunkyo-ku, Fax +81.3.38 18 08 64, e-mail: orders@svt-ebs.co.jp

Lightning Source UK Ltd.
Milton Keynes UK
UKOW06n0249230915

259075UK00003B/37/P